AF540286

PHARMACEUTICAL VALIDATION

PHARMACEUTICAL VALIDATION

By

Dr. G.P. Garg

&

Dr. M. Prakash

DISCOVERY PUBLISHING HOUSE PVT. LTD.

NEW DELHI-110 002

Published by:
Tilak Wasan
DISCOVERY PUBLISHING HOUSE PVT. LTD.
4383/4B, Ansari Road, Darya Ganj
New Delhi-110 002 (India)
Phone : +91-11-23279245, 43596064-65
Fax : +91-11-23253475
E-mail : discoverypublishinghouse@gmail.com
sales@discoverypublishinggroup.com
web : www.discoverypublishinggroup.com

First Published: **2011**

Reprinted: **2015**

ISBN: 978-81-8356-739-8

Pharmaceutical Validation

Printed at:
Infinity Imaging Systems
Delhi

Preface

The present title "Encyclopaedia of Pharmaceutical Technology" has been written for those in the pharmaceutical research and those responsible for the education and training in pharmaceutical science and technology of graduate and undergraduate students. Medicine is an ever changing science. As new research and clinical experience broaden our knowledge, changes in treatment and drug therapy are required. This branch of life science has progressed enormously in recent years and the significant advances in therapeutics and an understanding of the need to optimize during delivery in the body have brought about an increased awareness of the valuable role played by the dosage forms. This statement is as true as it was back in ninteenth century and perhaps more so, given the increasing emphasis being placed on discovery, development, and use of large molecular entities as therapeutic and diagnostic agents. Development of these abilities requires an integration of knowledge, skills, attitudes, and values that can be acquired only through structured learning process including independent study, hands on practice and the availability of advanced literature. This tittle has designed to meet such needs of learners in the health professions.

In the last two decades, the pharmaceutical industry has experimented and successfully adopted several integrated and multidisciplinary approaches in the research areas of dring compound screening, toxicological evaluation, and pharmaceutical product development. The book is written in a concise style that facilitates an in-depth level of understanding of the essential concepts. The objectives of the present title are three folds: (i) to serve as a useful tool to help guide scientists in research and development by outlining the theory and successful practice of in vitro - in vivo correlation, (ii) to help formulators apply the tool in designing and developing prototypes that enable selection of clinical formulations, and (iii) to help formulate strategy(ies) for product life-cycle management.

To make the work more comprehensive and informative, the author has consulted many authoritative books, research journals, abstracts, monographs etc., so there can be no claim to originality except in the manner of treatment.

The author expresses his thanks to his friends and colleagues whose continue inspirations have initiated him to bring out this book.

The author expresses his gratitude to Mr. Wasan and staff of M/s Discovery Publishing House Pvt. Ltd. for their whole hearted co-operation in the publication of this book.

Author

CONTENTS

1

INTRODUCTION

Biopharmaceuticals are drugs, vaccines, and pharmaceutical agents (typically therapeutic proteins or polypeptides) developed or produced using techniques of biotechnology. In many cases they are complex proteins exhibiting varying levels of heterogeneity, derived from recombinant gene expression or hybridoma production systems. These products of biotechnology generally are classified as biologicals by regulatory agencies. Specific categories of products include monoclonal antibodies and other recombinant proteins produced in cell culture, enzymes, hormones, soluble receptors, growth factors, imunogens, blood and plasma products, and animal-derived products. Biopharmaceuticals range in molecular weight from a low value of 22,000 for human growth hormone to about 150,000 for an intact immunoglobulin. These agents are among the most expensive products to manufacture, with typical inventory costs of hundreds to thousands of dollars per gram. There is also intense pressure to introduce a product to the market in a timely manner to recover research and facility investments. Consequently, the reliable production of quality biophar maceuticals is of the highest importance, translating into an intense focus on the creation of an effective and economical production process. Process validation is a key mechanism to successfully accomplish the task of process creation.

PROCESS VALIDATION OVERVIEW

Definitions

Validation derives from the Latin word *valere* meaning "to have the power", presumably referring to the power to prevent an unexpected and undesirable occurrence. It establishes that the process used is reliable and reproducible. The level of control implemented is supported by scientific knowledge of the culture and product, along with equipment capabilities. The U.S. Food and Drug Administration (FDA) definition of process validation (PV) is documented evidence to provide a high degree of assurance that a specific process consistently produces a product meeting predetermined specifications and quality characteristics. The International Conference on Harmonization (ICH) definition is similar, stating that process validation is documented evidence that the process, when operated within established parameters, performs reproducibly and effectively to produce an intermediate or active pharmaceutical ingredient (API) meeting predetermined specifications and quality attributes. Most simply stated, process validation provides a high degree of assurance that process will routinely achieve the stated goals. It accomplishes this goal by verifying product and process specifications to determine their weaknesses and reproducibility and by demonstrating at which steps contaminants are removed and the product stream achieves acceptance criteria. A verification of process consistency is conducted, highlighting the ability to produce essentially the same product (with the same safety and efficacy) over time, despite normal variability in operating conditions. Consistency of multiple batches is demonstrated at full scale, with specific focus on the process operating in a consistent manner, reproducible removal of contaminants to acceptable levels, and monitoring parameters that demonstrate this consistency.

Process validation for biopharmaceuticals is somewhat different in application from traditional pharmaceuticals because the technology is different, but the theory and principles are similar. Biotechnology quality control is defined by the individual production process and the product itself because quality cannot be tested into the product. The manner in which the biopharmaceutical is produced is part of its description: thus, biopharmaceuticals are characterized by chemical structure as well as by operational definition. Few doubt the need for process validation, but there is disagreement and confusion about what needs to be validated and how to perform it. Operational definitions of process validation have been developed to suit the philosophies of individual companies. Thus, there is increased interest in developing industry guidelines for the design and performance of validation studies.

The term *validation* has different implications under different circumstances, and thus, its use can be confusing. Furthermore, the term *validation* has been used interchangeably with other terms such as *performance qualification* and *process characterization*, when discussing process as well as equipment testing. Recognizing that individual firms distinguish among these terms differently, there has not been an attempt in this chapter to create strict definitions that artificially introduce restrictions where none exist currently. Rather, the terminology employed has remained flexible regardless of the specific terminology used in the source material, such that it reads as internally consistent. In addition, the focus of this chapter primarily is on process validation for steps required to produce bulk biological substances, but the principles discussed also can be applied to the final processing steps involved in formulation and packaging.

Purpose and Benefits

Validation has been a critical success factor in product approval and ongoing commercialization. It serves as a formal link of the process to the product, focusing on quality but often concurrently addressing critical business concerns. Each Good Manufacturing Practice (GMP) step must be controlled to maximize the probability that the finished product meets all quality and design specifications. In addition, each step must be evaluated for its function and effect on product identity, purity, potency, safety, or stability. An unvalidatable process is unacceptable and unreliable from both regulatory and manufacturing (i.e., business) perspectives.

There are two goals of process validation: (1) to support the safety, efficacy, and quality of the product; and (2) to identify major sources of process variability so appropriate controls can be implemented to provide consistency. Achievement of these goals demonstrates that potential risks have been adequately reduced and assures products consistently possess the required established quality attributes. Weaker points of the manufacturing process are uncovered and strengthened during the validation effort. Thus, process validation deepens process understanding, which in turn decreases the risk of processing problems/failures, defect costs, lot rejections, reworking/reprocessing, product shortages, or regulatory noncompliance. Assurance of process consistency maximizes productivity and increases cost efficiency. It influences process economics in many ways; one example is through the reduction of in-process control and endproduct testing by reducing the number and scope of quality control tests per lot.

Scope

Process validation is the culmination of all qualification and validation activities, representing process testing in its entirety. It is a dynamic process varying in depth according to the product life-cycle timeline, spanning from initial process design through ongoing commercial operation. Its execution can be envisioned as creating a "*design space*," a multidimensional space that defines how different variables interact. This design space (1) establishes the process ranges demonstrated to provide quality assurance, and (2) defines areas in which process adjustments and refinements may be undertaken without regulatory involvement. The dimensions of this design space are based on the scientific understanding of critical process parameters that has been created through development studies.

For a product, the overall list of subcomponent systems to be validated includes equipment, facilities, utilities, computers (including software and controls), processing environment, analytical methods, and operating procedures (e.g., cleaning and sterilization), as well as the process itself. Before process validation begins, these subcomponent systems are qualified. As process validation rests on the fidelity of the qualification of the subcomponent systems required for process operation, the undetected shortcomings of these efforts can compromise subsequent process validation. As with equipment qualification, process validation is most effective when conducted in combination with effective process and facility design efforts. Also, as with equipment qualification, predefined acceptance criteria and action plans in case of test failure are devised. The use of predetermined specifications serves to reduce the goals of a validation program to actual practice, assisting in implementation.

Process validation for the production process is only one means to assure product consistency. Other factors include quality control for the final product, in-process assays, raw material controls, appropriately designed facilities, personnel monitoring and training, and environmental monitoring. Additional factors that become concerns for multiproduct biopharmaceutical facilities include (1) segregation of materials, personnel, and equipment; (2) cleaning and product changeover; and (3) product cross-contamination. Characteristics of biopharmaceutical processing that generate specific areas of quality control concern are large, complex product molecules, complicated manufacturing systems, long production times, and pooling of fermentation lots before isolation. Other product quality concerns include genetic stability, product yield and stability, host and nonhost cell component contamination, and posttranslational processing, including glycosylation and folding. As biopharmaceutical manufacturing processes are complicated with multiple steps and extended production times, adequate in-process testing, thorough process validation, and appropriate measures to eliminate adventitious agents are necessary.

Regulatory

The completion of process validation represents the point at which the science of the process is ready to be explained to regulatory agencies. Process validation data are initially presented to the regulatory agency during application submission. These data set the bar by which the process is to be judged during future inspections, and consequently, one of most common FDA 483 observations is the lack of process validation. As manufacturing is a key factor in achieving the required quality and safety of biotechnology products, process validation is a regulatory requirement for product licensure, and limited process validation is considered essential even for product destined for clinical trials. Process validation is required in license submissions for all products regulated by either CBER or CDER. There are added challenges for biopharmaceuticals, however, as process consistency often replaces detailed product analysis as a key method of quality assurance, and biologically based production systems contribute biological contaminants that pose safety risks.

It has been stated that validation should be written as if the FDA were the customer, and this approach still is valid because worldwide harmonization efforts are well underway. Several guidance documents have been published in draft and finalized forms from various regulatory agencies and industry associations worldwide. New guidance, as well as interpretations of prior guidance, is continuously published, suggesting that there is not yet one consistent approach to process validation. Additional guidance leading to the improved definition of process validation requirements and reduction in marginally helpful studies is welcomed by industry. Several comprehensive publications describing the interpretation and application of process validation by industry are available, but terminology and definitions have become blurred and overlapping. Consequently, the use of the term selected must be fully and consistently understood by authors, reviewers, approvers, executors, and auditors in the context of its specific application.

Pitfalls

Validation (consisting of process, equipment, and facility systems) is a costly and time-consuming investment with more resources believed devoted to its completion than to the initial process development and production of clinical supplies. The actual cost of process validation is thought by some to be uncontrolled and excessive because there is no consensus on how much is enough. One key risk associated with bio pharmaceutical product manufacturing is the failure to gather sufficient information to support process decisions when faced with issues arising in process validation, failure investigations, product specifications, analytical methods, and equipment qualification.

Common pitfalls associated with process validation are numerous. They include a lack of overall strategy, insufficient planning/management, delay in early consultation with regulatory agencies, inadequate product definition, failure to observe current GMPs (cGMPs) and follow standard operating procedures (SOPs), poorly defined cell bank genealogy, inadequate analytical procedures, confusion over participant responsibilities, excessive process changes after process validation completion, insufficient prior process characterization or qualification, starting process validation too early and before process finalization, poor validation study design/definition, disagreement on evaluation/interpretation of results, and inappropriate acceptance criteria. When overall validation activities begin too late, the work required to validate methods, facilities, and/or processes typically has been underestimated, placing product launch at risk. When processes perform erratically during process validation, further investigation to uncover inadequate development or lack of control of one or more process variables is required, followed by additional validation studies. Validation must be science based. Sound science during process validation is the primary vehicle to reduce manufacturing costs while remaining compliant with regulatory expectations. Overly complex plans contradict desires to be efficient, lean, and cost-effective. More intensely planned projects produce more efficient, lower cost, and higher quality products in a faster time frame. Resulting risks for biopharmaceutical companies from ineffective process validation include patient (safety and efficacy), operational (safety, contamination, variability), financial (product loss, reputation, legal costs), and regulatory factors.

Evaluating Measures of Product Quality and Consistent Process Performance

A stream-lined, integrated, and comprehensive validation process is desired. The key to achieving a manageable process validation design is determining which process variables can be relegated to a noncritical status or maintained under tight control. Only when absolutely necessary should parameter ranges be validated. Thus development studies are required to identify critical parameters, limits to their operating ranges, and those process characteristics and equipment that enable their tight control. It is necessary to distinguish between measures of product quality and process performance (consistency) and to differentiate between release specifications (such as critical quality attributes, CQA) that are measures of product quality and process attributes that demonstrate consistent process performance. Validation studies are required to examine process parameter variations that cause yield losses by affecting product quality (i.e., critical parameters); they are not needed for process parameter variations that cause yield losses that do not affect product quality even though these losses can cause economic/ business concerns.

Critical Process Input Variables/Parameters

The basis of all process validation studies is the demonstration of control of critical process input parameters for reproducible operation of a commercial-scale production process. Critical parameters vary among processes so they must be separately assessed for each new process. As a typical process has hundreds of variables, critical process input parameters must be identified first, and then the extended range and normal (target) operating range for each critical parameter must be determined during process development and/or using historical data. Critical variables are identified using defined procedures combining elements of data analysis and scientific judgment and making maximum use of available data gathered during process development. Various companies have developed differing decision matrices to determine critical parameters, some of which are based on formal risk analysis exercises. A critical variable is defined as a parameter whose operating range lies near the edge of failure. Using this definition, in practice, most identified critical variables can be engineered out of the study. Critical steps are those steps that are difficult to control because they usually contain at least one or more critical variables that cannot be removed.

Critical control points (CCPs) are those locations within a process where control can be applied to protect product quality, specifically to prevent and eliminate quality hazards or to reduce them to acceptable levels. For controlling hazards, the appropriate CCP may be positioned in the subsequent step from the actual hazard location. In addition, more than one CCP can be used to control a single hazard and more than one hazard can be controlled by a single CCP.

Critical parameters are studied next to determine the effects of their outer limit values on important process characteristics. These critical outer limits must be attainable, accurate, robust, and scientifically based. The control parameter range is the span of values that lies between two outer limits or control levels of a parameter, and it represents the highest and/or lowest values of a given control parameter that actually are evaluated during validation. It is not usually necessary to test both ends of the control parameter range for all parameters because scientific judgment can help determine which end of the range (high or low) is more likely to generate an adverse effect. In other cases, testing of both the upper and the lower control limits for a large number of variables is required to identify worst-case conditions. Acceptable ranges are narrowed, and experiments are repeated until the acceptance criteria are met using an iterative process that requires substantial execution. The edge of failure is reached when an exceeded control parameter value adversely affects the process or the product in that process performance degrades or product fails; however, it is not necessary to validate the edge of failure when validating a process.

One strategy is to select worst-case conditions that encompass the upper and lower processing limits of critical input parameters, along with situations and circumstances over the entire process (rather than only a single step) that together result in the greatest chance of process or product failure compared with the ideal or target conditions. Worst-case runs are long and complex because the entire process must be run completely, usually at large scale or full scale. Because the worst-case approach comprehensively includes the direct effects and actions of all variables, if all experiments are successful, only a few studies are required. To mitigate the high likelihood of failure of a worst-case study that results in repeating lengthy runs using revised conditions, worst-case runs are performed after factorial experiments, usually conducted at a smaller scale and of a narrower scope, have confirmed a satisfactory outcome under the proposed worst-case conditions. A key philosophical weak point of the worst-case run strategy is that it is less probable in practice that all critical parameters experience simultaneous excursions to outer limits. However, because all critical parameters are tested at their extreme range, the worst-case approach can identify interactions that design of experiment (DOE) methods cannot detect.

Regardless of the strategy employed, worst-case conditions for critical parameters are established and process validation assures that the process yields an acceptable product when challenged under these worst-case conditions, even though full-scale validation runs may not have been conducted at many of these worst-case limits. Then operating ranges and control limits are set to establish a process robust enough to produce acceptable product, and full-scale validation runs are executed to demonstrate performance consistency. The assumption is that if the product is of acceptable quality when parameters are controlled at the outer limits of control ranges, then the quality also will be acceptable when these parameters are held within those control ranges. This strategy is analogous to the approach of using fractional cycles for validation and full cycles for actual operation when testing at cleaning and sterilization procedures.

For a controlled variable, several types of ranges exist around the set point. The normal operating range (NOR), or the alert limit, is established by trending performance during clinical material or qualification lot production, and then assigning usually two or three standard deviations to the set point. The proven acceptable range (PAR) encompasses all values of a given control parameter that fall between proven high and low worst-case conditions and constitutes the proposed operating range. The PAR should be greater than or equal to the MOR. The maximum operating range (MOR), or the action limit, is the range of the controlled variable within which product quality is acceptable, but not necessarily at the limit of failure; thus, if the variable value falls outside the MOR, it is not necessarily a failure. As MORs can lead to a decline in process .performance even if product quality remains acceptable, their frequent occurrence can become an economic or operational issue. The MOR should be sufficiently broader than the NOR to reduce the frequency of unplanned deviations. The MOR can be extended based on manufacturing experience when excursions outside the MOR occur without adverse quality effects. Overall, a demonstrated state of control is the condition when all operating variables that can affect performance remain within such ranges that performance is consistent and as intended.

Noncritical Process Input Variables/Parameters

Noncritical or operational parameters are process control set points that define the process recipe and show that the process can be executed consistently, but for which there is no established evidence of product quality impact. If the process performance is consistent when noncritical variables are controlled within their ranges and if minor deviations (e.g., instrumentation inaccuracy) from these ranges do not affect product quality, then the variable or step is classified as noncritical. Typical noncritical control ranges are wide and/or the variable/parameter is easy to control within the range. Although noncritical parameters do not require further study, they also are controlled and monitored during process validation to reduce variability and operator error. Recently, noncritical process parameters have been designated as key (ensuring operational reliability and desired process performance when maintained within a narrow range, significant impact but not failure within range) and nonkey (well-controlled within a wide range but a potential process or quality impact when outside range, no significant impact within range).

Process Control/Input Parameters (Xs)

Process control parameters are operating variables that have assigned values to be used for control. They usually are readily maintainable away from a point of failure and within a tested manufacturing range by a feedback control mechanism. Control parameters may also be thought of interchangeably as input parameters, defined as operational parameters that can be controlled. Control/ input variables are those operating parameters with set points or ranges that define process execution, e.g., pH, flowrate, temperature, raw material amounts and specifications, properties, and hold times for in-process streams of prior steps; thus, these parameters can be validated as a range or as set points. They are a subset of operating variables, all factors that potentially affect process control or product quality, that reasonably are expected to affect operation of a process step. Control/input parameters also are referred to as Xs, analogous to independent variables.

All input parameters must be identified and demonstrated to be in control for the product to be in a validated state and the more tightly the range is controlled, the less critical the parameter is considered.

Validation steps are (1) identification; (2) classification as critical or noncritical, subclassification of critical parameters into those to be validated over a broad range and those to be validated as a set point with a narrow tolerance range; (3) validation execution for those critical input parameters with a broad range; and (4) validation execution using target set points for all process input parameters both critical and noncritical. The complexity of process validation is dictated by several critical process input parameters requiring either a broad range or a broad set point. As fewer range testing studies are required if more parameters can be tightly controlled, one strategy is to design tight control set points for as many critical process input parameters as possible (e.g., pH and temperature).

Performance Uncontrolled Output Variables/Attributes (Ys)

Performance parameters reflect the outcome of a given step and indicate that the process gave the desired result or quality attribute. They are uncontrolled performance variables without a control action. Their natural variation is defined by operating history; specifically, their variability is characterized from known historical data or estimated based on similar process performance. Similarly, output variables reflect the step outcome and indicate performance was acceptable in terms of performance attributes for the step (e.g., titer and yield) or properties of the product stream (e.g., product homogeneity, purity, contaminant levels, and chromatography peak shape. Still another term used is critical Ys (analogous to dependent variables), defined as product and process output variables that relate to critical quality attributes (CQAs), which are measurable outputs of each process step that are used to provide evidence that the step performed correctly.

An input parameter value is directly related to an output parameter or quality attribute; specifically, the output parameter of one unit operation often is the input parameter for the subsequent unit operation. Equivalently stated, critical Ys (outputs or responses) from one stage often are inputs for next the stage. Input parameters are assessed as to whether they significantly impact critical output parameters (e.g., product safety, identity, and efficacy), although the definition of significant varies among applications. As all product quality attributes are not routinely measured during process development, some output variables are selected based on a hypothesis that they are linked to desirable product characteristics. An input parameter is determined as critical based on whether its operating point is located near the edge of failure and how well it can be controlled. Input parameters then are prioritized based on the (1) output sensitivity to input variations, (2) step proximity to the final product, and (3) technical difficulty controlling the input within the specified range.

A more formal approach involves listing all key process input variables (KPIVs), factors [both process (physical) and product (chemistry)] that could potentially affect the mean and standard deviation of critical Ys (outputs). KPIVs are identified using brainstorming to generate initial information. Then the identified factors are reviewed to select those that should be maintained constant based on scientific judgment. Next, a review of process development data and additional experiments using DOE are used to identify those KPIVs which influence critical Ys. Experimental results are inserted into a cause and effect diagram which statistically correlates input and output variables by constructing scatter plots.

Background and Requirements

Types of Process Validation

All three types of validation, prospective, concurrent, and retrospective, are part of most comprehensive process validation programs that occur throughout a product's lifetime. As a process approaches commercial status, validation approaches completion.

Prospective

Prospective validation is validation conducted before the dis tribution of either a new product or a product made under a revised manu facturing process where revisions may affect the product characteristics. Prospective validation assures that process quality attributes are met before manufacturing operations have commenced. It is based on a preplanned protocol. Usually process validation is prospective because a science-based, prospective validation is integrated as a continuous part of the development process. Validation performed prospectively is relatively less dependent on in-process or endproduct testing. Manufacturing lots can be released faster if prospective rather than concurrent validation is performed.

Concurrent

Concurrent validation is based on information generated during the actual implementation of the process, at the same time the marketed product is being manufactured. Concurrent validation reduces the load at the time of regulatory submission because experiments are delayed until the manufacturing process is operating, but it places marketable lots at risk if a failure is detected. Until process validation (e.g., useful resin lifetime) can be established at the manufacturing scale via concurrent validation, a thorough performance analysis of the step (e.g., chromatography) must be undertaken for each manufactured lot, which is quarantined until the results are evaluated. Thus, concurrent validation is based on batchwise process control and requires the use of validated in-process sampling and methods.

Retrospective

Retrospective validation is based on the review and analysis of historical information (e.g., batch records, in-process control testing, and stability testing) to reconfirm formally that control parameter ranges are appropriate. Validation protocols sometimes are not needed, but the final results are formally approved. As with concurrent validation, retrospective validation requires batchwise control of the process and usually depends on in-process testing. Retrospective validation has been found useful to augment (but not replace) premarket prospective validation for new products or changed processes. The proven acceptable range (PAR) can be developed using the principles of retrospective validation to link acceptable product lots to normal/permissible values for process operating parameters.

Retrospective analysis applies to a large number of batches that have been prepared similarly by evaluating input/output parameter variation and relating it directly to batch product quality. Specifically, it is most effective when many similar batches (e.g., tens to hundreds) exist. However, the observed range of some input parameters may be insufficient if they were tightly controlled during processing to effectively determine the impact of wider variations. In cases where disparate historical data sources may not be directly comparable or missing, a screening DOE might be appropriate to establish that existing specifications maintain CQAs at desirable levels.

Aspects of Process Validations

Process validation starts with the identification of product quality attributes and justification of acceptance criteria, followed by a review of the risk analysis, execution of process development runs, and compilation of clinical material manufacturing data to set specifications considering process variability. There is a greater focus on process validation for downstream steps rather than for upstream steps because downstream steps are associated with virus removal. Process validation is just one approach used to control virus contamination, however; others include cell bank characterization, in-process testing, inactivation procedures, control of raw materials, containment, and postmarket surveillance.

One significant source of variability in downstream process steps is changes in input streams between research/pilot-scale to full-scale. Thus, input streams of high and low quality are used when evaluating the performance of the subsequent step in a pair-wise validation strategy. Specifically, forward linkage studies are performed to understand downstream consequences for critical parameters. When process steps are studied individually in a factorial approach, forward linkage variables are the output variables of given step that affect the performance of the next step.

Fermentation

A validatable fermentation process demonstrates a controllable method of growing cells that reliably express the biopharmaceutical product that can be reproducibly recovered if broth is harvested within a set of specified conditions that allow the product to meet its quality specifications. The goals of fermentation process validation are to provide documented evidence that all aspects of the process perform as intended to generate consistent fermentation broths at harvest; this consistency in turn permits downstream steps to yield a purified product consistently meeting its predetermined specifications. Allowable ranges for culture conditions must be justified with scientific data. Typical components of fermentation process validation include the fermenter sterile medium hold, inoculum train, fermenter inoculation, sampling, feeding, fermenter growth and production phases, and harvesting. Specifically, the trigger for fermentation harvest (e.g., cultivation time, cell density, and viability) should be demonstrated to yield acceptable product. CQAs defined for fermentation include product yield, cell density, and culture purity; critical process parameters include inoculum state, nutrient feeding scheme, and harvest time. To ensure consistent broth quality, critical process parameters are best defined based on a culture physiological event rather than on elapsed cultivation time and are preferably those that exhibit distinctive online monitoring characteristics.

To link fermentation process input parameters to output parameters, specifically behavior in downstream isolation steps and ultimate product quality, usually a partial or total purification is necessary, which requires substantial labor to process samples. Sample evaluation also is limited depending on the level of product characterization. Consequently, fermentation process validation has been viewed as less rigorous compared with other forms of process validation.

Viral Clearance Studies

Requirements

Any biopharmaceutical product using animal-derived materials during the manufacturing process has the potential for virus contamination. The risk varies depending on the animal species and country of origin of the raw material and the safety concerns associated with expression and amplification of the production system. Process validation is conducted to determine the process capacity to remove and/or inactivate a virus using a wide variety of viruses in virus clearance studies. These studies complement analytical viral testing of product (at various stages of production, including the final product), starting materials (e.g., cell banks), and raw materials. Each process validation viral clearance study is reviewed individually to determine the log reduction performance versus requirements, which are set based on experimental limitations as well as on risk factors (i.e., number of patients and dosage). In practice, viral inactivation testing is less rigorous than microbial sterilization testing, viral test methods generally are cumbersome with variable results (although PCR technology has improved technical robustness), and viral inactivating agents less robust than saturated steam. Consequently, viral clearance studies are a substantial component of process validation.

Viral clearance can be demonstrated by two distinct mechanisms that both generate high clearance values. One mechanism is inactivation to reduce infectivity by chemical or physical means without affecting protein product stability. Methods include using pH (acidic, low pH conditions for pH inactivation for protein A, basic, high pH conditions for ion exchange resins), chaotropic agents (urea), ultraviolet irradiation, and solvent, detergent, or heat treatment. The second mechanism is removal or partitioning to effect a physical separation of virus from the product. Methods include using chromatography (adsorbing protein and leaving virus in the column flowthrough or vice versa) and filtration (depth filters with a 20–40-nm pore size or ultra-filtration membranes with a cutoff of <300 kDa).

Processing conditions significantly affect virus inactivation/removal performance. Specifically pH, buffer composition, protein concentration, flow rate, and product binding strength to resin influence chromatography steps. Membrane chemistry and pore size, geometry, velocity and pressure of process streams, transmembrane pressure, and product load per area (volume/area, concentration/area) influence filtration steps. When virus-inactivating buffers are used in chromatography, virus reduction is effected in the eluted product from a combination of removal and inactivation. Analytical methods that can evaluate infectious as well as inactivated virus distribution in process streams can assist in understanding virus removal mechanisms.

Steps to be Validated for Viral Clearance

Process validation for viral clearance is conducted only on robust steps that can (1) be scaled down accurately and (2) reproducibly and effectively remove and/or inactivate a wide variety of potential viral contaminants under a wide variety of process conditions. The number of steps selected for validation depends on estimated viral clearance effectiveness based on historical data and target clearance values. The FDA demands at least two different steps for virus reduction to guarantee safety and efficacy. Potentially only two steps are required for antibody processes that use serum-free medium, but additional steps might be required if viral contamination risk is increased by using serum-containing medium. Due to the use of live viruses to perform clearance studies, this work usually is outsourced to reduce cross-contamination issues.

The viral clearance reduction factor, the common logarithm of the ratio between the total virus loads before and after clearance, is established for viruses known to contaminate the production process. Individual step clearances are combined to obtain the total clearance reduction factor. This reduction factor is used in combination with an assessment of step robustness to classify the step as effective (≥ 4 reduction factor and unaffected by small changes in process variables), moderately effective ($4 >$ reduction factor > 1), or ineffective (≤ 1 reduction factor) with respect to virus clearance. Clearance factors are usually multiplied if the mechanism is different for two separate steps and sometimes are added if the mechanism is same. In other cases, if two independent steps have similar mechanisms of clearance, only one step is included in the summation because virus particles removed via that mechanism would only be expected to be removed in the first step. A total clearance of 12–15 logs is desired for lipid-enveloped viruses and fewer logs for nonenveloped viruses (e.g., polio).

Virus loads in unprocessed, prepurified bulk (harvest samples) are quantified, typically via transmission by electron microscopy or infectivity, to estimate actual virus load versus the expected virus removal capacity of the process. Total virus clearance should exceed measured levels by at least 3–5 logs. An example of a typical virus load is 10^5 to 10^7 RVLPs (retrovirus-like particles) per milliliter of unprocessed bulk from CHO cells. Clearance factors of 15–20 logs are typical for murine retroviruses and slightly more than for lipid-enveloped viruses. For most viruses besides endogenous retroviruses, however, there is no reasonable way to establish virus load in the bulk because these types of viruses should not normally be present. In addition direct testing methods are limited inherently because they are designed to detect only known and not known contaminants. Thus, the capacity of the downstream purification process to remove/inactivate known viruses should they be inadvertently introduced is defined for an extra degree of assurance.

Spiking studies

Often, if viruses are present in process streams, they are present at levels below analytical detection, so spiking-clearance studies are required for purification steps. Spiking studies are repeated so that their reproducibility and variability can be assessed. There are concerns that large spikes may not be representative of actual low-level virus behavior, however. Virus spikes are desired to contain as little protein as possible to reduce the impact of their addition on purification procedures. Addition of a virus spike can alter protein concentration and viscosity, which can change elution characteristics and prevent the small-scale model from accurately predicting full-scale performance. In practice, this goal is more readily achievable for non-lipid-enveloped viruses because enveloped viruses need a certain amount of protein to maintain stability. Maintaining the salt concentration constant or evaluating product resolution and purity are two ways to demonstrate that the virus spike addition had no significant effect. Consequently, there is a compromise between adding the highest amount of virus possible to more rigorously challenge and maximize the step clearance and maintaining the spike volume low (<10%) to avoid appreciable alteration of product composition and thus purification performance.

Virus selection

The goal of model virus selection is to demonstrate inactivation or removal of as many types of viruses as possible without compromising product activity and quality. One virus can act as a model for a group of viruses with similar physiochemical characteristics. Model viruses should be possible to grow in cell culture to high titers and detectable using a simple but sensitive assay. Some viruses that are known to potentially contaminate starting materials grow quite poorly in cell culture; thus, some model viruses have been tissue-culture adapted and consequently may not be truly representative of wild-type viruses. Another limitation of using model virus clearance studies is that model viruses may not behave similarly to actual viruses, but in many cases, model viruses are the only practical alternative.

Viral selection is based on (1) relevant viruses that are actual viruses (or of the same species as actual viruses and relevant to the host cell) that have been identified as contaminants (or potential contaminants) of the process, (2) specific model viruses that are closely related to actual viruses (e.g., same genus or family) and have similar physico-chemical properties, and (3) nonspecific model viruses believed to be representative of the spectrum of different virus physiochemical characteristics. Nonspecific model viruses are used to show inactivation/ removal of viruses in general and to characterize purification robustness. Virus clearance studies should cover emerging viruses and viruses currently believed to be absent in raw materials. These concerns are not addressed when relying on direct testing to ensure safety, specifically consideration of future virus removal requirements in anticipation of future regulatory changes.

Model viruses are selected that cover the range of physico-chemical properties of different virus species such as size (i.e., diameter and geometry), enveloped or nonenveloped, RNA or DNA, and single- or double-stranded genome. Examples of model viruses selected for various char acteristics are medium-to-large DNA/enveloped (Herpes Simplex I, pseu dorabies), small/DNA/nonenveloped (Simian virus SV-40), small/RNA/nonenveloped (Sabin Type I Polio, animal parvovirus), medium-to-large RNA/enveloped (Influenza Type A, parainfluenza virus, Sinbis virus 1), and retrovirus/RNA/enveloped for murine hybridomas (Moloney murine leukemia). Preference in the selection of specific model viruses is given to those viruses with significant resistance to physical removal/chemical agents. The number and type of viruses selected for spiking studies depends on the process materials (e.g., host cell) and product development stage. Before phase I, virus validation must be conducted. Typical viruses studied are the murine leukemia virus as a model virus for retrovirus-like particles produced by murine cell expression systems (if applicable to the process) and parvovirus. Before phase II, two to four additional viruses are selected that depend on the host cell and media origin. It is advised to solicit feedback on virus selection from the relevant regulatory agencies depending on where the trials are to be conducted before conducting viral clearance studies for product destined for initial clinical trials.

Starting and raw materials

Starting and raw materials are chemical, biochemical, or biological components used in a biopharmaceutical manufacturing process. Quality control strategies for these materials have been developed based on the assumption that these materials may be contaminated with a virus. Direct testing is limited by the fact that viral contamination can be nonhomogenously distributed in a raw material lot; thus, additional sampling has little value. In addition to being effective only if contaminants are homogeneously distributed, direct viral testing also only is effective if the contaminant is present at high titer, false positives can be investigated promptly, a broad spectrum of viruses are detectable by available assays, assays are adequately sensitive, and raw materials do not inhibit assay performance.

Cell substrate

Since the genetically altered cell substrate is considered the main component in the production process, complete characterization plus evaluation of genetic stability are primary concerns. Cell bank characterization in conjunction with product characterization (e.g., peptide mapping and amino acid sequencing) demonstrates the stability of the production process. Cell bank characterization in conjunction with process validation and endproduct testing demonstrate product safety. The most likely source of viral contaminations in a large-scale cell culture is the cell substrate. Process validation plus cell bank validation provides assurance that final product is free of contaminating viruses and other adventitious agents. There is little concern about viruses that do not replicate in the cell substrate, although nonreplication can be hard to demonstrate. As one of the most critical raw materials in production is the cell bank, defined acceptance/rejection criteria and parameters under which the bank will be used are required. Assays are performed on master and working cell banks to demonstrate stability and freedom from adventitious agents. Cells are analyzed both from master/working bank vials as well as from the end of the production run or a few doublings later.

During cell bank characterization, phenotypic characteristics of the master cell bank are established such as morphology, doubling time, product expression rates, karyology (for diploid cell lines), and isoenzyme analysis. Genotypic characteristics also are established, including a description of the vector and inserted gene, copy number, restriction maps, and the nucleotide sequence of a cloned gene. Tests are conducted for adventitious agents such as bacteria, fungi, mycoplasmas, and a wide range of potential viruses (e.g., retroviruses). Routine stability programs are undertaken to monitor genetic stability with respect to phenotype, expression, and nucleic acid integrity. A passage history (e.g., split ratio, storage conditions, and media used) is documented as well as the cell line origin. As a result of these regulatory requirements, cell banks must be prepared by those well versed in the technical processing steps, but also well aware of regulatory requirements.

Media

Basal medium and other supplemental components are tested in a scaled-down mimic of the production process to determine cell growth and product yield, and the product characteristics are compared against reference materials. It is necessary to assure that multiple lots of raw materials meet user specifications for performance and quality before selecting a vendor and that at least one backup vendor is available.

Step hold times

Documentation of bioburden and endotoxin control at the manufacturing scale over the entire hold time is accomplished via monitoring of intermediates using in-process samples. In addition, small-scale studies can provide relevant worst-case data. The cumulative worst-case hold times are obtainable from the summation of the maximum individual unit operation hold times. However, this worst case is not required to be validated because such a series of unexpected events is likely to cause adverse drug quality as well as high endotoxin or bioburden. Instead, hold time studies are conducted for process solutions over the maximum durations that they will be held in tanks used for manufacturing.

Real-time stability data are required for reliably assigning expiry periods. Stability data are obtained on the drug product stored in the proposed container under recommended storage temperatures, and this strategy has been applied for in-process streams. Although elevated temperature stability studies are used to accelerate product degradation rate to predict shelf-life, this acceleration methodology is usually not used to determine step hold times, which typically are a few days, weeks, or in rarer cases months. Additional stability and degradation concerns arise from the possible interaction of protein with stoppers and container closure systems and interaction of proteins with residual cleaning agents.

Contaminant/impurity clearance

Classes of contaminant removal include process-related, host-cell related, andproduct-related (e.g., aggregates, deaminations, and oxidations) substances. Contaminant clearance studies can be used to avoid lot-to-lot acceptance criteria because safety margins of several logs of excess clearance are demonstrated. In these studies, a contaminant is added to the input feed stream at the small scale, its recovery is measured at each stage of the process step (e.g., column flowthrough, product pool, and regeneration fractions), and mass balance measurements are performed. In a similar manner as viral clearance studies, each step's impurity clearance is challenged separately; then overall clearance is calculated by the product of individual clearances. Impurity clearance studies are similar in concept to viral clearance studies without many of the virus handling and personnel contact safety issues.

Process-related contaminants include cell substrate-derived (e.g., host cell protein, DNA, retroviral-like particles, and endotoxin for *E. coli* cultures), cell culture-derived (e.g., inducers, antibiotics, and serum/media components such as antifoam), downstream-derived (e.g., enzymes, processing reagents such as glycerol and guanidine, inorganic salts, solvents, leachables, and ligands), and adventitious agents (e.g., virus, bioburden, and endotoxin). Cell substrate-derived and adventitious agents have been discussed. For many process-related contaminants (e.g., antifoams and enzymes), the key to tracking and demonstrating their removal is the development of a robust, sensitive, and yet straightforward assay.

A documented methodology is required for how product-contact materials are selected and purchased for specific process use. Leachate process validation demonstrates that leachates are below limits of detection in each eluent pool; insignificant leaching occurs under severe chemical, time, and temperature exposure, and if significant leaching does occur, it is removed by the first few bed volumes of equilibration buffer. Product extractable testing evaluates product contact surfaces in terms of materials of construction, process solutions or solvents, duration of product contact with various surfaces, product contact surface areas, and potential for extractables at various process stages. Materials are prioritized to direct studies at the most critical, high-risk materials. High-risk materials are based on the proximity to the final API, extraction capability of solvent, length of contact, product contact surface area, cytotoxicity of extractables, temperature, and inherent material resistance to extraction. Example high-priority materials to assess are containers (e.g., stainless steel cans and plastic bags) for unfrozen and frozen storage of fermentation media/purification buffers/product intermediate streams, chromatography resins, valve diaphragms/transfer hoses, elastomers/ pumps especially on the final purification skid, filtration membranes, final sterilizing filter, gaskets/o-rings especially on the final bulk tank, and silicone boot/tubing for the filling machine. Material extractable data can be obtained in-house, or often it is available from the vendor.

Product-related impurities include truncated product forms, modified product forms (e.g., deaminated, isomerized, disulfide-linked, and oxidized), and product aggregates. One way these undesired forms arise is during freezing and thawing owing to product concentration and pH gradients; thus, the number of freeze/thaw cycles is minimized. Another way is from mixing liquids and dissoluting powders. The minimum mixing time until homogeneity is determined for which results vary only within assay variability; maximum mixing times are established to avoid shear, oxidation, and/or product degradation.

Reuse of chromatography resin

It is necessary to demonstrate that chromatographic media can be reused, cleaned, and sanitized. Used resins receive additional analysis not required with new resins such as the titration of small ion binding capacity, measurement of total protein capacity, comparison of flow versus pressure plots to indicate particle size (and attrition), particle size distribution, total organic carbon (TOC) removal by cleaning solutions, and microbial contamination/endotoxin (LAL) analysis. Exposure to cleaning/regeneration solutions, rather than contact with mild buffers and protein solutions during normal processing, is most likely to cause chemical degradation. Three types of studies thus apply to resins: Column reuse studies verify continued resin performance after multiple uses followed by small-scale carry-over runs to confirm cleanability with multiple uses, characterization studies prove the process is robust and defines acceptable operational limits, and another third study type demonstrates that regeneration sufficiently sanitizes the resin and that the storage solution is bacteriostatic and fungistatic.

Columns reused for many cycles may not provide the same virus clearance as new columns. Thus, virus spiking studies can be performed on new and aged resins to ensure clearance does not vary. Alternatively, virus clearance can be studied for new resins only, and performance attributes expected to decay before virus clearance ability can be monitored subsequently during actual reuse. Validation of the column resin cleaning and sanitization regime for virus inactivation also is necessary to demonstrate that bound virus does not accumulate and subsequently elute. The appropriate number of reuses is selected by balancing resin cost with the time required to conduct the reuse study and the expected annual number of production runs. Using resin to its functional lifetime maximizes its cost basis, which helps economics if the resin cost is high or the number of cycles is low. Virus removal filters also have the potential to be reused, and although less, if anything, has been published about their reuse, the performance characteristics necessary to demonstrate are expected to be similar to resin reuse.

Process Validation Execution Timing

The execution timing of key process validation elements varies according to the clinical phase of the product. As validation starts well before the last three lots before actual production, it is essential to consider the question of "how much process validation to do and when to do it" as early as possible. Creating the validation package too early might result in redoing substantial portions; creating it too late may delay product launch owing to an incomplete regulatory package. Process validation is a continual process and should be monitored closely for adherence to timelines, scope, and cost. It evolves along with the development of the process and should be complete at the end of phase III.

At the preclinical product phase, critical and noncritical classification of process input parameters should be initiated. Critical components of facility subsystem validation need to be essentially complete before phase I product manufacture. For phase I, it is necessary to validate aspects of the process related to product safety (e.g., sterility, mycoplasma, viral clearance, impurity removal, and stability). Abbreviated viral clearance studies for model viruses/retroviruses and impurity clearance studies for host cell DNA often are acceptable, resulting in fewer downstream steps validated at this product stage. If viral clearance results are available in sufficient time, the results can be applied to developing the phase I process steps. All assays do not have to be validated at this stage, but some (especially product-specific ones) should be at least qualified.

For phase II, no specific process validation activity is required unless process improvement changes potentially affect prior phase I validation work. Assay validation efforts should continue, however, so assays are ready for phase III validation and process development should be finalized before phase III. Most process and assay validation activities begin in phase II and often extend far into phase III, occurring in parallel with phase II and phase III clinical material production. Intensive process characterization often is delayed until after completion of phase II studies to conserve resources. About

12–15 months are allowed for its completion before the process validation runs. To minimize risk, if all phase II clinical data are not available, these activities can be ramped up slowly over the first few months. Raw material vendor audits should be performed between phases II and III before the manufacturing process is fixed.

Before phase III and process finalization, process robustness is evaluated via several scaled-down runs to quantify process variability. These studies form the basis for the process validation program if they are well documented, use operational range extremes, and test different resin/raw material lots. Based on the resulting data, additional optimization to improve robustness is conducted. Fully developed analytical assays are employed during these prephase III scale-down runs to ensure the process meets the quality acceptance criteria. Then during phase III, any remaining assays are validated.

The heavy-duty process validation occurs in phase III when the process is better understood, a commercial process is in place, and there are likely to be fewer changes, adjustments, and mistakes that can cause deviations. First equipment and other subsystem validation are completed and followed by process validation during three or more consecutive batches. The master validation plan usually is approved during phase III clinical material manufacture, and it sometimes includes manufacturing equipment validation in addition to process validation. Viral clearance studies are conducted with a greater number of model viruses possessing a greater range of virus characteristics, and the full range of impurity clearance and operating range validations is undertaken. Mass balances are attempted, duplicate runs are tested, and resin lifetime studies are conducted. Range testing validations typically are completed during phase III clinical production before the manufacture of qualification lots, except for viral clearance studies that are done earlier. Thus, the pivotal phase III clinical studies are conducted using a fixed process with refinements already incorporated to achieve a robust and cost-effective process. At this stage, operational parameters are defined and performance parameters are specified within wide limits until more extensive data are accumulated.

Process performance qualification typically is conducted during the production of qualification lots using target set points for all process input parameters to demonstrate consistency and reproducibility of input and output parameters. This process consistency is demonstrated by multiple full-scale batches, for example, three-to-five consecutive purification lots from three consecutive fermentation lots, during which yield and product concentration are monitored at each step. A failed lot can occur without resetting the count if it is due to a known assignable cause that is not process-related (e.g., operator error or equipment failure). The cause of noncompliance must be determined and corrected, the noncompliant product disposition designated, and any corrective actions taken recorded. At this stage, all assays are validated, all equipment and support systems are qualified, all personnel are trained, all critical input parameters with ranges are validated, and all critical input parameters with set points and noncritical input parameters are validated as a by-product of range-finding studies.

Development Support and Technology Transfer Activities

Process Development

Role, stages, and plans

Process validation is an integral part of process development. At the early stage of process development, the process is basic and unpolished with purity ill defined and poorly controlled. At the mid-stage, an optimized and more robust process exists, and by the end stage, the process is fully characterized, validated, and qualified. During process development and scale-up, critical variables either are removed or else highly understood to develop a robust process. Identification should start early and be based on literature knowledge, prior experience, or specific product information. Some critical variables are identified via close in-process monitoring and thorough investigation when unexpected results are obtained. Early, reliable, and accurate measurement of process variability increases the probability of operating and maintaining a robust, well-understood, and controlled process.

Successful process development establishes a clear logic path that streamlines subsequent validation design and testing. Process development serves to establish evidence that all key process control parameters and all control parameter ranges are validated and optimized to meet acceptance criteria before process validation. These acceptance criteria, specifically the critical process output parameters for scalability studies and range testing validations, in turn are derived from data obtained during development, preclinical, and clinical material production.

The greatest validation problems surface when insufficient resources and time are budgeted for understanding and optimizing production. Development personnel require sufficient time and financial support for thorough validation and technical transfer activities, specifically remaining involved in process validation activities along with manufacturing personnel. Consequently, development staff should understand compliance issues to accurately anticipate the appropriate level of quality assurance applicable to process development studies. Actual formal product development procedures have been recommended to ensure consistency, as well as capture best practices.

Process development documentation

As a considerable amount of relevant data is generated during process development, its documentation must be sufficient to support the selection of manufacturing steps. Development work and decisions made during development are captured in development reports that support future regulatory inquiries and demonstrate that regulatory requirements have been considered and addressed. Development reports should highlight potential weaknesses in the product and process design with the goal of suggesting which ones should undergo subsequent development and validation. They also include an analysis of critical process parameters. The first reports can be generated as early as before the initial product transfer to the process development group. Additional reports are generated after the end of process development and before the start of process validation. All of these reports need to be compiled and indexed so they are readily retrievable, perhaps stored in a database for easy access. They serve as a resource for the product's process development history if an employee leaves (or is reassigned) or as training for new employees.

An upfront listing of the titles and scope of expected reports felt to be necessary to support process scale-up, validation, and regulatory filings is created and reviewed within the multidisciplinary validation team. This listing helps identify required studies and form a process development plan that can facilitate future tracking of executed studies. Once the required component tasks and their execution order are established, this plan should be reviewed semiannually, adding accuracy and sophistication over time. Formal evaluation of the status of the process development plan demonstrates whether the project is on track and identifies deviations in time and cost. The interim goals, resources, and milestones listed in the basic plan focus efforts on priorities, permit staff to see how tasks are integrated, and reduce the likelihood of running out of time.

Process characterization

The terms *process characterization*, *robustness*, and *validation* are sometimes used interchangeably, and consequently, the distinction among these terms consequently is blurred. Process characterization is more encompassing than process validation because process validation uses only a subset of the data generated from process characterization. Characterization studies are similar in nature to validation studies except with less formal compliance to regulatory guidelines. It is the part of the process development examining manufacturing ranges, robustness, and the edge of failure for a limited number of critical parameters. For characterization studies, established scientific and engineering principles are used, along with methods that are not validated in the regulatory sense but are qualified scientifically with appropriate controls and written procedures. Typical causes of unexpected results in process characterization are inadequate procedures, or inadequate following of adequate procedures, and uncontrolled variables. Process robustness provides assurance that the process will not fail when operating within defined control limits for key process variables. This definition of robustness has been adapted from the ICH definition of analytical assay robustness, not from the guidelines for process validation.

Process characterization defines process capability and facilitates prospective process validation at the production scale. Full process characterization is valuable in maintaining smooth manufacturing operations and minimizing lost batches, and it provides supporting information for lot release justification for atypical batches. Its goals are to identify key operating and performance parameters, define control limits for key process parameters, demonstrate robustness of the commercial process, and provide technical information about the process. The steps involved in process characterization include risk assessments, scale-down model qualification, single-parameter ranging studies, parameter interaction studies, and worst-case studies. Process characterization is conducted initially during the preclinical through phase III product stages and continues during the ongoing commercial manufacturing product stage.

The overall goals of process characterization are to (1) understand the roles of each process step, (2) become aware of the effect of process inputs (operating parameters) on process outputs (performance parameters) and identify key operating and performance parameters, (3) assure that the process delivers consistent product yields and purity in all operating ranges, and (4) develop acceptance criteria for in-process performance parameters. Before beginning process characterization activities, advance preparation consists of examining available data and assessing risk, qualifying scale-down models, and developing process characterization plans. Execution involves four steps to achieving these process characterization goals: (1) characterize process performance ("*process fingerprinting data*") using screening experiments to eliminate additional parameters from further characterization studies, (2) identify interactions between key parameters, (3) establish process redundancy by determining the effect of feed quality on each unit operation, and (4) develop unit operation reports to document key operating and performance parameters and their respective ranges.

One recommended strategy for process characterization is to (1) measure as much as possible early in process development, (2) determine if changes in the magnitude of each variable/parameter are relevant to process (or process model) performance, (3) select the relevant variables to be controlled and documented, and (4) collect, organize, and archive all raw data. As the total number of factors to be tested can be very large, factors are combined and treated as single variables based on the experience gained during process development. Variables expected to have similar effects are linked so that their cumulative effect will be additive.

Assessment of Process Risks

Quality assurance (QA) groups often desire a 100% guarantee of quality, leading to risk avoidance and promoting "*over-validation*" in the form of additional testing and repetitive documentation that increases production costs. Although absolute safety is a theoretical concept just like absolute sterility or product purity, it can be approximated using established scientific and engineering principles. Risk analysis identifies the steps, critical factors, and parameters that affect product quality. A documented risk analysis determines the extent of process robustness, summarizes results in a form readily presentable to internal and external regulatory personnel, meets regulatory requirements, identifies critical parameters for monitoring, increases process understanding, assists in troubleshooting, and, most appropriately, focuses process validation efforts where they are most warranted and beneficial. It is first necessary to determine what level of each putative risk factor is considered safe, considering the intended clinical use of the biopharmaceutical (e.g., administration route, dose size and frequency, and total amount consumed).

The process design must include steps that reliably remove or inactivate potential risk factors. Rare, significant, and real risk factors must be distinguished from frequent, less significant, theoretical, or putative risk factors. In some cases, targets are more stringent for real and present risks than for putative ones, and reliance on removal/inactivation steps is less important if risks are purely theoretical. The list of putative risk factors is developed early in the process development cycle and then updated periodically as additional information and experience are obtained. Each potential risk is defined in experimental terms by assessing its biological, biophysical, and biochemical aspects. Two categories of risks are (1) potential pharmacological and toxicological effects of the product's active ingredient(s), and (2) other product components arising from the preparation process. Examples of specific risk factors are the presence of intact cells, adventitious agents (e.g., bacteria, fungi, mycoplasma, and viruses), endogenous retroviruses, residual cellular nucleic acid/proteins, microbial contaminants (e.g., endotoxin and proteins), and process chemicals (e.g., antibiotics, ligands, solvents, cleaning chemicals, inducers, and nutrients).

Risk assessment provides a systematic estimation and evaluation of the risk potential for all components used in the manufacturing process, including the origin and fate of each raw material [53]. Risk assessment also estimates potential risks associated with the application of certain procedures during the manufacturing process (e.g., isolation, validation, and testing) by quantifying a procedure's robustness and susceptibility to errors. It assesses which contaminants have the highest probability of being present and then provides a basis to establish a reasonable and economical testing scheme.

Each risk factor must be identified and quantified in terms of its likelihood of occurrence and its severity. After the initial first key steps of risk identification and quantification, the greatest risks then can be reduced. Reducing the probability of a risk's occurrence is achieved via implementations such as process automation, tighter controls, or removal of open processing steps. Reducing a risk's severity factor is achieved by process changes or product redesign. In contrast, raising the probability of failure detection by increasing sampling and monitoring activities has been found to be the least productive and most time-consuming solution with little opportunity for automation. If a significant risk cannot be reduced sufficiently, then the associated process step can be validated to provide additional performance assurances.

Risk assessment tools

Risk assessment tools (FTA, FMEA, and HACCP) can be used alone or in combination. They are tools for problem prevention, requiring failure anticipation rather than analyzing failures that have already occurred. After process characterization is completed, formal risk analysis exercises can be repeated so future focus can shift to newly uncovered unit operations and operating parameters requiring attention.

FTA

Fault tree analysis (FTA) is a deductive, top-down approach to failure mode analysis. Its open-ended structure is readily expandable, making it helpful for complex problems. The failure or hazard is assumed; then the combination of conditions or probable causes necessary for that event to occur is systematically defined by identifying how that high-level failure is caused by lower level, primary failures, specifically the failure of an individual component or subsystem. This information is presented in the form of a fault tree diagram with the assumed failure/hazard listed first at the top and the associated conditions/probable causes listed as branches with successive levels listed as further branches. Events at different levels of the tree are listed below the main failure event and connected by event statements and logic gates defined by Boolean logic. "And" is used if events need to occur together to cause the failure/hazard; "or" is used if the event alone would cause the failure/hazard. As a fully developed FTA can be complex, special symbols are used to describe events and gates to simplify graphical representation of casual relationships between branches.

FMEA

Failure mode and effect [criticality] analysis (FME[C]A) is a preventative, bottom-up approach to identifying potential failures that has been recently adapted to quantifying GMP risks. FMEA has been applied to audit preparation, batch record review, production validation, change control evaluation, retrospective validation, trend analysis, and validation master plan development. Although it includes identifying the effects or consequences of failure modes, it is a more practical tool and a structured guide to analyze major areas identified by the FTA. However, it is not considered as effective as FTA in identifying root causes for intractable process failures. FMEA uses its structured methodology to facilitate identification of critical variables, specifically reducing 20 or more to 2–3 to permit efficient further optimization. FMEA progresses over time, starting in the early stages of process development, and it is most successful if the process to be examined is clearly defined at the outset. Overall, FMEA serves to (1) readily identify potential problem areas where operators must be especially alert and where intensified test procedures may be required, (2) define operational constraints and preventative maintenance actions for equipment, (3) provide information for planning performance qualification, (4) prioritize corrective actions and improvements, (5) foster interdisciplinary teamwork and communication, and (5) facilitate decision making throughout the development process.

The first step in FMEA is to develop a working matrix that identifies all information categories that are intended to be studied. A flowchart describing process steps serves as the left column of the matrix. An accurate description of each step helps stimulate thinking about how the step might fail. A list of reasons is generated describing why each step might fail to complete its intended function (potential failure modes) and what would happen if failure occurs (potential downstream effects). All possible causes, however improbable, are identified that might result in failure; then the risk attached to each failure is evaluated using an established scale, for example, values from 1 to 5.

The next step is to rate the importance of the identified failure in terms of its probability of occurrence based on the controls in place (P), severity (S), and ability to detected (D), resulting in a risk priority number (RPN). It asks the following questions: What could go wrong, what is the probability of its going wrong, what are the consequences of it going wrong, and can in-process or final product testing detect it when it does go wrong? RPNs, also known as the criticality index, then are used to sort the identified causes/effects of failures, which enables FMEA to identify those failures posing the greatest threat to the manufacturing process. P, S, and D are all rated between the low and high values; P and S directly increase with numerical rating, and D inversely increases with numerical rating. The RPN value is calculated by the product, $P \times S \times D$. If P, S, or D is completely unknown, then a high value rating (e.g., 5) is assigned. Thus, in the worst case RPN = 125, and in the best case RPN = 1. In practice, RPNs only are calculated for the worst aspects of each failure to reduce workload and to permit identification of the most critical failures first without requiring detailed calculations for each identified cause. Frequently, the highest RPN steps are those steps involving human intervention because P is typically 3 or more.

The output of an FMEA study is the list of preventative and corrective actions necessary to improve the manufacturing process that now can be prioritized based on RPN values. An acceptable RPN should depend on the severity rating of the failure, specifically if S = 5 (high value), then the RPN should be ≤ 5, but if S is below 5, the acceptable RPN can be higher. The RPN then can be recalculated after corrective actions have been implemented providing measurable proof of impact.

HACCP

Hazard analysis and critical control points (HACCP) is a systematic approach that is system-based to determine high-risk steps. The definition of hazard includes both safety and quality concerns for biopharmaceuticals. An effective HACCP system reduces endproduct testing because sufficient validated safeguards are instituted. HACCP provides detail and documentation to show process/product understanding through identifying parameters to control and monitor. Its stages are to (1) conduct the hazard analysis, (2) determine critical control points, (3) establish critical limits, (4) establish monitoring procedures, (5) establish corrective actions, (6) establish verification procedures, and (7) establish record-keeping and documentation procedures.

Validation of Assays

Purpose

As biopharmaceutical products are large and complex molecules and no single test method is sufficient, product analysis uses multiple, different analytical methods strategically designed to be complementary with respect to selectivity and specificity. More sensitive test methods allow proof of greater removal of a putative risk factor, and the more key parameters that can be measured assure that process variability is understood and controlled. However, it is important to avoid setting product specifications at the assay's limit of detection. Assays provide adequate in-process testing via process validation and a comprehensive assessment of the final product using a variety of analytical methodologies for identity, purity, potency, strength, safety, and stability.

Assay validation characterizes the assay performance so that the significance of the measured assay values obtained is readily understood. Test methods should be validated when important decisions are to be based on the data generated. Thus, the extent of method validation depends on the stage of clinical supply manufacture. The key elements of assay validation for a method are to establish reliability, the intra- and interlaboratory test variation, and relevance, the meaning of the results for a specific purpose. The robustness of an analytical procedure is its measured capacity to be unaffected by small variations in controlled parameters and reliability under normal usage.

Scope

The scope of assay validation is to assess the essential test method performance characteristics of accuracy, reproducibility, repeatability, linearity, and limit of quantitation/detection. A test method is evaluated for its readiness for assay validation against the following criteria: (1) description of the test basis and scientific purpose, (2) case for relevance, (3) proposed practical application, (4) statement of limitations, and (5) acceptable intra- and interlaboratory precision. Before actual validation, the test method should be optimized and standardized, specifically controls necessary to invalidate inappropriate out-of-specification results should be incorporated. Assays must be validated for each matrix in which samples will be run and for its capability on a protein-by-protein basis.

Assay ruggedness also is measured in terms of the similarity of results from different laboratories, manufacturer's equipment, and analysts. Interoperator, interday, and intraassay variations can be quantified by comprehensive validation. Interassay (intermediate) precision is the precision of multiple determinations of a single sample analyzed in various runs. Intra-assay precision or repeatability is the precision of multiple determinations of a single sample within one assay run. Interlot precision tests analyze values of aliquots from a single sample run using lots of different assay components. Finally, lot-to-lot precision is the precision of multiple determinations of a single sample analyzed using different lots of assay components. These multiple types of variations must be considered so that release criteria ranges are not set too tight. The limit of quantitation (LOQ) is the lowest concentration that produces a signal 10-fold above background, whereas the limit of detection (LOD) is the lowest concentration that produces a signal threefold above background. The assay sensitivity and achievable concentration limits of additives define a "*window of clearance*," which is the difference (on a log scale) between the highest attainable initial contaminant/impurity concentration and the lowest detectable concentration (LOD) of that additive. This difference is the amount that can be measured and thus the amount that can be claimed to have been removed by the process.

A low-level sensitivity is required for viral test methods to maximize reduction factors. However, the ability to detect low virus concentrations is limited by statistical sampling. The probability of detection (POD) for low-level virus concentrations depends on test volumes, batch volumes, and test sensitivity. The POD is high when sample virus concentrations are well above the test method sensitivity, the POD is lower when concentrations are at or below the test method sensitivity, and the POD is even lower for very low concentrations due to the low probability of obtaining a virus in the sample as described by the Poisson distribution. Test method sensitivity should be based on a POD ≥ 95 %.

In-process and release (endproduct) parameters, both critical and operational controls, are controlled and monitored during production using assays. In-process controls generate data at critical process steps, which serve as a basis for specification development for product intermediates. Specific in-process controls, routine sampling, and monitoring at specific process steps are established to monitor key process outputs. Information only tests are used postvalidation without preestablished acceptance criteria until sufficient data have been collected to statistically establish clear limits or else omit the testing. Thus, sampling and obtaining data for information only is an important part of process validation that must be recognized.

Assay types

Potency

Binding assays for quantitation use the binding of at least two molecules to form an interaction that withstands multiple washing steps, and they are the least variable. Cell-based bioassays for potency use a cell line mixed with a sample to generate a cellular response that is quantified. They have more variability and are tricky to use to measure potency because the CV often is >30%. Whole animal assays for potency are time-consuming and highly variable, and they have the typical disadvantages of *in vivo* tests in that they are expensive, inaccurate, slow, and raise animal ethics issues.

The development and validation of *in vitro* tests that correlate with potency, typically desirable for vaccines, is tedious and rarely successful, requiring thorough knowledge of the immune response after infection or vaccination. An alternative approach is to demonstrate batch comparability and then assume identical properties *in vivo*. For an increasingly greater number of vaccines, no routine animal potency testing is being conducted because the product is well characterized, critical production process steps are controlled, immunology knowledge permits functional test development, analytical knowledge permits antigen characterization, and test procedures are becoming harmonized and validated.

Impurities

Analytical methods for impurity clearance require sensitivities capable of demonstrating sufficient clearance to well below safety margins. rDNA technology has stimulated the development of a wide variety of assay types. Specifically, PCR is used to understand how manufacturing steps impact retroviral clearance due to its high precision, high throughput, and low cost. Typical testing for in-process impurities includes endotoxin, host cell and other proteins, DNA, viruses, and altered protein forms (e.g., proteolytic clips, deamination, oxidized methionines, and amino acid substitutions). Clearance of host cell proteins is measured using immunoassay. Host cell DNA is radiolabeled by nick-translation and then measured in column fractions (also radiolabeled host-cell proteins), and it is measured directly in production streams. Cytotoxicity and interference testing using non-virus-containing samples are performed to ensure that sample matrices in a viral clearance study do not adversely affect the ability to titrate virus. These tests are performed well in advance of the actual validation so that conditions may be found for which dilution is not required, and thus, assay sensitivity is not reduced by dilution.

There is a lack of practical laboratory assays to detect bovine spongiform encephalopathy (BSE) - like agents so the potential introduction of these agents into the process must be controlled by avoiding bovine-based materials, using materials from low-risk bovine tissues, and/or sourcing materials from countries with good BSE control measures. Typical testing on final purified bulk includes those tests conducted with in-process testing plus total protein content and potency. The final product (sterile filtered, filled and sometimes lyophilized, then packaged into vials and ampoules) is tested for sterility, pyrogenicity, particulates, content uniformity, identity, excipient chemical content, potency, and protein content.

Standards

Key to the success of any assay method is the availability of a reliable standard. A primary standard is one recognized by a national or international agency, whose characteristics have been established by collaborative effort. Secondary standards are calibrated against primary standards. Reference material is used for the evaluation of other materials to generate comparative data. Primary reference material has been thoroughly characterized, and it is the purest material available in quantities large enough for use. Biochemical reference standards are used for all product tests and for process-specific tests both for material release as well as for upstream/downstream process monitoring and assay development. They are unique to a specific product in its amino acid sequence and glycosylation but different for each manufacturer. To ensure compatibility with the matrix of the intended assay, different standards can be required for different process steps. It can be challenging to provide sufficient quantities of the various types of reference material early in the product development cycle. A working reference material is required to validate analytical procedures. It should be stable for at least 2–4 years, and its stability should be monitored regularly.

Change Control and Ongoing Process Validation

Validation maintenance, an ongoing activity for manufacturing processes, continues through the life cycle of the process with a changing focus as the process matures. There is a need to address the process life cycle as a whole and not to suspend process validation after three production scale runs are completed. To support this life-cycle approach, process expert teams are created to rapidly resolve process deviations, determine trends toward loss of control, comply with regulatory requirements, assess process change impact, and identify areas for process improvement.

A validation program is specific for a product manufactured by a given process. A strong change control program needs to be established once the process is validated. Changes to process equipment, operation, or facilities should be reviewed carefully before the change is approved to determine the potential validation impact and if repeating validation studies are required. Such changes include process improvements, raw materials changes, step substitutions, and scale-up. Changes that are expected to shift the value of a performance parameter require revalidation. Specifically, if the purity is decreased at a specific step, then recovery of this purity must be demonstrated downstream. In general the potential quality impact of process changes is higher with glycosylated rather than with non glycosylated proteins.

The process change is documented in a proposal with its justification, along with the number of batches necessary and strategy (e.g., samples and data needed, extent of validation testing, and acceptance criteria) to evaluate the change. In some cases, the original risk assessment (e.g., FMEA) is revisited or a new one conducted to ensure an unintentional new failure mode has not been created. A formal change control report is written and approved.

Revalidation is the repetition of the validation process or specific part of it, and it has some conceptual overlap with retrospective validation. Periodic revalidation has been conducted in some cases even if nothing has changed. Specific elements of most validation programs are repeated (at least partially) at regular, appropriate intervals (e.g., every 6–24 months) to verify that the original parameters are still effective. In other cases, if there have been no changes, process revalidation can consist of a formal review of operating and performance parameters, along with the nature and frequency of excursions, which can be executed as part of the annual product review. When existing processes are reassessed, some input parameters may be more tightly controlled than previously permitted or a noncritical parameter may be found to be critical. Product failures occurring within validated ranges of a process might be due to simultaneous excursions of several variables not studied during the initial process validation or from the use of an inadequate scale-down model.

Trending of process variables is used to refine range limits. Manufacturing data can lead to superseded NORs and/or MORs, which are justified by the associated operational trends and product quality achieved. Extreme parameter values subsequently can become acceptable in process validation if the acceptability of final product has been confirmed by multiple observations.

Process Validation Documentation

Documentation of process validation serves to establish that its goals are reasonable and achievable, as well as to ensure that the study design is based on solid scientific and engineering principles. The process validation master plan defines the scope and rationale of process validation, giving an overview of the validation, its philosophy, and general testing strategy. It describes how the validation is to be done, including the schedule, studies to be performed, systems to be validated, responsibilities, and approvals required.

The process validation protocol is a preapproved written plan stating how the validation will be conducted and identifying acceptance criteria as well as sampling and assay requirements and other testing details. It is a prospective experimental plan that when executed produces documented evidence that the system has been validated. The protocol defines the system to be validated, identifies operating variables and probable control parameters, and indicates the number of replications required to provide statistical significance. There is a major savings of cost and time realized by adopting potential streamlining measures, for example, combining resin reuse and chromatography step characterization studies into a single protocol. The entire process validation study protocol is reviewed and approved by manufacturing and quality personnel as well as by process development representatives. The process validation report includes the validation protocol, deviations from protocol, validation results, and conclusions about validation status of the step. Copies of most critical validation reports and summaries of other reports are included in the license application, so their careful assembly, clarity, and accuracy is critical. Common validation submission deficiencies include the lack of data or protocols, inadequate data summaries, missing acceptance criteria, and inadequate monitoring or sampling.

Process Validation Strategies

Several value-added, science-based, best practices are evolving for process validation, which are appropriate from both business and regulatory viewpoints. For a biopharmaceutical process, the potential number of variables and possible interactions among variables is large. One possible approach is to conduct a worst-case test to evaluate each known critical variable separately, and if necessary to run steps more than once if they possess more than one critical variable. Although the use of simple experimental designs to develop the relationship and describe the link between input and output parameters is straightforward, it can result in high numbers of experimental runs, which are impractical. Potential streamlined approaches include retrospective analysis, qualified scale-down studies to identify critical parameters and important interactions, and worst-case runs. In addition, more than one variable can be coupled together into a single variable if they are believed, based on science, to have a predictable effect on output variables. Scouting studies then are used if process development data are limited regarding one or more variables or if the ranges previously studied were insufficiently large.

Historical Data Review

Retrospective analysis of historical data can be used to assess process reliability. The initial process capability specifications are established based on a few runs (usually less than around 5–10) with acceptable results. This number of runs often is too small to accurately define and characterize actual process variability. It can be difficult to claim that the previously set process capability specifications were flawed after validation runs fail to meet them. Thus, the selection of acceptance criteria must consider the benefits of broad versus narrow tolerance ranges.

It is best to develop acceptance limits for parameters such as yield and purity using statistics applied to historical data. The difficulty in setting acceptance criteria depends on the availability and quality of historical data. Small datasets tend to underestimate process variance because they contain only a limited number of historical production runs. If historical data are used, excessively large ranges are difficult to defend.

Process variability is determined using available tools such as preparing historical trends of the mean ±3 standard deviations SDs to demonstrate agreement of manufacturing scale runs with clinical manufacturing/development runs. After 15 or preferably 30 data points are obtained, a control chart based on a moving range is the best tool for monitoring process stability. Statistical process control (SPC) and multivariate analysis can be applied to historical data to identify strategies for improving yield through investigation of cause-and-effect relationships using correlation tools and process knowledge.

Statistical Design of Experiments (DOE) and Analysis for Process Characterization

Experimental designs are used to efficiently identify those input variables that significantly affect output. The use of DOE to easily screen a variety of operating parameters provides a framework for the design and interpretation of experiments, identifies those factors with the greatest effects, segregates key from nonkey parameters, identifies interactions and synergistic effects, and models how outputs relate to inputs. DOE is a powerful, prospective method compared with retrospective analysis. Its ability to determine interactions between key parameters leads to the identification of other weak spots in the process not observed during initial screen experiments. DOE is limited to assessing interactions among input parameters that can be tested within the same experiment. Usually there are more variables than can be tested in single experiment. To prepare for successful characterization via DOE, there is a need to design for simplicity by removing non-value-added experiments and to remove as much experimental variation as possible.

DOE modeling can be used early in process characterization to set guard bands, ranges for key process input variables where no statistical change to output is observed. These guard bands are set to locate optimal settings that maximize output and minimize variation. Subsequent validation consists first of experimental design to screen key process input variables set at the guard bands previously determined and then to confirm that the output is within specification. Modeling DOE helps understand the relationship between key input factors and critical Ys, relates input factors to responses (critical Ys) via a model (transfer function) that essentially is process characterization, determines input factor settings that optimize responses, and uses a model to set a limit on input variation such that no statistical changes in KPIVs are observed. This approach is consistent with the PAT initiative.

The maximum information per experiment can be obtained by combining studies and varying factors (i.e., variables) using fractional factorial design. A set of fractional factorial runs provides an estimate of each variable's effect and interactions, but no single run can be compared with a control run. This design permits a large number of variables to be tested with lower number of experiments. Often variables are tested at a low and a high level that permits only linear interpolation (i.e., assumes a linear process response). If center points (i.e., mid-point of the tested range) are added to the experimental design, nonlinearity or curvature can be detected if present. Replication of low- and high-level test conditions increases the precision of the estimate of that factor's effect. Two-way variable interactions are tested with factorial design, but additional experiments may be necessary to deconvolute the effects of two factors that are confounded (i.e., indistinguishable effects from one another). Fractional factorial designs test the extremes of all variables and then generate the bestfit model with an evaluation of the statistical confidence of the model response predictions. If no process failures are predicted by the best-fit model, then the process step is considered robust over the ranges of control parameters tested.

Statistical analysis demonstrates which input parameters are important contributors to output parameters. JMP statistical software (SAS, Cary, NC) can be used to analyze data and generate separate analyses for each response variable of interest. A difference of 3 SDs often is selected as the criterion for significance corresponding to a 95% confidence level, and the test acceptance criteria range typically are set as the mean plus/minus 3 SDs (industry standard).

Family/Matrix Validation and Platform Technologies

Common validation studies are required across different processes to demonstrate capabilities for viral clearance, resin and membrane reuse/sanitization/storage, buffer stability, filter extractables, and resin leachables. Furthermore, many biopharmaceuticals are being developed using common platform technologies (e.g., cell line, medium, unit operations) to reduce development time. Thus, templates can be developed that identify key input and output parameters for a certain unit operation and then customized to address unique process or product specifics. Generic validated assays can be used for impurity removal, if a platform cell line and similar culture conditions are used that then are qualified for each new product. In addition, generic validation can be developed in which the supplier and potential industry users define generic operating conditions under which the technology is to be used, and the equipment manufacturer conducts much of the testing for every industry user. This reduces additional user validation testing to only product- or user-specific applications (e.g., product compatibility).

To significantly reduce the number and extent of new studies associated with new products processed using similar or identical process operations (i.e., platform technologies), family and matrix validation approaches are applied to reduce repetitive work. In a family approach, one piece of equipment is validated by three consecutive runs and other similar equipment is validated by one confirming run in each unit. This approach can be applied to the process validation for a product with several distinct, different but similar, components (e.g., antigens for a multivalent vaccine) by (1) treating different product components as a product family, (2) classifying product components into groups based on their similarities, and (3) selecting one component from each group to validate, possibly based on worst-case experience during process development. This strategy is facilitated when (1) the final product can be fully analytically characterized, (2) there is significant prior manufacturing experience with similar production processes and significant process development experience with the new production process, and (3) clinical trial data show comparable safety and efficacy profiles for some product components.

In a matrix approach, validation is conducted at the full range or extremes of process parameters, and then values in between are assumed validated. This generic strategy is used to support a wide range of bracketed conditions that include the most common operating parameters for more than one product, as long as process streams and key step components (e.g., resin type) are similar. The matrix approach reduces the extent of process validation required for successive products, at the expense of only a limited impact on the initial product's process validation, as long as the platform technology is reasonably maintained. Example applications have been retrovirus inactivation via low pH treatment and viral clearance using anion exchange chromatography.

Scale-Down Models

Although the most reliable data are obtained from actual production runs, determination of operational ranges at the manufacturing scale is laborious, time- consuming, and costly. Thus, typical manufacturing scale validation is limited to impurity clearance (e.g., proteins, DNA, and small molecules) and resin/membrane cleaning. If the process step cannot be scaled down successfully, then range definition validation studies are required at the large scale.

Small-scale process models are an essential and valuable tool for process validation and ongoing trouble-shooting. Scale-down factors ranging from 10- to 10,000-fold are employed with the extent of scale-down depending on the actual production scale and smallest scale that can reliably reproduce the process. Small-scale equipment is permissible only if the scalability of the unit operation is demonstrated. The same technical principles for scale-down are used as for scale-up for the step of interest.

The scale-down model should represent the large-scale model with respect to input parameters and typical values for output parameters. Data are collected under conditions relevant to full-scale manufacturing GMP process. Qualified scale-down models are used in combination with strong statistical tools like DOE, but sample handling at the small scale is easier than during GMP manufacturing runs. Multiple validation experiments can be conducted in parallel employing several identical scale-down units, thereby shortening the experimental time expended. Also a hybrid approach can be instituted where samples from full-scale process streams are used as feed streams to scaled-down steps. Overall the amount of resources used in small-scale validation is likely to be less than that needed for manufacturing scale validation, although in manufacturing scale validation, resource utilization is spread over a longer period of time.

Scale-down studies have been used for a wide variety of process validation studies, including resin lifetimes, in-process stream hold times, buffer stability, virus clearance, harvest criteria, filter extractables, resin leachables, and cell age at harvest. The ease of scale-down differs depending on step and should be considered in selecting those steps to be validated. In fact, certain validation issues can be addressed only via small-scale models (e.g., virus clearance evaluation, nucleic acid and other impurities/additives removal, cleaning and storage procedure evaluation, and column lifetime estimation) because their use increases worker safety, reduces costs, and permits use of higher titer samples for improved accuracy of prediction. Specifically, viral clearance studies can only be performed at the small scale because virus introduction into cGMP manufacturing scale equipment is impractical and inappropriate. For viral clearance studies, the ideal scale-down factor is 10- to 100-fold.

Although scale-down models have been used largely in purification, they also have been used in fermentation. Fermenter scale-down models use the same set points for volume-independent operating parameters (e.g., temperature, pH, and DO) and adjust the set points for volume-dependent parameters such as mixing and gassing (e.g., dCO_2 stripping). The inoculum split ratio for cell culture scale-down is maintained constant. Characterization studies are performed in small-scale fermenters, and then it is demonstrated that the ranges established are insensitive to scale-up. Only the critical process parameters found to be sensitive to scale-up require range studies at the manufacturing scale.

There is increased regulatory concern over the accuracy of results obtained from small-scale models. Consequently, the scale-down model must be validated to be consistent with full-scale manufacturing before validation studies begin. For chromatography steps, it is necessary to determine that product purity and yield are the same or demonstrate comparable HETP, peak asymmetry, and retention time. Any product streams tested should be representative of a commercial-scale process feed stream.

For chromatography steps, the scale-down model consists of a column with system and auxiliary components (e.g., distributor, monitors, and fraction collectors). Scale equivalence for chromatography columns maintains constant column bed height and linear flow rate, while varying column diameter, buffer, and load amounts, which are scaled to column volume. Specifically, the column diameter is decreased, but the bed height is maintained to maintain residence time, and the volumetric flow rate is reduced, but the linear flow rate is maintained. Constant residence time is important if viral clearance is due to inactivation rather than removal. Configuration, transport distances (tubing diameters as well as tubing lengths), and materials of construction are similar to the commercial-scale system. The same methods of preparing buffers are used, including the same quality of water, buffer, and salts. The chromatography medium has the same base matrix, functional groups, and degree of substitution, as well as the lot used should meet approved specifications. Finally, the product mass loading and relative buffer/load volumes between scale-down and production systems are similar.

Although chromatography scale-down is extensively studied owing to its use for viral clearance validation, the scale-down of other purification steps also is conducted. Virus filtration scale-down maintains the same linear or filtration pressures, product feed concentration, ratio of feed volume to filter area, and temperature as the production system. Other steps such as solution inactivation (e.g., pH and heat treatment) are relatively easy to scale down because it is simply necessary only to maintain buffer composition, pH, protein concentration, and temperature consistent with production conditions. The time course of the inactivation is quantified along with the upper tolerable range of inactivation agent concentration and minimum exposure time. Residence time differences between the production and small scales might change parameters such as buffer temperature, which might affect solution as well as chromatography inactivation steps.

Well-Characterized Biotechnology Products

A well-characterized biological (biopharmaceutical) is a chemical entity whose identity purity, impurity, safety, potency, and quality can be determined and controlled. To be well characterized, the drug substance must be >95% of the main component and/or related isoforms. Well-characterized molecules are evaluating using sensitive and discriminating tests that are quantitative and relevant *in vivo* and *in vitro* potency assays. The recent explosion in the availability of sophisticated, reliable, analytical instrumentation, combined with extensive, sensitive product analysis methods has resulted in great advancements in defining *"well-characterized"* biopharmaceuticals.

Although for a well-characterized biological the FDA trend is to rely on reduced final product testing, process validation must be present to assure product quality and consistency. There has been an elimination of regulatory agency lot release for specific well-characterized biopharmaceuticals. In addition, process-related impurities (e.g., host cell protein and DNA) are controlled by process validation *in lieu* of lot-release testing. Furthermore, many process changes are justifiable using analytical data and process validation studies without a clinical trial. The following principles can be applied to the manufacturing and testing of a well-characterized product: (1) The manufacturing process should be robust, reproducible, validated, and designed to produce active drug substance; (2) the safety of the final product is assured through process validation using validated analytical testing to demonstrate removal of impurities to safe levels; (3) tests for identity, purity, and potency should be sensitive, quantitative, and validated; and (4) specifications should be quantitative and based on historical manufacturing data and clinical experience.

The more characterizable the biopharmaceutical product, the more emphasis is placed on validating that the correct molecule is being produced than assuring that the cell biology is being controlled.

However, the difficulty of characterization increases in direct proportion to the complexity of molecule. When less is known about the product, a greater reliance is placed on product and process consistency. Most vaccines used today are not well-characterized biologicals, so batch release must be performed by the manufacturer and by the appropriate national control laboratory. The quality of vaccines is increasingly guaranteed by the use of robust and reproducible production processes, and thus, a high reliance is placed on process validation.

FUTURE TRENDS

Future developments in the biopharmaceutical industry are likely to impact the scope and execution of process validation activities. The nature of process validation is continuously changing to meet the requirements of biopharmaceutical development and manufacturing. The understanding and implementation of new strategies based on future developments is key to maintaining an effective process validation methodology.

Process Analytical Technologies (PATs)

PAT is a system for designing, analyzing, and controlling manufacturing through timely in-process measurements of critical quality and performance attributes, leading to the goal of ensuring final product quality. The implementation of PAT potentially minimizes the number of tests that need to be performed at the time of lot release, or in the future for certain products, it might eliminate lot-release testing by the manufacturer entirely. Its precedent was the dropping of lot-release testing for certain impurities when validation of their removal was able to be assured.

Online and automatic methods have been demonstrated to be more accurate and precise compared with manual methods because (1) sampling and sample pretreatment artifacts are eliminated, minimized, or reproduced; (2) measurement frequency is increased; and (3) results are independent of personnel availability. Continuous, real-time monitoring is preferred when feasible. PAT is used to implement in-line controls to increase productivity and reduce costs. In addition, accumulated data from numerous commercial batches are used to generate trend analysis profiles showing high and low control limits for process parameters. These limits then are used to predict when processes may be deviating from their validated control ranges, although they are currently operating within them.

Relationships among manipulated (controlled) variables, online measured variables, and product (uncontrolled) variables in most biosystems are nonlinear to some extent. A forward model is when parameters, starting conditions, and relevant equations governing behavior are known, readily measurable inputs and the outputs are variables; an inverse model is when the inputs are readily measurable variables and the outputs are difficult to measure parameters. The forward model is most applicable to process validation, whereas the inverse model is most applicable to metabolic pathway analysis. Modeling systems such as neural networks have been used to describe the characteristics of extremely complex bioprocess systems.

Mathematical models can be used to simulate the controlled process variables and thus predict the effect of variations on the uncontrolled process variables. Linking online sensing to modeling is effective when there is product yield and biomass variation among optimal values, optimal values may vary over time for processes that are not stationary, parameters can be measured directly or otherwise, the cost of online control is a small fraction of capital and expense costs to run a process, and historical data combined with mathematical methods provide identification of key parameters and their optimal values to achieve rational process improvement. Achieving good modeling is not always easy and involves correct identification of parameters and variables, and selection of the type of model (forward or inverse) along with key inputs and outputs, showing the relationship between predictions and actual data to assess model effectiveness.

A solid understanding of a product's critical quality attributes and what aspects of the manufacturing process control them is necessary to fully gain the benefits of PAT. Furthermore, the inherent complexity of protein-based biopharmaceutical products makes it difficult to use PAT to assess product characteristics critical to safety, efficacy, and stability. In addition, it is difficult, compared with small molecules, to directly monitor the desired product concentration during upstream/early downstream processes in a background of protein impurities deriving from medium components or host cells. However, PAT can be used for process monitoring and control that then indirectly results in improved productivity, process consistency, and product quality.

The pharmaceutical industry lags behind other automated industries in manufacturing quality analysis because it is mostly lab-oriented with little closed-loop, real-time control, and limited enterprise-wide data availability. There is a fear of potential regulatory agency reprisals if PAT is implemented for existing processes, and its use detects behavior that would not have been detected using conventional process monitoring. Before PAT is widely implemented, the risks associated with data variability need to be evaluated and reliable methods need to be instituted to distinguish among signal, process, and product variability.

Process Reliability

More increasingly, the supply capability of a commercial organization depends not only on manufacturing but also on process reliability, GMP compliance, and operational metrics. Process reliability lies at the heart of lean manufacturing and Six Sigma programs because it ensures that the manufacturing process can be maintained in a compliant, validated state. Performance factors are measured and monitored on an ongoing basis so that improvement efforts can be targeted at the most significant opportunities leading to the removal of variation from the manufacturing process. The greatest threats to process reliability are production variances and associated investigations. Variance analysis identifies systems prone to problems, and then it uncovers the root causes of these variances, strengthening the mechanical and operational aspects of the process. Process reliability is the ability of the process to consistently produce required results as measured through the primary dimensions of uptime, dependability, and first run yield. Uptime is the time the process is in operation compared with the available time the process is scheduled to be in operation. Dependability is the repeatability of a process' actual run rate compared with its scheduled run rate. First run yield is the ability to produce quality outputs the first time through production run without any rework. Reliability losses are measured in terms of unscheduled downtime, run rate losses, yield losses, and reprocessing.

Process reliability is improved most effectively using cross-functional teams by the following process: (1) identification of the opportunity; (2) collection of reliability loss data regarding uptime, dependability, and first run yield; (3) analysis of loss data and determination of the root cause of the problem; (4) brainstorming of solution alternatives; (5) selection and implementation of solutions considering solutions that are safe, feasible, implementable, and cost-effective; and (6) monitoring of results and repetitions to assess the impact of solutions and to prioritize remaining opportunities. Six Sigma states these concepts for continuous process improvement as DMAIC: define, measure, analyze, improve, and control, which are readily applicable to process validation. Measurable benefits of improved process reliability include increased customer service (e.g., timely delivery), increased schedule adherence, reduced lead time, reduced inventory levels, increased effective capacity (i.e., greater process uptime and reduced unplanned down-time), decreased cost, creation of time available for predictive maintenance, incremental capacity for new products or increased volume without additional capital investment, increased process dependability, improved quality and first run yield, and reductions in setup and changeover time.

Process flexibility is needed for rapid turnover and reduced inventories that are key to lean manufacturing, which in turn are crucial to making more customized drug products and remaining competitive. Flexibility losses are when time, people, and material waste are consumed by product changeovers. Flexibility is improved by mapping the changeover process, analyzing steps, and then eliminating, resequencing, or improving activities. In addition, standardizing procedures and setup locations and advance preparation for changeovers improve efficiency.

Biogenerics

Biogenerics, also known as *"follow-on"* biologics, are pharmaceutical preparations, using a generic name, that are based on drug substances arising from recombinant technology (complex structure and high molecular weight) that have been demonstrated to be essentially similar to an original pharmaceutical with an expired patent. The main features of biogenerics processes (such as reproducibility, validation, and controls) need to be maintained similar to the patented biopharmaceutical product and should include quality, safety, and efficacy. Key scientific issues for biogenerics are product characterization, demonstration of bioequivalence, and manufacturing issues (e.g., lack of ownership or access to a contracted facility, incomplete disclosure of patented product processes, and difficulty obtaining a suitable cell line and raw materials). The process as well as the strain for biogenerics are different from those of the original product, and the impact of even small changes on biopharmaceuticals is not clear.

The potential world market for biogenerics has been estimated at $5.4 billion/ year by 2008, assuming the evolution of a favorable regulatory environment, compared with a total biopharmaceutical market of $30 billion/year. These estimates may be too high for the market potential for biogenerics because patients often are switched to the next-generation versions of branded products due to rapid innovations in these products. In fact, the main barriers to entry are the fast pace of existing product enhancement or new product introduction, and an illdefined regulatory framework. In addition, due to the expense of biomanufacturing and developing a biomanufacturing process, the cost reduction of biogenerics may not be as significant as with non-biopharmaceuticals. One estimate is that biogenerics will sell for 10–20% less than branded counterparts rather than 40– 80% less as with small-molecule drugs. Generic biopharmaceutical products, possessing a similar complex structure and high molecular weight as the original product, are harder to characterize than small-molecule generic drugs; thus, they are harder to prove equivalent. To show bioequivalence, that the biogeneric is *"essentially similar"* to the patented biopharmaceutical, sophisticated analytical analysis is required. Comparability studies are required to prove the similar nature of the generic product, and the nature of these studies is product-class specific. Prior experience is that even small changes in the product can result in significant safety or efficacy differences.

Biogenerics are currently in a state of *"regulatory purgatory"*. Key regulatory issues are that the approval process is not well defined and is uncertain, particularly in the United States. The FDA says creating a regulatory pathway for biogenerics is a top priority (Europe already has a biogenerics regulatory framework), but little resolution has been reached. Regulatory authorities are requesting extensive demonstrations of biological activity, which translate to lengthy and costly clinical trials. Proof of identity is difficult for biopharmaceuticals because they are difficult to analytically characterize. "The process defines the product" notion still exists when there is limited knowledge and experience regarding cause-and-effect relationships. Extensive oversight of biogenerics manufacturers is expected because the entire manufacturing process is as important as the final product and needs to be carefully regulated. These requirements make development timelines and costs substantially higher than for small-molecule generics.

Outsourcing

As biopharmaceutical companies redefine their goals and priorities, outsourcing of workload can maximize investment and assure an ability to meet capacity demands. Previously, outsourcing has been done in clinical research development and fill/finish manufacturing steps. Now it is being done for

QC/QA functions because every quality function except final release responsibility for bio-pharmaceutical drug product for human clinical trials can be outsourced. Outsourcing also is occurring in many areas such as process development, clinical material production, and marketable production. Specific areas such as cell line development (high producer screening) and scale-up also can be out-sourced. Risk management systems are used to proactively identify the risks and liability between the organizations.

Contract companies can provide more than simply additional capacity. They can provide translation of bench-scale operations to cGMP compliant manufacturing, technology transfer, and process validation. Contract services also are provided by equipment suppliers to optimize/develop processes using their equipment. These services can be more cost-effective than third-party laboratories, contract manufacturing, or in-house.

Risk-Based GMPs

In the future, when manufacturing processes are developed and understood, there will be increased innovation and regulatory oversight proportional to risk. The major goals of risk-based GMPs are to focus GMP attention on potential risk areas, ensure regulations do not impede innovations, enhance GMP inspection consistency, and encourage the use of the latest scientific advances in manufacturing. To accomplish these goals, work is progressing based on several major principles, including risk-based orientation, science-based policies/standards, integrated quality systems orientation, international cooperation, and strong public health protection. The advent of risk-based GMPs provides a timely opportunity for industry to prospectively evaluate ways to streamline the complexity of existing and proposed processes using sound and defendable methodologies for risk assessment.

Overall, process validation is a methodology to permit organizations to take advantage of process improvement opportunities presenting themselves over the course of a product's lifetime. Process validation continues to be a formidable undertaking, requiring extensive resources and time for full execution. Improvements in efficiency are likely to arise as technologies for high-throughput scale-down units and fast-turnaround, sensitive analytical assays become more readily available. Focused guidance on process development, characterization, and validation also should be beneficial to evaluate and align varied industry practices.

2

Macromolecular Validation

Before implementation of analytical methods for routine use, careful validation is required to demonstrate that the method is suitable for the intended purpose. Analytical methods employed for the quantitative determination of drug substances and their metabolites in biological media play a significant role in the evaluation and interpretation of pharmacokinetic data. To define the requirements and procedures for the validation of bioanalytical methods, a conference was held in 1990 in Crystal City in the Washington, DC, area, which was co-sponsored by the U.S. Food and Drug Administration (FDA), The Canadian Health Protection Branch, the American Association of Pharmaceutical Scientists (AAPS), and the Association of Official Analytical Chemists (AOAC), bringing together scientists from regulatory authorities, industry, and academia. Upon evaluation of the results of the first meeting, another conference was held 10 years later that ultimately led to the publication of the FDA guideline "Guidance for Industry: Bioanalytical Method Validation" complementing the general guidelines on method validation such as guidelines Q2A and Q2B by the International Conference on Harmonization (ICH) or pharmacopeial regulations. From the beginning, it was realized that each analytical technique has its own characteristics, which will vary from analyte to analyte. Despite the fact that some similarities exist, a general difference between chemical methods, such as chromatography, and biological assays, such as immunoassays and microbiological assays, was acknowledged.

Small, "*conventional*" drug molecules are preferentially analyzed by chromatographic techniques, specifically by liquid chromatography-mass spectrometry (LC-MS) and liquid chromatography-tandem mass spectrometry (LC-MS/MS), and, to date, most emphasis has been on the validation of bioanalytical methods for such molecules, which is also reflected in the FDA guideline. However, because of the progress in recombinant DNA technology, the number of protein pharmaceuticals has increased dramatically. From 1996 through December 2005, the FDA has approved 253 so-called "*biologics*" for 384 indications. Most of these products are proteins. As a result of their high potency and subsequent low applied doses resulting in extremely low concentrations in biological media, chromatographic techniques are not sensitive enough for bioanalysis. Thus, immunoassays are primarily used for the bioanalysis of protein drugs.

This divergence in analytical techniques for small molecules and macromolecules has triggered workshops and conferences on bioanalytical method validation of macromolecules focusing on issues such as quantitative immunoassays for therapeutic proteins, biomarkers, and drug neutralizing anti bodies as well as bioassays. The results are documented in several publications of meeting reports, and these publications currently serve as quasi-guidance as no complete official document by the regulatory authorities of the United States or Europe on bioanalysis method validation of macromolecules exist to date. The FDA guidance on bioanalysis acknowledges differences between the assay formats but does not cover all necessary topics for bioassays. A guideline by the European Agency for the Evaluation of Medical Products (EMEA) on pharmacokinetics of pharmaceutical proteins also states specifics of immunoassays and lists points that should be addressed during method validation, but it provides no general guideline. Chromatographic assays are commonly applied to the analysis of protein drugs, but almost exclusively during product characterization release. Method validation of chromatographic techniques is basically identical for small molecules and macromolecules and is addressed in the ICH guidelines, FDA guidelines, as well as in publications and books. This chapter focuses on validation issues for macromolecule bioanalysis summarizing the current opinion according to the meeting reports and further publications on method validation for macromolecules. If possible, all terms related to assay validation are used in the sense of the ICH guideline Q2A.

Method Validation

Relevant macromolecular analytes in biological media can be classified into three categories: (1) pharmaceutical proteins administered as therapeutic agents; (2) biomarkers (i.e., endogenous substances that reflect physiological or pathophysiological processes or pharmacological responses to a therapeutic intervention); and (3) drug neutralizing antibodies that are generated as the response of the human organism to the application of a therapeutic protein. The primary assay formats for these molecules are ligand-binding assays (i.e., immunoassays and receptor-binding assays). Method validation of immunoassays will be the focus of the following discussion whereas cell-based assays will be only briefly addressed. Immunoassays can be roughly divided into competitive assays and sandwich assays. Validation will be discussed for immunoassays for the determination of pharmaceutical proteins in detail and, in subsequent sections, differences with regard to biomarkers and anti-drug antibodies will be mentioned. Not specifically addressed here, but evident in a good laboratory practice (GLP) environment, is the fact that proper documentation and standard operation procedures (SOPs) have to be written.

Ligand-Binding Assays

The term "*ligand-binding assay*" refers to methods that depend on the specific binding of an analyte to a biomolecule. Generally acknowledged inherent differences exist between bioanalytical chromatographic techniques and ligand-binding assays. Whereas chromatography is based on physico-chemical principles, ligand-binding assays are based on a biological response because of the interaction of a ligand with an antibody or a receptor. Consequently, the reagents are derived from living organisms with the attendant variation typical for such reagents (i.e., poor batch-to-batch reproducibility). High-purity, well-characterized reference standards are most often not commercially available. Although specificity in chromatography is obtained by isolation of the typically small molecules from the matrix combined with analytical separation from other sample components and probably even detection by mass spectrometry, the isolation of macromolecules from biological media is impractical in most cases because of the low concentrations and the structural or physico-chemical similarity between the analytes and endogenous compounds. Thus, detection of the macromolecule analytes occurs in a complex physiological milieu and, therefore, highly depends on the specificity of the reagents and detection systems. Finally, whereas chromatographic assays display linear relationships between analyte concentration and detector response over a broad range covering 2–3 orders of magnitude, calibration curves of ligand-binding assays are typically nonlinear covering a rather limited range requiring dilution of very concentrated samples. On the time scale, the development of an immunoassay will be longer compared with high-performance liquid chromatography (HPLC) methods because of the need of the generation of antibodies. Once these antibodies have been obtained, the time frame for method validation between the assays is comparable. Sample throughput of immunoassays is excellent.

Standard immunoassays

Validation is a continuing process through the whole life cycle of an assay. After selection of the assay format, preliminary data are obtained during method development, which are confirmed during prestudy validation and consequently applied during in-study validation. This scenario is considered a "*full validation.*" Partial validation is conducted when changes of a fully validated method occur that are considered minor, such as changes in the anticoagulant or changes in the used reagents. Partial validation can range from a single intra-assay accuracy and precision determination to nearly full validation. Method transfer from the developing laboratory to another laboratory or a production site requires at least partial validation. Cross-validation is conducted when two or more validated bioanalytical methods are used within the same study. Test samples (spiked samples or incurred test samples) should be used and the data should be evaluated using appropriate predefined acceptance criteria. Some, but not all, validation issues have been addressed in the FDA guideline on bioanalytical method validation.

Assay format

Assay format selection is the first step in method development. Assay formats include competition, sandwich, direct and indirect binding, inhibition, solid-phase, and solution phase assays. Reagents, first of all, include the antibodies; but diluents and additives such as detergents also have to be considered. For solid-phase assays, selection of the solid support as well as the chemistry used for the immobilization of the antibody may be critical. Consideration should also be given to the selection of the assay detection system to provide good signal-to- noise ratio. Detection may be improved by switching from colorimetric detection to fluorimetric or chemiliminescesence or, seldom, to radiometric detection. All these variables are evaluated during method development and confirmed during prestudy validation. In addition to the individual components, the manner in which an array is set up and run should already be considered during method development. The assay configuration (i.e., the number and placement of standards) of quality control (QC) samples, and study samples on a plate in an attempt to mimic the anticipated size of the run batches during routine use should be established as early as possible and confirmed during prestudy validation. It is recommended that at least 5% of the total samples of a given batch consist of QC samples.

Reagent selection and stability

Probably the most critical components of the assay are the antibodies used. These antibodies are produced by living organisms with the inherent variability of such reagents. They must be acquired in adequate amounts and sufficiently characterized. As antibodies are prone to lot-to-lot variations, ideally, different lots are evaluated during method development and prestudy validation. When an antibody (reagent) lot has to be changed during routine application, in-study validation must demonstrate comparable performance of the lots.

Assay performance and sensitivity will deteriorate upon degradation of the antibodies and other reagents. Therefore, it is important to investigate storage conditions to ensure the integrity of key reagents for the estimated period of time that they will be used. Stability testing is not addressed in the regulatory guidance documents, but it is an important aspect of method validation. If manufacturers provide expiration dates of reagents, they may be used instead of in-house stability determination. Reagent and antibody stability does not only concern storage at low temperatures (refrigerated or frozen), but standing times in laboratory equipment have to be considered. Thus, storage and handling conditions usually include bench-top stability, short-term and long-term storage, and stability to multiple freeze–thaw cycles. As it may also be desirable to store batches of assay microtiter plates for later use, the performance of a stored plate batch should be evaluated testing positive and negative samples. Stability is typically assessed during method development and confirmed during prestudy validation. It should be monitored during routine use.

Reference material

In contrast to small molecules where reference standards are well characterized and certified standards are often commercially available from sources such as the U.S. Pharmacopeia, the European Pharmacopoeia, or the World Health Organization (WHO), proteins are often not as rigorously characterized and their purity may vary from supplier to supplier. Variation in posttranslational modifications such as glycosylation and deamidation may be present. Thus, the proteins can vary in their potency and immunoreactivity. As the reference compounds are used as standard calibrators, validation sample and QC sample variation of the reference will have a profound impact on the assay performance. Therefore, it is important to clearly document the source of the material and to characterize the proteins as thoroughly as possible. Comparability between lots or sources should be evaluated if possible. If the analyte is not a new drug entity, the innovator company is typically the most reliable source of authentic material. As stated for the reagents, stability of the reference compounds is an issue that has to be ensured.

Specificity and selectivity

With regard to antibodies, specificity is the ability to specifically bind to the protein of interest in the presence of related endogenous and exogenous components (i.e., without cross reactivity). Selectivity, a related concept, describes the ability to determine an analyte in the presence of other constituents in a sample. Chromatographic methods are selective because they separate and detect analytes in a complex sample, typically after sample preparation steps for compound isolation. In contrast, ligand-binding assays measure analytes in biological matrices without prior isolation. Thus, high specificity may be desirable. With regard to interferences with other sample and matrix components and nonspecific binding of an antibody to such components, the terms "*specific nonspecificity*" and "*nonspecific nonspecificity*" are also used sometimes as synonyms for the ICH terms. Specific nonspecificity is the interference caused by compounds with structural similarity to the analyte of interest. Such compounds may be metabolites, degradation products of the analyte, isoforms and variants with posttranslational modifications, as well as endogenous substances. Causes for nonspecific nonspecificity may be unrelated matrix components, (patho) physiological factors interfering with ligand binding such as serum proteins and lipids, hemolysis, or anti-IgG antibodies. In addition, nonspecific adsorption to the microtiter plate may occur.

As macromolecular analytes often have structural elements in common with endogenous compounds, specificity may be difficult to achieve. Variant forms of proteins may not be available at the time of method development. In such cases, retrospective assessment may be acquired for the assay as more data become available over time. Rather than investigating specificity during method development, it is recommended to focus on reliable quantification of the analyte against a background of interfering matrix components.

Assay selectivity (nonspecific nonspecificity) is evaluated during method development by assaying spiked samples. Multiple lots of matrix should be evaluated, at least six to 10 lots are recommended. As selectivity problems occur, mostly at low concentrations, spiking should be performed at or near the lower limit of quantification (LLOQ). However, it may also be advisable to investigate higher concentrations. In case of interferences, it may be necessary to adjust the LLOQ before validation.

During prestudy validation, specificity and selectivity are confirmed. Selectivity may be expressed as acceptable recovery, applying the same principles as for the assessment of accuracy. Acceptance criteria should be predefined. Acceptance criteria for selectivity and specificity typically do not exist for in-study validation. If potential interference may become a problem caused by the matrix from persons with the disease, specificity and selectivity should be confirmed by repeating suitable experiments once those disease-state matrices become available.

Matrix selection

Matrix selection occurs in the development stage. Typically, biological fluids such as urine, plasma, serum, or cerebrospinal fluid as well as tissue samples may be collected. Additives such as anticoagulants, protease inhibitors, antioxidants, and so on may be present. It is necessary to document collection, processing, and storage conditions. The assay format may influence the choice of the matrix. For example, automated pipetting systems may be clogged by fibrin clots from plasma. In the absence of an endogenous signal, simple spike recovery experiments will determine the suitability of the matrix. In contrast, when the therapeutic protein is a recombinant version of an endogenous constituent, quantifiable amounts of the endogenous protein will be present in the matrix. Various strategies may be employed to limit or eliminate such interferences. If the endogenous concentration is very low, and subsequently the percentage of the area under the curve obtained in pharmacokinetic studies caused by the endogenous compound is below 5%, the endogenous protein will introduce only a small bias and can be neglected. Alternatively, the endogenous level is determined from blank samples (no spike added) of a number of subjects and subsequently subtracted from the spiked samples. As already stated, 6–10 lots of the matrix should be evaluated. Further strategies include "*stripping*" of the matrix from the endogenous analyte either by nonspecific adsorption on charcoal or specific removal by affinity chromatography, the use of surrogate matrix from other species, or the use of protein- containing buffers. However, one has to keep in mind that the QC samples have to be prepared in the "original," unprocessed matrix. The presence or absence of matrix effects should be demonstrated by analyzing spiked samples at least at one concentration level. Differences between matrices obtained from healthy and diseased individuals may have to be considered. In prestudy validation, the matrix selected during method development will be used to construct the calibration curves and validation samples. Once the effect of the matrix has been determined in method development, no further validation in later stages is required unless changes in the matrix occur.

Minimum required dilution

The minimum required dilution for an assay is the minimum magnitude of dilution of a sample with a defined diluent to optimize accuracy and precision in an assay. In many cases, dilution may not be necessary when analyzing plasma, serum, or other body fluids. Calibrator and validation samples are directly prepared in the matrix. For example, dilution may be required for samples with a background signal that is not caused by the endogenous version of the analyte. In the interest of a high signal-to-noise ratio (i.e., good accuracy and precision), sample dilution should be kept at a minimum. Once established during method development, this parameter should not be changed in later stages.

Assay range

The assay range is defined as the validated concentration range between the LLOQ and the upper limit of quantitation (ULOQ), for which the results have an (predefined) acceptable level of precision and accuracy. The LLOQ and ULOQ are determined by the lowest and highest validation samples that show precision and accuracy of at least 25% expressed as relative error. The range is estimated during method development and validated by samples in the area of the anticipated LLOQ and ULOQ during prestudy validation. During routine use, samples that are above the ULOQ must be diluted ("*minimum required dilution*" above). Samples that are below the LLOQ must be reported as "below LLOQ." The LLOQ during a batch run must be revised to higher concentrations if the QC samples at the lowest concentration fail to meet the 25% precision criteria.

Calibrators and standard curve

Standard calibrators are prepared by spiking known amounts of the (ideally, well-characterized) reference material into the matrix to obtain a standard curve from which the sample concentrations will be calculated. One of the major differences between chromatographic methods and immunoassays is that immunoassays display nonlinear relationships between the concentration and the measured response, which makes selection of the mathematical calibration curve model more complicated. Selection of the optimum calibration function is important to define the correct quantification range, to maximize accuracy and precision, and to achieve the quality control criteria.

The mathematical model most widely used for immunoassay calibration curves is the four-parameter logistic function. If the curve is asymmetric, inclusion of a fifth parameter (i.e., using a five-parameter logistic function) may improve the fit to the data. Algorithms that linearize the function such as logit-log may be used if goodness of fit is demonstrated, but such models are not recommended. Proper weighting of the data points in a calibration curve is also important to minimize bias and imprecision of the interpolated values near the LLOQ and ULOQ. Replicates with smaller variances are given greater weight compared with those with larger variances. The latter are normally found at the asymptotic ends of the curve.

As the standard concentrations should not be changed once validation has started, detailed investigation during method development is recommended using a greater number of data points and replicates compared with later validation stages. In the method development phase, the calibration curve should be constructed from a minimum of 10 non-zero standard points in duplicate spanning the anticipated concentration range about equally spaced on a logarithmic scale. Curve fit is achieved by a four-to-five-parameter logistic function. Whether to weight or not weight the responses should be supported by an evaluation of the relationship between the standard deviations of replicate values and the mean values at different concentration levels. A minimum of three independent runs should be used to establish the calibration model with duplicate curves included in each run to estimated intrabatch standard curve repeatability. The absolute relative error for back-calculated standard point should be ≤ 20% ("*intracurve*"). Acceptability of a model is verified by evaluating the relative error (relative bias) between back- calculated and nominal concentrations of the calibration samples. A model is considered acceptable if the relative error for all back-calculated standard points does not exceed 10% ("*intercurve*") and the precision (coefficient of variation) for each calibrator is ≤ 15%. Lack of fit may be caused by the use of an inappropriate mathematical function such as applying a four-parameter logistic function to asymmetric curves or inappropriate weighting of calibrators.

During prestudy validation, a minimum of six non-zero standards in duplicate are spaced evenly on the logarithmic concentration scale to fit the four-to-five parameter logistic function. At this point, additional calibrators outside the range of quantification (so-called "*anchor points*") may be included to facilitate curve fitting. This approach is in agreement with the FDA guidance on bioanalytical method validation. The regression model should be confirmed using at least six independent runs. Typically, the same runs are used to determine accuracy and precision. For acceptable curves, the back-calculated values for at least 75% of the standard points not including the anchor points should be within 20% of the theoretical value (except at the LLOQ, where 25% are acceptable), and upon completion of the validation, the cumulative relative error and coefficient of variation for each calibrator should be ≤ 15% and ≤ 20% at the LLOQ.

The standard curve should be monitored during in-study validation with at least one set of calibrators per patch run. As for prestudy validation, the curve should be constructed from six concentrations in duplicate. Anchor points may be used. The final number of points used for curve fit must be either 75% of the total number or a minimum of six calibrator samples not including the anchor points. The relative error of the back-calculated samples should be ≤ 20% (≤ 25% at the LLOQ). If either the high or low calibrator standards have to be deleted, the range for this particular run must be limited to the next standard point. Samples out of range must be repeated.

Precision and accuracy

Precision and accuracy are assay performance characteristics that describe the random (statistical) errors and systematic errors (bias) associated with repeated measurements of the same sample under specified conditions. Precision is typically estimated by the percent coefficient of variation (% CV, also referred to as relative standard deviation or RSD) but may certainly also be reported as standard deviations. Method accuracy is expressed as the percent relative error (% RE) and is determined by the percent deviation of the weighted samples mean from samples with nominal reference values.

Spiked samples are analyzed over multiple runs with replicate determinations during method development and prestudy validation. QC samples are used during in-study validation to monitor the performance of the assay. Limits for minimum acceptable precision and accuracy should be established before or during method development and used throughout the life cycle of the assay.

It is recommended to determine accuracy and precision during method development with at least three batch runs using a minimum of eight sample concentrations analyzed in duplicate. The concentrations should span the whole validation concentration range of the assay. Recommended target limits for intrabatch and inter- batch precision (% CV) are ≤ 20 %, bias (% RE) should not exceed ±20%. At the LLOQ, a maximum of 25% for % CV and % RE is acceptable. These values are more lenient compared with the typical target values of chromatographic assays (% CV; 15% and 20% at LLOQ) because immunoassays are inherently less precise than chromatographic assays. In prestudy validation, at least six batch runs with a minimum of five different concentrations, one at the LLOQ, one at the ULOQ, and three concentrations in the lower, medium, and high range, analyzed in duplicate should be used for accuracy and precision determination. For each validation sample, the repeated measurements from all runs have to be statistically analyzed together.

The target values for intrabatch and interbatch precision as well as accuracy (bias) are the same as the values applied in method development (20%, except for LLOQ, where 25% is acceptable). The total error of the method (i.e., the sum of % RE and % CV) should not exceed 30% (40% at the LLOQ). Further, for each in-study run, precision and accuracy are monitored by QC samples. Recommended run acceptance criteria are based on the total error, specifically on the deviation of the measured values from the nominal values, and not on statistical calculations such as the means or standard deviations. As QC samples, one set of at least three concentrations, one each in the low, medium, and high concentration range, are analyzed in duplicate in each batch run. As for small molecules, at least two thirds of the measured values of the QC samples must fall within a certain percentage of the corresponding nominal values and at least 50% of the results for each concentration of the QC samples must be within the specified limit. Thus, not all samples of a specific concentration are allowed outside the specifics. For chromatographic assays for small molecules, 15% has been adopted as limit (i.e., the "4–6–15 rule"). At the LLOQ, 20% are acceptable. As a result of the lower precision of immunoassays, the error margin has been widened, a 6-4-25 rule is recommended by Findley et al., whereas a 4–6–30 rule has been proposed at the macromolecule bioanalysis workshop. The 30% margin is identical with the maximal acceptable total error of the method (sum of % RE and % CV) of the prestudy validation. Other statistical methods as acceptance criteria have been published and can also be applied.

Dilutional linearity

As the range of an immunoassay is usually limited, it may be necessary to dilute concentrated samples. Therefore, it has to be demonstrated that the analyte can still be reliably quantified upon dilution of high concentration samples so that they fall within the validated range of the assay. Moreover, a so-called prozone or "*hook effect*" can be identified. A hook effect is present when high concentration samples above the ULOQ display a lower response than ULOQ samples because of signal suppression caused by the high concentration of the analyte. Dilutional linearity should not be confused with parallelism.

Dilutional linearity is evaluated during method development, typically with spiking 100-fold to 1000-fold greater concentrations into the sample matrix followed by dilution with the assay matrix. Dilutions should be made so that several dilutions fall within the standard curve in the lower, middle, and upper parts of the curve. Dilution samples above the ULOQ can be included to evaluate a hook effect. The dilutions are further confirmed during prestudy validation. The back-calculated concentration for each diluted sample should be within 20% of the nominal or expected value. The precision of the cumulative back-calculated concentration should be ≤ 20 %. If a sample has to be diluted during routine use of the method to a higher extend than assessed during prestudy validation, dilutional linearity should either be repeated or a dilutional QC sample should be included in the assay.

Parallelism

Parallelism is a characteristic that is typically assessed during in-study validation. It is conceptually similar to dilutional linearity with the difference that it is determined by dilutions of actual study samples (incurred samples). In some cases, samples from a preclinical pilot study may be available during prestudy validation so that assessment of parallelism may be performed at that time. Moreover, when an assay is validated with the aim to replace another assay, incurred samples from a previous study may be available for evaluation of this performance characteristic.

Parallelism is assessed using C_{max} samples from an actual study. Commonly, samples from several individuals are pooled to create a suitable validation sample. Using pooled samples eliminates the need for generation of multiple values for individual study samples. It is recommended that the relative standard deviation between samples of a dilutional series should be ≤ 30%.

Sample stability

Experiments demonstrating sufficient stability of the analyte in the sample matrix must be included in prestudy validation. Such experiments should mimic as closely as possible the conditions under which study samples will be collected, stored, and processed. Assessment should include bench-top stability, refrigerator stability, whole-blood stability, freeze–thaw stability, and long-term freezer stability. Stability samples can be prepared by spiking the analyte reference at high and low concentrations into the sample matrix.

Bench-top stability refers to the conditions under which the samples are handled during processing of the samples at the analytical site and should be examined at room temperature for at least 2 h and at 2–8°C (refrigerator temperature) for a minimum of 24 h. The stability in whole blood can be determined by spiking the analyte into freshly collected whole blood followed by incubation for up to 2 h and processing to obtain plasma or serum samples at certain intervals. The samples are subsequently processed and analyzed. Typically, freeze–thaw stability evaluation includes three freeze–thaw cycles with at least 12 h between the thaws. The rate of freezing and thawing should mimic the manner in which samples will be handled as they are thawed before the assay. Long-term stability should demonstrate that the samples are stable throughout the lifetime of the study. The necessity to conduct studies on samples stored at −20°C and −70°C to −80°C may depend on the duration of the study.

Assessment of the stability is typically performed during prestudy validation and continued during in-study validation. If changes in sample handling or storage occur, additional stability evaluations must be carried out to reflect the altered conditions. The acceptance criteria for the stability evaluations, with the exception of the whole-blood stability, will be the same acceptance criteria applied for accuracy and precision of QC samples. If the measured value is within the acceptance criteria for accuracy, the sample is considered stable.

Robustness and ruggedness

Robustness is the ability of an assay to withstand small but deliberate changes that may affect the assay. Such factors may, for example, include incubation temperature and duration, number of washes, light exposure, and lot-to-lot differences in key assay reagents or microtiter plates. Changes that may have an impact on the assay have to be clearly identified in the method description (SOP). The term ruggedness is not mentioned in the IHC guidelines, but it is included in the USP monograph on validation. The term describes the consistent performance of an assay under routine changes (i.e., different analysts, instruments, batch size). Such changes should have no significant impact on the consistency of an assay.

The extent of the assessment of robustness and ruggedness depends on the anticipated application of the method, the current status of the assay's life cycle, industry standards, and, last but not least, common sense. The majority of robustness testing will be conducted during method development to facilitate the early identification of factors that affect assay performance. Prestudy robustness and ruggedness validation may be limited to the conditions demonstrating acceptable performance under the anticipated in-study conditions, such as incubation temperature and time tolerances, batch sizes, and so on, but more formal evaluation can also be applied. Acceptable robustness and ruggedness during routine use are assumed when monitoring in-study QC samples demonstrating acceptable intraassay and interassay precision.

Run acceptance criteria

Run acceptance criteria are used to accept or reject a run because of its performance. As a consequence, no defined run acceptance criteria are applicable during method development. Prestudy validation runs are accepted based on the standard curve acceptance criteria. No run can be rejected because of poor performance of a sample during precision and accuracy evaluation; all data from prestudy validation runs are reported unless there has been a clearly recognizable error during sample preparation or measurement. Despite the fact that the standard curve must satisfy the criteria described for standard curves above, in-study runs are accepted based primarily on the performance of the QC samples. As stated above in the paragraph on precision and accuracy, the 4–6–30 rule is recommended (i.e., at least four of six QC samples must be within 30% of their theoretical values and at least 50% of the values for each level must satisfy the 30% limit.

Biomarker assays

A biomarker is defined as an endogenous substance that reflects physiological or pathophysiological processes or pharmacological responses to a therapeutic intervention, with a few exceptions such as viral load biomarkers are endogenous substances. It is a diverse class ranging from electrolytes to small molecules and macromolecules and a wide variety of analytical methodologies is used to quantify such substances. Although many assay characteristics apply to other analytical techniques and analytes as well, the following discussion will only touch on ligand-binding assays for the determination of macromolecules. As for the bioanalysis of therapeutic proteins, no official guidance documents are currently available for biomarker analysis. Moreover, differences exist between validation approaches according to GLP regulations, which are the basis for documents of the FDA and other regulatory agencies and the National Committee for Clinical Laboratory Standards (NCCLS) guidelines for diagnostic assays.

Besides, in clinical diagnostics especially, novel biomarkers play an increasing role in drug development for the investigation of the pharmacologic response to drug treatment or as surrogate markers for clinical endpoints. Clinical and drug development decisions will depend on the quality of biomarker data. Thus, the utility and value of such data is ultimately determined by the validity of the assay and requires demonstration and documentation of performance characteristics, as mentioned in the previous subsection, for immunoassays such as accuracy, precision, specificity, range, stability, and so on. However, in contrast to bioassays for drug compounds, where quantitative results are achieved by calibration typically using well-defined reference standards, biomarker assays may differ considerably depending on the type of analytical measurement, the type of the analytical data that develop from the assay, or the intended use of the assay. Subsequently, different assay types and validation levels may apply. Rigorous method validation for a novel biomarker is not necessary for drug discovery-phase work. However, the design of the validation must change when the assay is transferred from screening to quantitative determination in later phases of drug development.

Biomarker assays (as other bioassays) may be classified into "*definitive quantitative assays*," "*relative quantitative assays*," "*quasi-quantitative assays*," and "*qualitative assays*" with varying degrees of validation requirements. For definitive quantitative assays, a well-defined or characterized standard of the biomarker is available. In the case of relative quantitative assays, calibration is performed with a standard that is not well characterized, not available in pure form, or not representative of the endogenous biomarker. Results from these assays are expressed as numerical values. Currently, most biomarker assays fall into the relative quantitative category. In quasi-quantitative assays, no reference material is available for the construction of a calibration curve. Nevertheless, the analytical result is expressed in numerical units. Examples are the measurement of enzymatic activity (expressed as units per volume) and vaccine or anti-drug antibodies where the response is reported as percent binding or titer. Qualitative assays use no standard either, and the results are reported non-numerically (i.e., "low, medium, and high" or "+, ++, and +++").

Although with respect to validation criteria a lot of similarities exist between ligand-binding assays for pharmaceutical proteins and biomarker assays, significant differences have to be noted, especially for novel bio markers, in which a suitable reference standard is not present. If the intended reference is a recombinant protein, one should keep in mind that such proteins often have glycosylation patterns different from the endogenous equivalents. The glycosylation pattern of endogenous proteins is often heterogeneous so that it is virtually impossible to prepare glycoprotein standards that are identical to the natural circulating proteins. In the ideal case, a purified endogenous protein from the target species is used as a reference. This standard should be characterized in terms of analytical purity as thoroughly as possible. If a well-characterized standard is not available, the assay results will provide rather "relative" than "true" numerical values. As a result of the presence of endogenous biomarkers, no analyte-free matrix exists for the preparation of calibrator standards, which makes the establishment of the LLOQ particularly challenging. Standard curves may be prepared using pooled matrix from individuals with low baseline concentrations of the compound. Alternatively, (affinity) stripped matrix, a protein-containing buffer or matrix from an alternate species with negligible concentrations of the analyte, may be considered. Further strategies for minimization of interference from endogenous biomarkers can be used. The preparation of calibrator standards not in the actual sample matrix is one major difference of biomarker assays from assays of protein drugs. When using such approaches, it has to be ensured that the use of the surrogate matrices does not introduce a bias in the assay. In contrast to calibration samples, QC samples must be prepared in an authentic matrix. In this case, matrix samples containing low basal levels can be selected and the middle and upper QC concentrations can be prepared by the addition of known biomarker amounts. Moreover, the disease state can have an impact not only on endogenous biomarker levels but also on the composition of the matrix itself. High concentrations of the marker produced during disease can cause a hook effect. A disease state may also alter the heterogeneity of the biomarker with altered cross reactivity to the antibody relative to the standard. The modified matrix composition can result in increased nonspecific binding (i.e., nonspecific nonspecificity).

The stages of validation of biomarker assays include establishment of the biomarker (development), so-called prevalidation, prestudy validation, and in-study validation. The following short discussion will focus on the "GLP-like" definitive and relative quantitative assays. As the development and validation of an assay for novel biomarkers is quite diverse, the application of strict validation procedures appears problematic. Therefore, upon establishment of the prototype assay in the development phase, a formalized validation plan should be developed that defines the scope and purpose of the assay. Further activities during method development include the establishment of the reference standard, selection of antibodies and the assay format, as well as evaluation of key reagents. As mentioned above, selection of the matrix for the preparation of the calibrator concentrations may be challenging because of the presence of endogenous biomarker. Subsequently, the calibration curve model will be established. As for other immunoassays, nonlinear calibration using the four-to-five-parameter logistic model is the commonly acknowledged model for data fitting.

The prevalidation phase may be regarded as a method optimization phase where the calibration model is confirmed; range, LLOQ, and ULOQ are defined; and matrix interference is evaluated. The use of anchor points for the calibration curve may be feasible. As mentioned above, determination of the LLOQ may be difficult because of the presence of the endogenous analyte. Dilutional linearity may be evaluated as well. It is also considered useful to assess the biomarker in healthy and diseased individuals. For this purpose, at least 25 individuals should be tested to account for intrasubject variability caused by circadian and seasonal fluctuations and intersubject variability.

Prestudy validation will additionally evaluate standard and reagent stability as well as matrix stability during collection processing and storage of the samples, will determine dilutional linearity and parallelism, and will confirm assay range and the calibration model. These criteria can be determined as described for immunoassays for pharmaceutical proteins above. In addition, accuracy and precision have to be determined. It is recommended to use validation samples at five different concentration levels analyzed at least in duplicate and in a minimum of six runs. One concentration should be at the anticipated LLOQ, one about 2–4 times the LLOQ, one in midrange on the log scale, one about 70–80% of the anticipated ULOQ, and one at the anticipated ULOQ. The following method acceptance criteria have been recommended: Both accuracy (% RE) and precision (% CV) should be within 25%, except at the LLOQ where 30% is acceptable. Even more lenient criteria may be required in some cases, depending on the analyte or the type of assay and its limitations. It is important to note that such QC samples must be prepared in the actual matrix. The use of buffer, surrogate, or stripped matrix is not feasible, except for rare matrices such as cerebrospinal fluid or tears, where a surrogate matrix may be the only practical option. Spike recovery experiments should be performed on multiple individual lots of matrix to assess the accuracy, matrix effects, and interference. It may also be favorable to include a pilot study into prestudy validation runs.

As for immunoassays for pharmaceutical proteins, in-study validation of biomarker assays should include one set of calibrators to monitor the standard curve as well as a set of QC samples at three concentrations analyzed in duplicate for the decision to accept or reject a specific run. Recommended acceptance criterion is the 6–4–30 rule, but even more lenient acceptance criteria may be justified based on statistical rationale developed from experimental data.

Anti-drug antibody assays

Basically, the protein sequence of biophar-maceutical therapeutics can be nonhuman, chimeric, humanized, or fully human. Most such therapeutics elicit some level of antibody response against the product leading to potentially serious side effects or loss of drug efficacy. Thus, the immunogenicity of therapeutic proteins is a concern for clinicians, manufacturers, and regulatory agencies. For the detection of anti-drug antibodies, a number of assay methods including enzyme-linked immuno-sorbert assays (ELISA), immunoblotting, surface plasmon resonance, and bioassays are available, each technique having its own advantages and disadvantages. Whereas binding assays identify the antibodies, immunoblotting provides information on the specificity. Surface plasmon resonance can show the antigen-antibody interaction in real time, whereas bioassays demonstrate the neutralizing potential of the antibodies. To date, microtiter plate-based ELISAs are still the most widely used format for testing for anti-drug antibodies because of their simplicity, sensitivity, and high-throughput capability. Generally, the validation parameters outlined for standard immunoassays as required by the regulatory authorities apply to immunoassay-based anti-drug antibody assays as well. These parameters include specificity, selectivity, accuracy, sensitivity, precision, robustness, ruggedness, and stability of reagents, analyte, and matrix. However, some differences exist because of the nature of the antibodies.

As a result of the lack of reference material, anti-drug antibody assays are generally quasi-quantitative assays. In addition, the target analyte is generally polyclonal, consisting of antibodies of various isotype classes, specificities, and affinities (i.e., the analyte is not a defined molecule). Thus, no single positive control exists that accurately represents the target analyte. During the early validation phase, no clinical studies have typically been performed, so it may be a challenge to obtain a representative positive sample for method development and validation. When establishing specificity, accuracy, and sensitivity, several control analytes from different individuals or sources representing the test population should be investigated. Specificity of analyte binding can be assessed using immunodepleted samples.

Selectivity is a critical parameter determining the reliability of an antidrug antibody assay. In this context, one has to keep in mind that selectivity can vary between test samples because of the heterogenous nature of the antibodies. For the evaluation of selectivity, immunoglobulins and other potential interfering substances can be spiked into positive and negative samples at high but physiologically relevant concentrations. No substantial interference can be concluded if the recovery is 80–125%. The influence of different sample matrices, typically serum and plasma, should also be evaluated if both matrices may be analyzed with the same assay. The type of the matrix should not change the outcome of the assay. Furthermore, a com parison of specificity between normal- and disease-state matrices should be conducted to detect interfering substances that may be present in certain populations or disease states. Another unique property of anti-drug antibody assays is that the drug itself can act as an interfering substance, which can be mimicked with addition of the drug in varying concentrations to positive controls.

As a result of the quasi-quantitative nature of anti-drug antibody immunoassays and the lack of a reference standard a threshold value, the so-called "*cutoff*" or "*cutpoint*" is used to identify positive samples from nonspecific background noise. The assay cutoff is preferably determined by analyzing samples from healthy individuals and those affected by the disease. The data are subsequently used to calculate the cutoff value yielding 5% of false positives. Moreover, one should consider that a low optical readout increases imprecision so that the cutoff level should not be too low for optical assays.

The sensitivity of an immunoassay is typically defined by its LLOQ, which can only be determined when a reference standard is available. Alternatively, a detection limit of qualitative assays is used where a distinction is essentially made between positive and negative results only. Typically, the antibody data are reported as "titer," the titer being the reciprocal of the highest dilution of a sample in which the instrument response is greater than the cutoff response. At least two positive control analytes should be used. If a positive control antibody is available, a pseudo- calibration curve can be generated by a series of dilutions. However, one should keep in mind that "true" quantitation is impossible because of the lack of a true reference compound. Determination of the dilutional linearity is not so important when the result is reported as a titer. However, if the determination of positive samples is based on the interpolation from a reference standard curve, it is essential to demonstrate that the QC samples fall within the (limited) linear range of the calibration curve and not on a plateau or a region that may include a hook effect.

Precision should be assayed using positive controls, negative controls, and a diluent sample. Positive controls should be prepared at a high and a low concentration to demonstrate precision within this assay range. Typically, precision (% CV) of ≤ 30% is considered acceptable. In-study monitoring of a batch run using QC samples consisting of at least one positive control, a matrix negative control, and a diluent negative control should be used to estimate assay performance.

Validation of Cell-based Bioassays

Bioassays use living systems that measure the biological activity of a therapeutic agent. Such assays may be used to study the effects of hormones or growth factors, but such systems can also address drug toxicity and side effects. Moreover, bioassays may also be applied to bioanalysis of biopharmaceutical proteins. Only *in vitro* assays using cell culture systems measuring a discrete response such as cell proliferation, differentiation, or survival will be briefly addressed. Bioassays may generate quantitative or quasi-quantitative data. Only a few considerations for bioassay method validation will be mentioned, as this type of assay is not frequently applied. Most validation procedures for quantitative assays, such as calibration and reagent and matrix stability, accuracy, and precision, are essentially identical to the procedures described for standard immunoassays above.

For a validated assay, an established immortal cell line is typically used. Thus, during method development, not only must a suitable reference standard be established, but also documentation of the cell line with respect to characteristics such as origin of the cell line, culture and passage history, morphology, surface markers, and receptors is required. It is advisable to study the effect of cell age (number of passages) on the measured response. Specificity may be another issue as cell lines proliferate, differentiate, or senesce and die in response to alarge number of biomolecules that may be present in the samples obtained for bioanalytical studies. In addition, macromolecules can be metabolized leading to metabolites that may also be biologically active, which is not relevant when a pure compound is applied to the cell culture to study its effect on the cells. However, bioanalytical methods based on bioassays may not be specific for the analyte of interest. In this case, extensive study of interference because of nonspecificity should be conducted during prestudy validation using samples from a number of representative individuals.

Conclusions and Future Considerations

Despite the wide availability of chromatographic techniques hyphenated to mass spectrometry, immunoassays remain the most important methods for bioanalytical applications for monitoring macromolecules such as therapeutic proteins, biomarkers, or drug-induced antibodies. Current guidelines of regulatory authorities focus on chromatographic techniques with no or little reference to the specifics of ligand-binding assays. As some differences with respect to assay validation exist between chromatographic and ligand-binding assays, a number of issues require special attention. Reference material of the target analyte(s) is not always available in pure form, which is especially true for biomarkers and anti-drug antibodies. In addition, key reagents such as the antibodies for the immunoassay are frequently not commercially available. Stability issues of those key reagents, the reference material, and the biological matrix have to be considered.

The calibration curves of immunoassays are nonlinear, so that special attention should be paid to the selection of the correct calibration model. Anchoring points out of the validated range may optimize the curve fit. Selectivity of an immunoassay depends on the specificity of the antibody directed toward the analyte. Non-specific interferences from the matrix as well as specific interferences (cross reactivity) from related compounds have to be considered. Special challenges occur if the analyte is an endogenous compound. In this case, analyte-free matrix may not exist, so that alternative strategies for the preparation of validation samples have to be explored. However, QC samples should be prepared in the original matrix if possible. Pathological states may alter the composition of the matrix or, in the case of biomarkers, the respective concentration, which has to be considered for an appropriate selection of the calibration standards and QC samples. Assays for anti-drug antibodies are quasi-quantitative so that complete GMP-like validation is normally not possible. Finally, as ligand-binding assays are inherently less precise than chromatographic assays, more lenient acceptance criteria for accuracy and precision as well as for run acceptance should be applied. The current opinion according to conference reports recommends as target values for precision (expressed as % CV) and accuracy (expressed as % RER) a maximum of 20% (25% at the LLOQ). Despite known disadvantages, application the 6–4–30 rule as run acceptance criteria during in-study validation has been adopted.

The current gap between the need for validated immunoassays according to GLP compliance and the lack of official guidance documents will certainly be closed in the near future because ongoing efforts at conferences between scientists from regulatory authorities, pharmaceutical companies, and scientific organizations will ultimately result in such guidance documents. However, technological advances in instrument automation and new technologies will continue to create new issues that have to be considered when developing and validating methods for bioanalysis. As each technique has and will have unique features, the challenge is the implementation of a dynamic, yet standardized and systematic approach for analytical method validation.

3

Physico-chemical Methods

To the pharmaceutical world, the meaning of analytical methods validation is the process to confirm that a method does what it purports to do, that is, to document through laboratory studies that the measurement procedure can reliably assess the identity, strength, and/or quality of a bulk drug substance, excipient, or finished pharmaceutical product. To provide consistent, worldwide regulatory expectations, previously unavailable, the International Conference on Harmonization (ICH) has defined the methods validation process for the release and stability testing of all new products. This chapter interprets these ICH regulatory definitions and requirements, as well as provides direction toward rational and efficient validation.

Regulatory methods can be compendial or noncompendial. Wherever possible, methodologies are to be employed which are documented, generally recognized as official pharmacopoeia or compendial. Compendial methods are considered valid; however, suitability must be verified under actual conditions of use. Non-compendial methods require validation, and must be selected if a compendial method does not exist. A non-compendial method can be chosen over an existing compendial method, if it can be demonstrated to be superior to the compendial test.

Before a product dossier has been submitted to an agency for regulatory market approval, analytical laboratories have utilized validated methods to support toxicological, clinical, stability, development, scale-up, optimization, process, and cleaning validation studies. Unreliable data for any of these studies have the potential to completely undermine the speed and success of approval. A method's "*life cycle*" parallels the drug development process. Starting with early (preclinical) development projects, the related methods for drug substance and finished drug product require only some rudimentary validation to provide sufficient confidence in the results, eventually leading to a complete methods validation package for the final stages of product development and commercialization. The methods life cycle concludes with methods transfers, monitoring of routine quality control (QC) usage, and revalidation. We define revalidation as repeating those parts of validation that are affected by a modification, for example, specificity, if the column has changed. Repeating the whole validation periodically is superfluous; instead, continuous monitoring of the performance of the analytical procedure should be performed (see section "Maintenance of the Validation Status"). Many tests may be specified in the early development of a product or process that will not be ultimately selected for routine release testing. Clearly not all products reach the approved and marketing stage, due to toxicology, efficacy, or even business conditions. Multiple other changes can occur along the way toward approval such as active pharmaceutical ingredient (API, drug substance), synthetic route changes, drug product formulation, and process changes, as well as newly identified degradation pathways. All of these affect the method applied. Therefore, methods (development) validation requires efficient planning of resources to match the accuracy and precision requirements needed to assess product quality.

Methods Selection and Applicability for Routine Use

The target laboratory [development (R&D) or QC] where the methods will be utilized and the stage of development are just as important as the analyte/sample to be measured when considering the selection of a method as these will affect the accuracy and precision requirements, as well as laboratory economic, environmental, and ergonomic factors. Methods should be selected that are adequate for testing the attribute to be measured. They must be sufficiently selective, accurate, precise, and robust to demonstrate conformance to proposed specifications. It should be noted that a precise method is an extremely important attribute in QC. A precise method permits a fluctuation in the manufacturing process to be detected before it can cause an out-of-specification (OOS) event. With a sufficiently precise method, subsequent tightening of the specification should not necessitate modification or revalidation of the test method.

Additionally, these procedures should be devised with the explicit objective of transferring the methods to a qualifiable laboratory. The development laboratory should specify test techniques, parameters, and other details in the final dossier submission that have the highest likelihood of being transferred successfully to a QC site. Methods shall be selected that experience shows will likely be reproducible. Reproducibility is assessed late in the validation process. Methods should be designed to minimize direct analysis and turn-around time, to maximize efficiency, and to shake the convenience, safety, health and environmental impacts of the test as consistent with the other primary objectives of method development. Development considerations should include equipment and expertise limitations of the receiving laboratory, expected sample volumes, and achieving a balance between acceptable traditional validation parameter values (accuracy, precision, etc.) and analysis time and robustness. The receiving laboratory should participate in the early review of these methods to provide and prepare for the transfer (e.g., purchase equipment) and should also assess safety, meaningful system suitability parameters (derived from robustness studies), and overall clarity of the written method. Automated tests may be desirable. Where a method has been developed and performed on automated equipment, an early assessment should be made as to whether automation is critical to the accuracy, precision, reproducibility, and robustness of the method compared to a manual method.

Validations and Specifications (Limits)

Method validations and drug substance or finished pharmaceutical product specifications are intimately linked. To ensure transferability of the method and to ensure the method will operate successfully in a QC site, the method variation (from the intermediate precision) should be known and monitored. The method variation is an estimate of the variation that will be experienced in routine use of the method. More method variation will create unacceptable random failure rates, and provide no room for reasonable product variation or even minor stability changes. The method variation should be less than one-third of the interval from the mean or target (typically the midpoint of the upper and lower specification limit) value to the nearest specification limit, or one-sixth of the in-specification operating range of the method, whichever is smaller. Otherwise, OOS results may occur, even for product that was produced at target and with zero process variation. If a reasonable opportunity exists (based on common belief and experience) to improve the method variation to one-fourth or preferably less of the specification interval, this effort should be made. In the example of a drug product where the specification is 95%–105% with a target of 100%, then the maximum method variation must be less than 1.67%; however, if the method variation is above 1.25%, efforts should be made to reduce its variation. Ideally, the method variation should not be greater than 2.0% even if the specification range is wider than 10%.

The 2.0% maximum method variation requirement does not apply to tests where the variation of the method is substantially confounded with variation of the product being measured.

Validation as a Good Business Practice

While compliance to legal requirements is paramount to the pharmaceutical industry and its associated regulatory bodies, it is by far not the only reason to judiciously develop and validate analytical procedures. Well-developed and validated methods represent good business practices, as haphazardly chosen and/or poorly validated methods can haunt a company financially for the short and long term.

Extensive sample preparation with long cycle times, and excessive hazardous solvents usage and disposal are easily calculable financial and safety losses. Imprecise stability data can easily lead to erroneous or shortened expiration dating assignments. Poorly validated methods increase the chances of OOS results and investigations absorb costly laboratory resources. Incapable methods (inadequate precision for the associated specification) cannot readily discriminate passing from failing products: therefore, one can release unacceptable product, leading to product recalls. Inaccurate methods can lead to sub- or superpotent products. Non-reproducible methods do not transfer quickly or efficiently and can become limiting factors of pre-approval inspections with potential to affect product launches.

Regulatory Requirements

Due to the importance of demonstrating the suitability of new analytical procedures described in submission dossiers, in the 1980s many regulatory agencies published requirements for analytical validation, in varying details. The U.S. Food and Drug Administration (FDA) issued two guidelines, one for the applicant, the other for inspectors and reviewers. The first one is also intended to ensure that the analytical procedure can be applied in an FDA laboratory and requires, therefore, a detailed description of the procedure, reference materials, discussion of potential impurities, etc. With respect to validation, data should be provided to demonstrate an appropriate accuracy, precision, linearity, selectivity, and quantitation limit (QL) for impurities and degradation products. For drug product, recovery, lack of interference from placebo, and variability with respect to time, laboratory, operator, and column should be demonstrated.

The second guideline is focused on reversed-phase chromatography and gives details regarding critical methodological issues, as well as acceptable results for parameters. A revised draft for the first guideline, published in 2000, focused on providing raw data in detail. However, this has nothing to do with validation and should be an inspection issue, as there is a real danger to burden the validation documentation with huge amounts of data, which make it difficult to concentrate on a scientifically justified demonstration of suitability. Additionally, there are some inconsistencies with the ICH documents, which are not helpful for the harmonization process.

The same validation characteristics were described in the *U.S. Pharmacopoeia* (USP). Three categories of analytical procedures were distinguished: quantitation procedures for main components in drug products, procedures for determination of impurities, and procedures for pharmaceutical–technical characteristics (e.g., dissolution). The guidance on validation of the European Community was rather general and incorporated in the respective sections of the submission documentation. In the Canadian guideline, a very detailed discussion is provided for requirements and especially acceptance criteria. Although this gives some orientation, the given acceptance criteria were sometimes a bit ambiguous, for example, the intermediate precision/reproducibility of below 1% for drug substances.

International Conference on the Harmonization of Technical Requirements for the Registration of Pharmaceuticals for Human Use (ICH)

This process was initiated in 1990 in order to harmonize the submission requirements for new pharmaceuticals in the three main regions of Europe, the United States, and Japan and to avoid duplication, inefficiencies, and delays. A forum was created for a constructive dialogue between regulatory authorities and industry. The six cosponsors of ICH were the European Commission, the European Federation of Pharmaceutical Industry Association (EFPIA), the Japanese Ministry of Health (MHW), the Japanese Pharmaceutical Manufacturers Association (JPMA), the Food and Drug Association (FDA), and the Pharmaceutical Research and Manufacturers of America (PhRMA). Several organizations such as the Canadian Health Protection Branch (HPB), the USP, and the European Pharmacopoeia (EP) participated as observers. Within the Quality section, seven topics were taken into account: stability, validation, impurities, pharmacopoeial harmonization, biotechnological products, specifications, and good manufacturing practice (GMP).

The ICH was very valuable in harmonizing terms and definitions as well as basic requirements for analytical validation. Of course, due to the nature of the harmonization process, there are some compromises and inconsistencies, but the importance of a proper validation is currently widely known and accepted. In the following, the main ICH requirements for the validation characteristics are summarized. However, the ICH guidelines must not be regarded as a checklist. "It is the responsibility of the applicant to choose the validation procedure and protocol most suitable for their product."

Specificity

"Specificity is the ability to assess unequivocally the analyte in the presence of components which may be expected to be present. Typically, these might include impurities, degradants, matrix, etc." For identification, discrimination between closely related compounds likely to be present should be demonstrated by positive and negative samples. For assay and impurity tests, available impurities/ degradants can be spiked to the corresponding matrix or degraded samples can be used. Specificity can also be demonstrated by verification of the result with an independent analytical procedure. The overall specificity can (and often will) be obtained by a combination of several analytical procedures, for example, in case of a partly specific titration with a chromatographic impurity determination. In case of chromatographic separations, resolution factors should be obtained for critical separations. Tests for peak homogeneity, for example, by diode array detection (DAD) or mass spectrometry (MS) are recommended. All tested substances should be documented including the rationale of their selection. All relevant results, e.g., as tables or chromatograms, should be provided, discussed, and evaluated.

Linearity

"The linearity of an analytical procedure is its ability (within a given range) to obtain test results which are directly proportional to the concentration (amount) of analyte in the sample." It can be distinguished between the linearity of the detector/instrument, obtained from a dilution of the analyte and the linearity of the analytical procedure, obtained from independent preparations (spiking, weighing) including (as far as possible) the complete sample pretreatment. At least five concentrations over the whole working range should be analyzed. Besides a visual evaluation of the analyte signal as a function of the concentration, appropriate statistical calculations are recommended, such as a linear regression. The parameters slope and intercept, the sum of squares, and the coefficient of correlation should be reported.

Range

"The range of an analytical procedure is the interval between the upper and lower concentration (amounts) of analyte in the sample (including these concentrations) for which it has been demonstrated that the analytical procedure has a suitable level of precision, accuracy and linearity."

The following minimum ranges are required:

1. Assay: 80–120% of the test concentration.
2. Content uniformity: 70–130% of the test concentration.

3. Dissolution: 20% below to 20% above the specified range.
4. Impurities: reporting level to 120% of the specification.
5. 100% method: reporting level of the impurity to 120% assay specification.

Accuracy

"The accuracy of an analytical procedure expresses the closeness of agreement between the value which is accepted either as a conventional true value or an accepted reference value and the value found." This validation characteristic is an indication of systematic errors (bias). Accuracy can be demonstrated by the following procedures:

1. Inferred from precision, linearity, and specificity.
2. Comparison of the results with those of a well characterized procedure.
3. Application to a reference material (drug substance).
4. Recovery of drug substance added to placebo (drug product).
5. Recovery of the impurity added to drug substance or drug product (impurities).

For the quantitative approaches, at least nine determinations across the specified range should be obtained, for example, three determinations at three concentration levels. The percent recovery or the difference between the mean and the accepted true value together with the confidence intervals (CIs) are recommended.

Precision

"The precision of an analytical procedure expresses the closeness of agreement (degree of scatter) between a series of measurements obtained from multiple sampling of the same homogeneous sample under the prescribed conditions. Precision may be considered at three levels: repeatability, intermediate precision, and reproducibility." Precision measures random errors and should be obtained preferably with authentic samples. As parameters, the standard deviation, the relative standard deviation (RSD) (coefficient of variation), and the CIs should be calculated for each level of precision. Repeatability reflects the analytical variability under the same operating conditions over a short interval of time (within-assay, intra-assay). At least nine determinations across the specified range or six determinations at 100% test concentration should be performed. Intermediate precision includes the influence of additional random effects according to the intended use of the procedure, i.e., within laboratories variations, for example, different days, analysts, equipment, etc. Reproducibility, i.e., the precision between laboratories, is not required for submission, but can be taken into account for standardization of analytical procedures. The variations should be selected according to the intended use of the analytical procedure.

Detection and quantitation limit

"The detection limit (DL) of an individual analytical procedure is the lowest amount of analyte in a sample which can be detected but not necessarily quantified as an exact value. "The QL of an individual analytical procedure is the lowest concentration of analyte in a sample which can be quantitatively determined with suitable precision and accuracy." Various approaches can be applied:

1. Visual definition.
2. Calculation from the signal-to-noise ratio (DL and QL correspond to the 3- or 2- and 10-fold of the noise level, respectively).
3. Calculation from the standard deviation of the blank.
4. Calculation from the calibration line at low concentrations.

$$DL; QL = \frac{F \times SD}{b} \quad ...(1)$$

where *F* is the factor of 3.3 (DL) or 10 (QL): SD is the standard deviation of the blank, standard deviation of the ordinate intercept, or residual standard of the linear regression; and b is the slope of the regression line.

The estimated limits should be verified by analyzing a suitable number of samples containing the analyte at the corresponding concentrations. DL or QL and the procedure used for determination as well as relevant chromatograms should be reported.

Robustness

"The robustness of an analytical procedure is a measure of its capacity to remain unaffected by small, but deliberate variations in method parameters and provides an indication of its reliability during normal usage." During the development phase of the analytical procedure, susceptible parameters should be identified, for example, stability of analytical solutions, extraction time, pH and composition of mobile phase, column lots and suppliers, temperature, flow rate, etc. A factorial design is encouraged.

System suitability tests

"System suitability testing is an integral part of many analytical procedure...." Suitable parameters depend on the type of analytical procedure; reference is given to pharmacopeias.

Rational and Efficient Validation

As analytical procedures are used throughout drug development and the manufacturing and release of drug substances and drug products, the reliability of their results is essential. Important decisions such as the establishment of the shelf-life from stability studies, the need for additional toxicological trials if new impurities appear or if known impurities exceed the qualified levels, and the reworking of batches and batch release or rejection are based on analytical results. Therefore, an appropriate validation to demonstrate the performance and suitability of the analytical procedures is much more than a formal requirement.

Suitability of the Analytical Procedure

What does "suitability for its intended purpose" mean? Basically, suitability is determined by the specification limits (or the aim of the analytical investigation) and the design of the given test item. For some applications, the requirements are explicitly defined in the ICH guidelines. For example, the reporting level for unknown impurities in drug substances is set to 0.05% or 0.03%; thus the corresponding test procedure must be able to quantify impurities at this concentration with an appropriate level of precision and accuracy. A maximum permitted analytical variability can be calculated from assay specification limits, based on the concept of CIs to describe analytical and manufacturing variability. At least, the compatibility between specification limits and analytical variability should be verified. Preferably, the limits are established taking the analytical and manufacturing variability into account. In this case, an analytical variability normally expected for the given kind of analytical procedure (analytical state of the art) can be defined as acceptance criterion. Of course, the

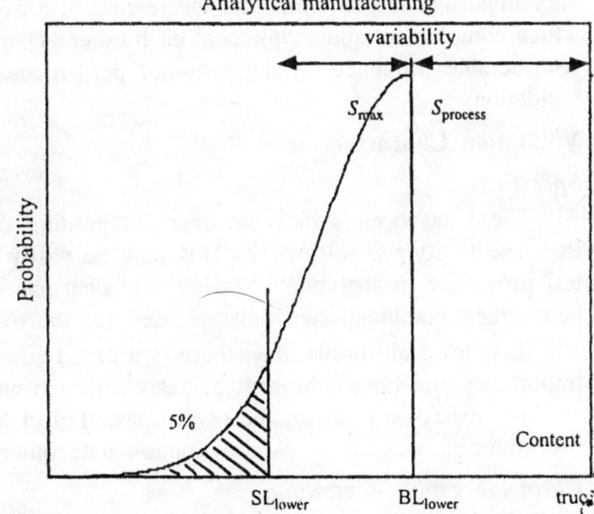

Fig. 3.1. Construction of specification limits from 95% CIs of the probability distribution of experimental results.

thus-obtained limits must primarily meet necessary quality and safety requirements. However, if this is satisfied, limits can reflect analytical variability. With respect to assay determinations, the variability of the analytical procedure is often larger than the variability of the manufacturing.

$$S_{max} = \frac{|(BL - SL)|\sqrt{n}}{t_{n-1,0.95}} \qquad \ldots(2)$$

where BL is the basic limit, obtained from the theoretical content and the manufacturing variability, with respect to the critical "half" of the specification range; SL is the (overall) specification limit with respect to the critical "half" of the specification range; n is the number of repetitions in the assay; t is the Student's t-factor for $(n - 1)$ degrees of freedom in the validation and 95% statistical confidence (one-sided).

It must also be demonstrated that the design of the analytical procedure, for example, the intended calibration mode, the number of repetitions, etc. is suitable. Therefore, suitability is strongly connected with the given, individual analytical procedure. The performance parameters are of varying importance and have different acceptance criteria. In consequence, a "checklist" approach to validation must be avoided. The analyst has to identify critical parameters, which are of importance for the required performance of the individual analytical procedure, to design the experimental studies accordingly and to define acceptance criteria for the results.

Statistical tests should only be carefully (directly) applied as acceptance criteria due to the small number of data normally obtained. Sometimes, because of abnormally small variabilities in the analytical series, differences are identified as significant which are of no practical relevance. In addition, when comparing independent methods for the proof of accuracy, different specificities can be expected which add a systematic bias, thus increasing the risk of the aforementioned danger. The analyst must decide whether detected statistical differences are of practical relevance. On the other hand, a large variability can also obscure differences which are not acceptable. If validation software is used, it must be flexible enough to meet these precautions. The analytical state of the art should be taken into account, although it is not the ultimate goal to optimize an individual analytical procedure as well as possible. It is also very important to recognize that the release of a given batch is based on a whole set of test procedures which complement and supplement each other. Their selection in the specification design has, therefore, considerable influence on the required performance of the individual control test and, hence, on its validation.

Validation Characteristics

Specificity

There has been some controversy regarding the technical term for this validation characteristic, i.e., specificity vs. selectivity. This may be partly attributed to the fact that in contrast to an isolated test procedure in analytical chemistry, in pharmaceutical analysis, the sum of various control tests and hence their combined specificity is used for the overall evaluation.

In spite of all discussions, there is a broad agreement that this validation characteristic is of crucial importance and builds the critical basis for each analytical procedure. As no absolute and quantitative measure exists (at least for the overall specificity), the requirements depend on the individual analytical procedure as well as on its combination with others.

Chromatographic separation

With respect to chromatographic techniques, specificity can be demonstrated by a sufficient separation of the substances present. For the assay, appropriate separation means an adequate resolution between the peak of interest and other peaks (e.g., impurities, placebo or matrix components), which need not to be separated from each other. In contrast, universal procedures for the determination of impurities require a sufficient separation of all relevant impurity peaks. The required resolution is strongly dependent on the difference in the size of the corresponding peaks as well as on their elution order. Therefore, if separation factors are determined, the typical concentration levels or the specification limits (as worst case) of the impurities should be maintained. Resolution factors can be calculated according to EP and USP at half height and at the baseline, respectively. However, this is only sensible for baseline-separated peaks. The USP approach is less sensitive toward tailing, but more complex to determine.

$$R_S = \frac{1.18(t_{Rb} - t_{Ra})}{w_{0.5a} + w_{0.5b}} \qquad \ldots(3)$$

$$R_S = \frac{2(t_{Rb} - t_{Ra})}{w_a + w_b} \qquad \ldots(4)$$

where $t_{Ra,b}$ is the retention time of peaks a and b with, $t_{Rb} > t_{Ra}$, $w_{0.5a,b}$ is the peak width a and b at half height, and $w_{a,b}$ is the peak width a and b at baseline.

In case of incomplete separations, especially for peaks of different magnitude, calculations according to Eqs. (3) and (4) are not possible or are biased due to the additivity of the peak curves. Here, other separation parameters such as the peak-to-valley ratio (p/v) should be used. This approach, which measures the height above the extrapolated baseline at the lowest point of the curve separating the peaks with respect to the height of the minor (impurity) peak, is directly related to the peak integration and independent on tailing or "smearing" effects in the elution range behind the main peak.

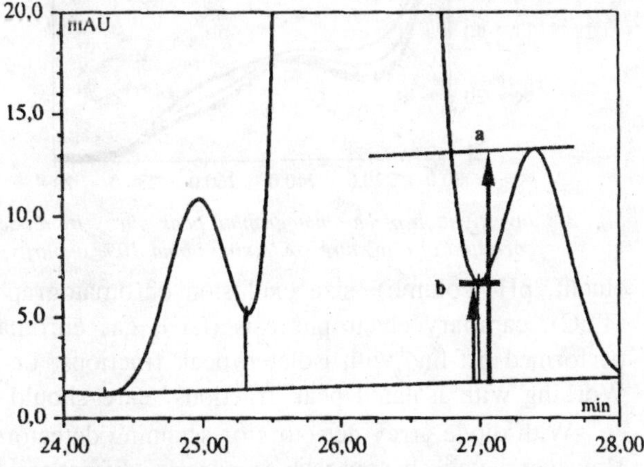

Fig. 3.2. Peak separation indices: peak-to-valley ratio p/v = a/b.

Besides a "physical" improvement of the separation, it can also be optimized "visually" if the spectra of the two concerning peaks are different. Then, a suitable wavelength can be selected to suppress interferences. However, such an approach has to be balanced with respect to the QL and the robustness of the quantitation if the detection wavelength does not correspond to a stable region of the spectra, such as (relative) maxima or minima or shoulders.

Peak purity investigations

In order to be able to detect the coelution of unknown substances, peak homogeneity (also termed peak purity) investigations should be performed. In case of not too large concentrations differences of the coeluting peaks, simple methods of one-dimensional detection can be applied. For normal eluting pure substances, the peak width at half height is proportional to the retention time. Therefore, performing isocratic chromatography with different concentrations of organic modifier, a plot of the peak width vs. the retention time will give a linear relationship for homogeneous peaks. For a single chromatographic separation, the symmetry factor is independent on the height of pure substance peaks.

In case of small amounts of coeluting impurities, rechromatography of suspected peaks represents a simple, universally available and sensitive approach. The more the two applied chromatographic methods differ, the greater is the power of the investigation. Various combinations can be taken into consideration such as coupling of reversed phase (RP) chromatography with another RP method (different

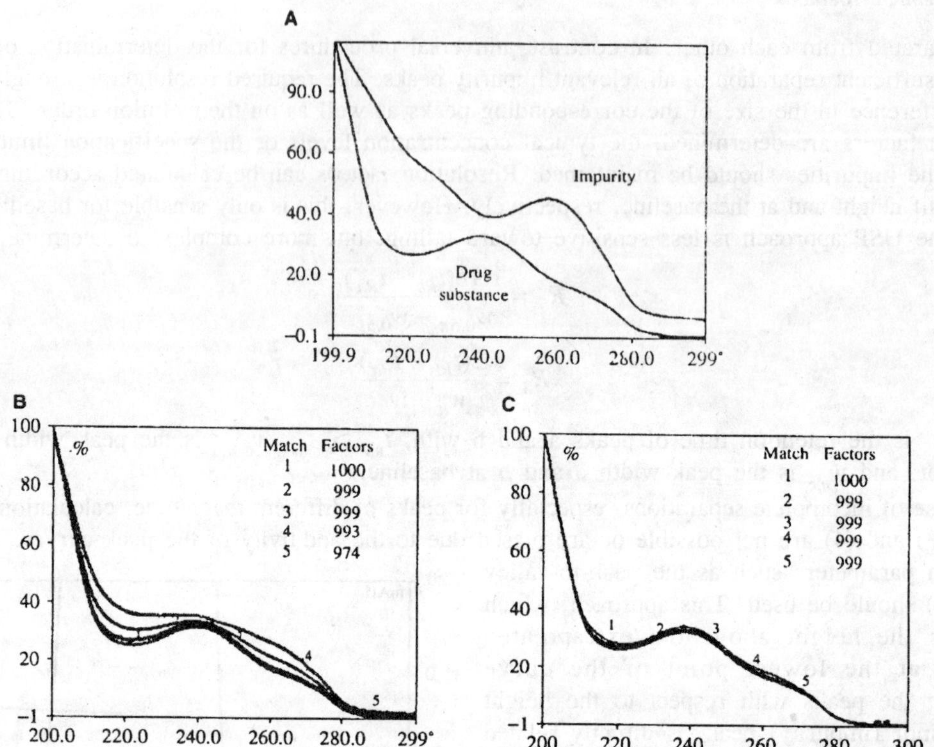

Fig. 3.3. Investigation of chromatographic peak purity by diode array detection. A–spectra of drug substance and impurity; B–coelution of a mixture containing about 10% impurity; C–coelution of a mixture containing about 0.5% impurity.

eluent, pH, column), size exclusion chromatography, ion chromatography, thin layer chromatography (TLC), capillary electrophoresis (CE), gas chromatography (GC), etc. The rechromatography can be performed off-line with isolated peak fractions, or as a direct orthogonal coupling of the two methods. Working with isolated peak fractions, care should be taken to avoid artifacts due to degradation.

With diode array detectors or scanning detectors, the spectral peak homogeneity can be investigated. However, such an approach requires a difference in both the spectra and in the retention time of the coeluting substances. If this is fulfilled, detection of inhomogeneities with commercially available software is easy, if the concentration difference is not too large. However, impurities below 1% are difficult to recognize.

The most discriminating technique for investigation of the peak purity is mass spectrometric detection. Using on-line LC–MS coupling, mass spectra are taken over the whole elution range of the suspected peak. In a first step, the obtained signals (mass-to-charge ratio, *m/z*) must be assigned to the main substance. In the given example, *m/z* 275.8 and 295.6 belong to the drug substance and represent the doubly charged molecular ion and a cluster formed by the doubly charged ion and acetonitrile (from the eluent). If during the spectra "scrolling" additional masses are detected such as *m/z* 324.9, the corresponding mass chromatogram is extracted. Differences in the retention time or elution behavior with respect to the UV peak is proof of a coeluting impurity. Even peaks with identical retention can be attributed to impurities if a change in the mass-to-charge ratio cannot be explained by the drug substance itself. In the given example, the impurity amounts to 0.5%. Of course, the DL depends on the individual MS response of the concerned substances and diastereomers cannot be detected. If LC procedures with non-volatile buffers are validated, the corresponding peak fractions can be isolated and rechromatographed under MS-compatible conditions. Alternatively, the coupling can be performed on-line. Although not often applied in routine (pharmaceutical) analysis, MS detection offers tremendous gains in efficiency and reliability of the procedures, such as highly specific detection (largely) without interferences, for monitoring of impurity profiles and identification.

If samples from stress testing are used to demonstrate appropriate separation power, care should be taken to avoid over-degradation as this would result in secondary (or even higher order) degradants which are of no practical relevance. Therefore, degradation should be restricted to about 1 0%. Alternatively, samples from regular stability studies (accelerated storage conditions) may be used.

Linearity and range

Although a linear relationship between the analyte concentration and the measured signal will exist for most methods used in pharmaceutical analysis, there are some exceptions such as TLC and fluorescence detection. Therefore, the term "*analytical response*" would be more appropriate.

Prerequisites for the calibration types

It depends on the design of the analytical procedure as to which regression parameters are meaningful and which results are acceptable. In other words, the model to be used for quantitation must be justified. For a single- point calibration (external standardization), a linear function, zero intercept, and the homogeneity of variances are required. The prerequisites for a linear multiple-point calibration are a linear function and in case of an unweighted calibration also the homogeneity of variances. A non-linear calibration requires only a continuous function. With respect to the 100% method (area normalization for impurities), both for the main peak and the impurities, a linear function and a zero intercept are required, within their working ranges. The required linearity range must be obtained from the working range of the analytical procedure. It may be useful to extend the minimum concentration range when applying a single-point calibration in order to avoid an extensive extrapolation to zero. This might cause problems in the evaluation of the significance of the intercept. If the calibration for an analyte determination in a complex matrix (drug product, impurities, and degradants by external standards) or with a complex sample preparation is intended to be performed with a simple solution of the reference standard, this linearity should be compared with the linearity of the whole procedure using reconstituted (spiked) samples.

The homogeneity of variances over the whole range (homoscedasticity) is a prerequisite for an unweighted linear regression in order to ensure the same influence of all concentrations. This can be verified by performing a suitable number of repeated measurements (n = 6-10) at the minimum and the maximum of the required linear range, and comparing the variances with an F-test. However, in pharmaceutical analyses, as the concentration range of interest is usually not very large, it is not required to perform a separate test for the homogeneity of variances. In general, the homogeneity of variances is maintained over about two orders of magnitude when using UV absorbance (within the linear range of the detector/ instrument). If a calibration is extended over several orders of magnitude (which is more common for bioanalysis; but may also be considered for impurity determinations), variances are not likely to be homogeneous. As an unweighted linear regression minimizes the absolute residual sum of squares, higher concentrations with larger absolute scattering dominate and are better fitted to the regression line. Consequently, large deviations will occur if such a regression line is used for quantitation of small concentrations. For a better representation of the lower concentrations, additional weight must be given to their signals performing a weighted linear regression. As weighting factors, the reciprocals of the individual standard deviations or variances can be used or, as an approximation the reciprocals of the concentrations themselves or of their squares. The equations can be found in statistical textbooks or in corresponding software products.

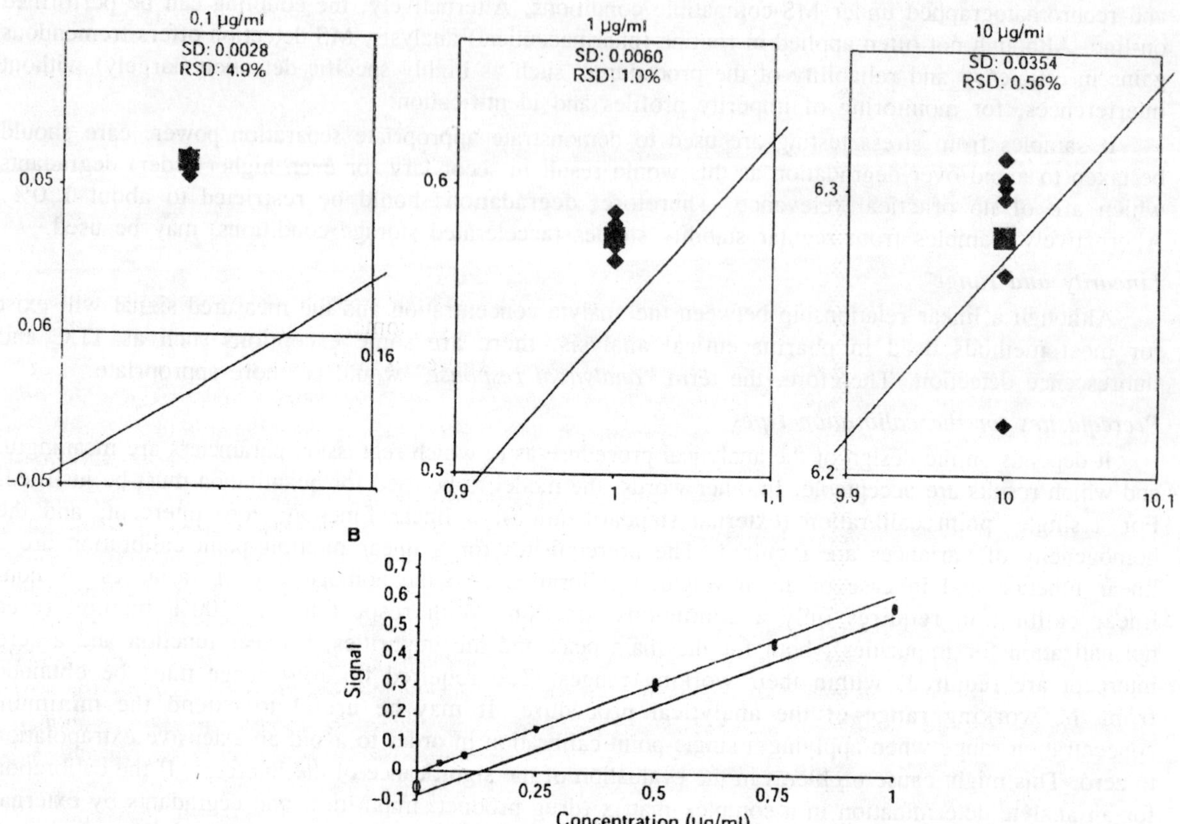

Fig. 3.4. Dependence of the variability on the analyte concentration (A) and its influence on the regression line (B).

If deviations from linearity are detected or known, non-linear response functions must be applied, for example, quadratic regressions. However, these models should be used carefully if a linear relationship is normally assumed for the analytical procedure. Otherwise, it would also fit erroneous experimental values due to the larger flexibility of the regression curve. According to the principle of Ockham's blade, the model should be kept as simple as possible. Even in the case of intrinsic non-linear response functions, it can be investigated if deviations resulting from linear regression are acceptable in the required working range. In the example, the difference between the results obtained by the quadratic regression and a linear regression from 400 ng to 700 ng analyte (to represent a multiple-point linear calibration) is calculated to 0.4% and 0.55% at the lower and upper limit of the range, respectively. This must be evaluated with respect to a precision of about 2% for this type of procedure.

Evaluation of linearity

In the ICH guideline, there are only scarce hints how to evaluate linearity. Primarily, a qualitative statement is sufficient for the evaluation of linearity (linear function): Does a linear relationship exist in the required working range? When aiming at a single-point calibration, a positive answer is sufficient (in addition to a zero intercept) because the regression parameters obtained during validation are not used further in routine testing. In pharmaceutical analysis, this is also the case using a multiple- point calibration. However, relevant parameters may be selected to define acceptance limits for a system suitability test in routine calibration.

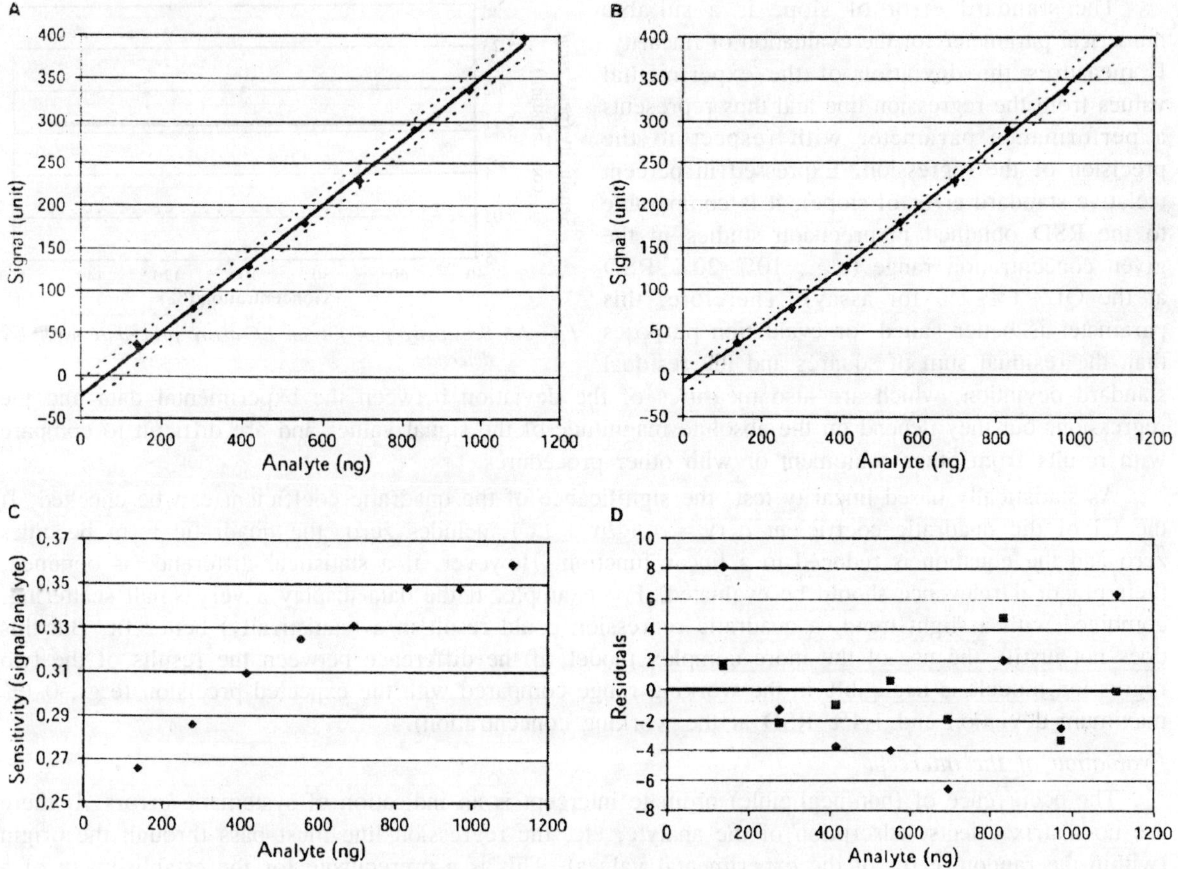

Fig. 3.5. Deviation from a linear response function.

The coefficient of correlation is generally expected (and also mentioned in the ICH guideline), but it is not a quantitative measure for the degree of linearity. It just gives an indication of whether a relationship exists between two sets of data. The coefficient of correlation for a linear regression was calculated as 0.99916. However, the more narrow 95% prediction interval of the quadratic regression as a measure for the expected deviation of (future) experimental data from the regression line indicates a deviation from linearity. This is also easily recognized by investigation of the sensitivities, i.e., the ratio of analytical signal and the corresponding concentration. Their graphical presentation as a function of the concentration results in a horizontal line for the linear range of the procedure. The ASTM recommends an interval of $\pm 5\%$ around the sensitivity mean. This interval should be adjusted to the concentration range in question; an acceptable precision can be used for orientation purposes. For concentrations around the QL, a wider interval can be accepted than for an assay procedure (e.g., $\pm 2\%$). Plotting the differences between the experimental values and the values calculated using the regression function vs. the concentration (residual plot, scatterplot) is another possibility of graphical linearity evaluation. With the proper response function, the residuals display a random (and narrower) scattering around the zero line; otherwise a systematical pattern is observed. However, in case of only few data (e.g., five according to ICH), a systematic pattern might be difficult to recognize. Here, the sensitivity plot is preferable as trends are better detectable as an upward or downward sloping of the data points.

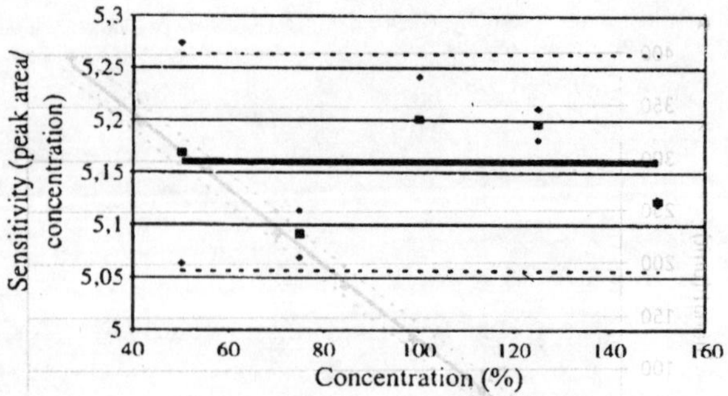

Fig. 3.6. Sensitivity plot for an LC-array procedure with UV detection.

The standard error of slope is a suitable numerical parameter for the evaluation of linearity. It measures the deviation of the experimental values from the regression line and thus represents a performance parameter with respect to the precision of the regression. Expressed in percent (relative standard error of slope), it is comparable to the RSD obtained in precision studies in the given concentration range (e.g., 10%–20% RSD at the QL, 1%–2% for assay). Therefore, this parameter is better suited for evaluation purposes than the residual sum of squares and the residual standard deviation, which are also measures of the deviation between the experimental data and the regression, but they depend on the absolute magnitude of the signal values and are difficult to compare with results from other equipment or with other procedures.

As statistically based linearity test, the significance of the quadratic coefficient can be checked. If the CI of the quadratic coefficient c ($y = a + bx + cx^2$) includes zero, the quadratic term becomes zero and the equation is reduced to a linear function. However, if a statistical difference is obtained, their practical relevance should be evaluated. For example, if the data display a very small scattering, combined with a slight trend, a quadratic regression could result in a (statistically) better fit. But this does not justify the use of the more complex model, if the difference between the results of the two regression models is negligible in the working range compared with the expected precision (e.g., 0.1% maximum deviation and 1.4% RSD at the working concentration).

Evaluation of the intercept

The occurrence of (non-negligible) ordinate intercept is an indication of systematic errors. If there are no matrix effects, adsorption of the analyte, etc. the regression line must pass through the origin (within the random error of the experimental values). This is a prerequisite for the establishment of a single- point calibration and of the 100% method for the determination of impurities. The so-called single-point calibration represents, in fact, a two-point calibration line where one point equals zero and the other the standard concentration. The zero intercept can be demonstrated statistically when the CI (usually at 95% level of significance) of the intercept includes zero. Again, such a statistical test should be interpreted carefully and a statistical significance should be evaluated with respect to its practical relevance. On the other hand, a large variability can obscure a substantial deviation of the intercept from zero. Therefore, as an absolute parameter, the intercept should be expressed as a percentage of the analytical signal of a 100% working concentration. For the acceptance limit, a basis for orientation may be sought in an acceptable value for the precision (e.g., 1%–2% for assay). In fact, this approach can be regarded as an extrapolation of the variability at the working concentration to the origin. In order to avoid weighting effects, very large extrapolation may be disadvantageous. Even if the required range for an assay determination is 80%–120%, the linearity for a single-point calibration should be validated starting with approximately 10%–50%.

Accuracy

Accuracy by comparison

For drug substance, the only possibility of a quantitative assessment of accuracy is the comparison to the results of another analytical procedure or to a reference (if established with other procedures and/or additional characterization). This can be performed statistically with a t-test. However, the shortcomings of these statistical tests (or better the justification of their use) are especially important here. It must be taken into consideration that two independent analytical procedures most probably differ in their specificity. This may lead to a systematic influence on the results. If the effect can be quantified, the means should be corrected before performing the statistical comparison. If a correction is not possible, the presumptions of the statistical test are violated and the *t*-test should consequently not be performed. Instead, it should be evaluated if the absolute magnitude of the difference is below an acceptable value (e.g., 2%).

Accuracy by recovery

Interferences between the matrix (placebo) and the analyte, adsorption within the equipment, incomplete extraction of the analyte during the sample treatment, degradation, etc. can be verified by spiking known amounts of the analyte to the matrix (placebo). For example, drug substance is spiked to placebo (reconstituted drug product) or impurities/degradants are added to drug substance or drug product and are subsequently analyzed. This should be performed as near as possible to the authentic conditions. Ideally, the drug product is prepared with different contents of active ingredient. The least authentic approach would be the addition of standard stock solutions to a placebo solution. The recovery can be calculated either at each level separately as a percent recovery, or as a linear regression of the found analyte vs. the added one (recovery function).

In the former case, it can be tested, whether the recovery mean differs significantly from the theoretical value of 100% (e.g., by the inclusion of 100 within the 95% CI). However, again it should also be taken into consideration if the absolute magnitude of the difference is acceptable, especially with respect to impurities in low concentration ranges.

With respect to the recovery function, the slope and intercept can be tested vs. the theoretical values of 1 and 0 (by their 95% CIs) or vs. acceptable limits for deviation. Due to the different weighting effects, the two approaches might lead to different results. The percent recovery calculation gives easily interpretable results and should therefore be preferred, at least for narrow working ranges.

It is absolutely essential that the accuracy be validated with the same quantitation method that is used in the control test procedure. Recovery deviations from the theoretical values while performing a calibration with a drug substance alone may indicate interferences between the analyte and placebo components. In such a case, the calibration should be done with a synthetic mixture of placebo and drug substance standard. Such interferences may also be detected by the separate determination of linearity for dilutions of the drug substance and for a spiked placebo.

Precision

Precision should be measured using homogenous, authentic samples. According to the ICH recommendation of nine determinations over the whole range, it may also be measured using artificially prepared samples or sample solutions, combining the validation characteristics linearity, accuracy, and precision in one experimental series. However, it should be noted that a larger variability can result due to the additional preparation steps. On the other hand, problems of the sample homogeneity and of the sampling itself cannot be detected.

It is essential to be absolutely aware of the different levels of precision, especially if acceptance limits are defined or if the resulting variabilities are used for further calculations. Often, the real uncertainty of results is underestimated, especially with respect to long-term applications. The large variability of the experimentally determined standard deviation has also to be taken into account.

In addition to the ICH levels repeatability and intermediate precision, the system precision, i.e., repeated injections/determinations of a single sample solution (also referred to as injection repeatability or injection precision), provides valuable information. Evaluation of these data will help us to show that the chosen equipment is suitable for its intended use. Injection precision will also become part of the system suitability requirements of the method and an acceptance criterion should be appropriately set. In the EP, a procedure is described which links the maximum permitted injection precision with the specification limits, thus allowing a specific evaluation of the suitability. However, this approach requires that the specification limits are established appropriately, i.e., taking the analytical and manufacturing variability into account.

The various levels of precision may be calculated by means of an analysis of variances. The overall variation is divided into the contributions within and between the series, allowing us to assess the most sensitive part of the analytical procedure as well as the robustness. Acceptance limits for assay determinations can be derived from specification limits established on the basis of experience and the analytical state of the art. With the former approach, the suitability of either the specification limits or the precision of the analytical procedure is tested. Typical RSDs for system precision of LC assay procedures should range below 1%, for repeatabilities up to 1–2%, and for intermediate precision/reproducibility twice the value for the (average) repeatability can be expected (depending on the amount of variations, time period, etc.). For impurity determinations, the variability is strongly dependent on the concentration level. The reproducibility of the sum of impurities can sum up between 10% and 30%.

Detection and quantitation limit

One should be aware that the determined QL (or DL) is strongly related to the equipment used at the time of determination. They may represent more system parameters than characteristics of the analytical procedure. They are also dependent on the calculation procedure applied.

In cases where a general QL is required, as in pharmaceutical analysis, it is essential to define a realistic QL (or DL) for the analytical procedure, independently from the equipment used, because this limit has important consequences (e.g., for the consistent reporting of impurities or for method transfer). They may be derived by taking QL (or DL) from various instruments into account ("intermediate QL," during the development process) or can be defined taking the requirements of the control test (specification limits imposed by toxicology or by a qualified impurity profile) into consideration. For example, a QL which amounts to 50% of the specification limit would allow an appropriate quantitation. For unknown impurities, the ICH reporting thresholds of 0.05% or 0.03% can be defined as QL. During validation, it is just verified, that the actual QL is below the defined limit. For this purpose, each of the approaches described in the ICH guideline can be used.

Calculation from noise

For chromatographic methods, DL and QL can be calculated from the noise. Here the (random) fluctuations of the baseline performing a blank injection is regarded as "noise." It is recommended to obtain the difference between the highest and the lowest signal (amplitude) in a range corresponding to at least 20 peak widths of the (expected) analyte peak. This is a very straightforward procedure, but is dependent on the operator. Care should also be taken to avoid the interpretation of baseline trends as "noise." Only noise signals with a "peak width" similar to the analyte to be determined can influence its detection and determination. It should also be taken into account that the results represent signal (peak) heights.

Calculation from linearity

For approaches based on a regression line, it must be taken into account that the residual standard deviation is strongly influenced by the absolute magnitude of the signal values (weighting effect, homogeneity of variances) and therefore by the concentration range used for the linear regression. This range should not exceed the 10-fold of the DL. In this range, the variances can be expected to be

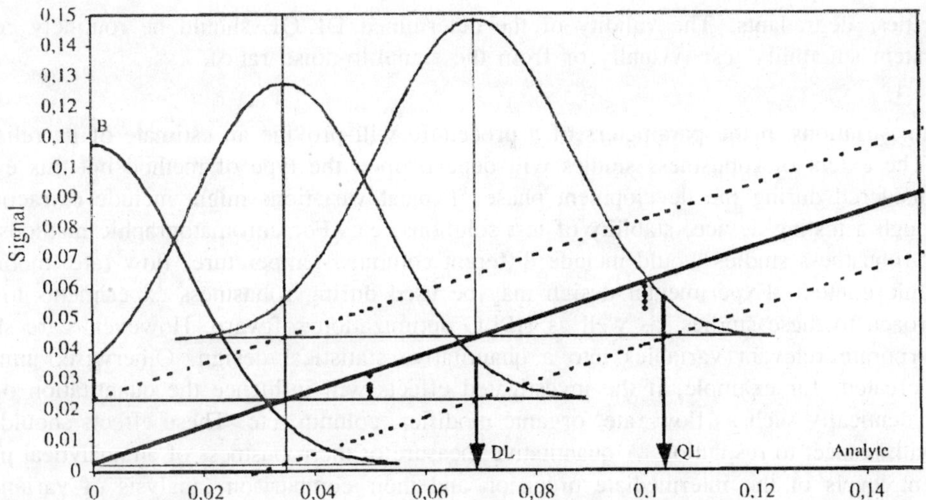

Fig. 3.7. Calculation of the detection and quantitation limits from the 95% prediction interval of the regression line. LC peak areas were obtained for six analyte concentrations between 0.05 µg/ml and 1 µg/ml with six repeated injections each.

homogeneous. Another approach is directly based on the dispersion of the experimental data in the low concentration range, represented by the prediction interval of the regression line. This interval can be interpreted as the probability distribution of (future) determinations, which can be experimentally expected. The upper 95% limit of the analyte concentration, whose probability distribution has a 50% overlapping with the distribution of the blank (and therefore a 50% error rate), is defined as the DL. With respect to the QL the overlapping is reduced to 5%. Hence, a reliable quantification is possible in the latter case.

Estimation from precision

The QL can also be obtained from precision studies. For this approach, decreasing analyte concentrations are analyzed repeatedly. The RSD is plotted against the corresponding concentration. If a predefined limit is exceeded (e.g., 10% or 20%), the corresponding concentration is established as the QL. However, a sufficiently large number of analyte concentrations must be analyzed due to the large scattering of the standard deviations in the low concentration range. This approach can be simplified if a defined QL is to be verified. Then, a sample containing the impurity at the defined QL is repeatedly analyzed. If the obtained RSD is below the predefined limit, the analytical procedure has a suitable sensitivity. If varying concentrations are used to obtain DL and QL, available impurities and degradants should be spiked to the drug substance or drug product. Different contents can also be obtained by mixing impurity-free and impurity-containing batches. The concentration of the active or matrix components (placebo, cleaning solutions) should be maintained at the nominal level of the test. The QL of unknown substances can be obtained using representative peaks or inferred from the QL of

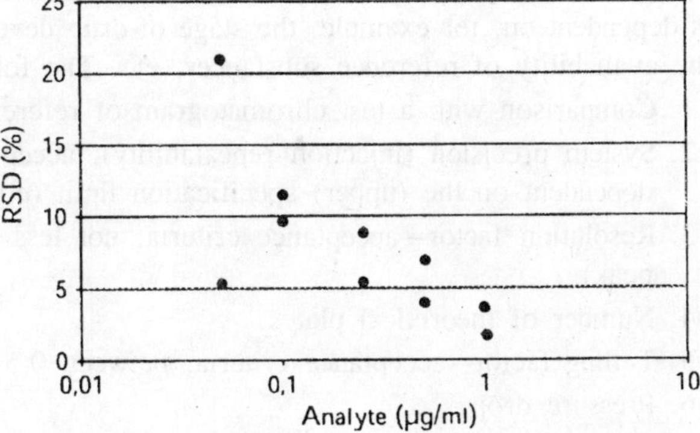

Fig. 3.8. Relative standard deviations obtained from six repeated injections of analyte concentrations from 0.05 µg/ml to 1 µg/ml.

known impurities/ degradants. The validity of the determined DL/QL should be routinely confirmed within the system suitability test (visually or from the signal-to-noise ratio).

Robustness

Deliberate variations in the parameters of a procedure will provide an estimate of its reliability in routine use. The extent of robustness studies will depend upon the type of method but this evaluation should be considered during the development phase. Typical variations might include extraction time, flow rate through a testing device, stability of test solutions, etc. For chromatographic methods, typical variations for robustness studies would include different columns, temperature, flow rate, mobile phase pH, and organic content. Experimental design may be used during robustness experiments to develop a matrix approach to these studies, as well as HPLC optimization software. However, care should be taken to incorporate relevant variables into a quantitative statistical design. Otherwise, unnecessary work-load is created, for example, if the investigated effects will influence the quantitation of sample and standard identically such as flow rate, organic modifier, column, etc. These effects should only be investigated with respect to resolution. A quantitative measure of the robustness of an analytical procedure is the different levels of the intermediate precision and their comparison (analysis of variances). Of course, this approach only addresses random effects, which depend on the extent of variations designed in the intermediate precision studies. In case of insufficient robustness, it will be often not possible to identify its source. In these cases, a systematic investigation is required. If the robustness studies indicate that the experimental data are susceptible to variations in the method parameters, the appropriate system suitability requirements should be established to ensure the validity of the analytical procedure during routine use.

System suitability tests

The validation of an analytical procedure produces performance parameters of a "well-behaved" and "well-conditioned" system/instrument which are more or less "snapshots" of the combination procedure/system. In order to routinely confirm the suitability of the integrated measurement instrumentation used with a given procedure, system suitability test parameters should be defined on the basis of the validation results and robustness studies. Larger variations under routine conditions or multiple laboratories should also be taken into consideration. The extent of the system suitability testing is dependent on, for example, the stage of drug development, the objective of the analytical procedure, the availability of reference substances, etc. The following parameters may be considered:

1. Comparison with a test chromatogram of reference standard (cf. retention times).
2. System precision (injection repeatability); acceptance limit for LC: 2% RSD, for drug substance dependent on the (upper) specification limit (e.g., 102.0% and $n = 6$: 0.85%).
3. Resolution factor—acceptance criteria: not less than 2.0 (recommended with respect to the main peak).
4. Number of theoretical plates.
5. Tailing factor—acceptance criteria: between 0.5 and 2.0 (recommended).
6. Pressure drop.
7. Baseline drift.
8. (Detector) linearity or sensitivity at different concentrations.
9. DL/QL (e.g., as signal-to-noise ratio—acceptance criteria: not less than 3 and 10, respectively).

Validation during Drug Development and Manufacturing

The ICH requirements are intended for the submission of new pharmaceuticals. Good manufacturing practice regulations, which include analytical procedures for in-process controls, QC of excipients, starting materials, intermediates or during drug development prescribe no details of validation requirements. In these applications, the ICH guidelines should be used for orientation with an increasing expenditure of effort and requirements as development or manufacturing progresses. For validation purposes, three distinct levels can be described for which validation requirements can be defined.

Level I

Level I is intended for analytical procedures during the early development (preclinical phase), for starting materials and in-process controls. At this stage of development, relatively small quantities of drug substance are available, analytical reference standards have not been established, and little information is available regarding synthesis or degradation impurities. Also, frequent changes/ improvements in drug substance and formulations are expected. As such, the validation that is conducted is at a minimum. Validation data may be extracted from routine testing. The specificity can be demonstrated using available batches and samples from stress testing in combination with simple variations in the chromatographic conditions (gradient, elution time, pH). For demonstration of linearity, a dilution of the analyte is performed (detector linearity). Accuracy is inferred from specificity, linearity, and precision. A system precision is performed with six injections. QL is defined visually. The results are summarized and evaluated in order to make a statement on the suitability.

Level II

Level II is applied for drug substances and products during the early clinical phases and for intermediates. At this stage of development, drug substance synthetic processes are becoming finalized and higher quality material is available in larger quantities. A drug substance reference standard is established and information is increasingly available on synthetic and degradation impurities. Formulation development activities are giving rise to finished products to be used in clinical studies. It is at this stage that formal control tests must be established. The validation effort is significantly extended from Level I. Specificity is investigated using various batches, available impurities, excipients, and samples from stability testing. Investigations on peak purity may be performed. The linearity of the detector or of the procedure, depending on the complexity of the latter, is validated. Accuracy is inferred (drug substance) or obtained from three determinations of the recovery at the working concentration. A repeatability study ($n = 6$), or depending on the application of the procedure, an intermediate precision is performed. Quantitation limit is obtained visually or verified with one of the quantitative approaches. The documentation consists of a short summary of the performed investigations and an evaluation of the results.

Level III

Level III is applied during clinical phase III and for the submission, as well as for important intermediates, and corresponds to the ICH requirements. At this stage of development, the commercial synthetic process for drug substance is established, and important process and degradation impurities have been identified and synthesized. The final formulations and dosages have also been established.

A full validation report is required with description and justification of the design of the experimental studies, and a detailed discussion and evaluation of the results.

In all levels, validation software can be used to standardize and to improve the efficiency of documentation of the data and calculations. However, it should be flexible enough to allow the necessary case-by-case (or type-by-type) design of the validation.

Maintenance of the Validation Status

In several guidelines, the term revalidation is mentioned, sometimes in more detail. However, one should be aware that validation is always more or less a "snapshot" of the actual state of the overall system equipment—analytical procedure. Therefore, it should be regarded as a basis, i.e., the proof of the general suitability. If adjustments of the analytical procedure are restricted to the validated and recommended ranges, there is no rationale, for a repeated validation. Only if a procedure is changed, a new validation is required. Of course, it must be guaranteed that the analytical procedure is consistently in a validated state. This can be achieved by monitoring appropriate SST results. Another possibility is to perform (regularly) supplementary investigations such as further intermediate precision studies, which can be included in the routine analysis. With this approach, it is possible to supplement and extend existing information and to take the very important time factor into proper consideration. Information can be obtained on the long-term behavior of an analytical procedure and therefore on the reliability in routine use, for example, better estimates on the true (long term) analytical variability.

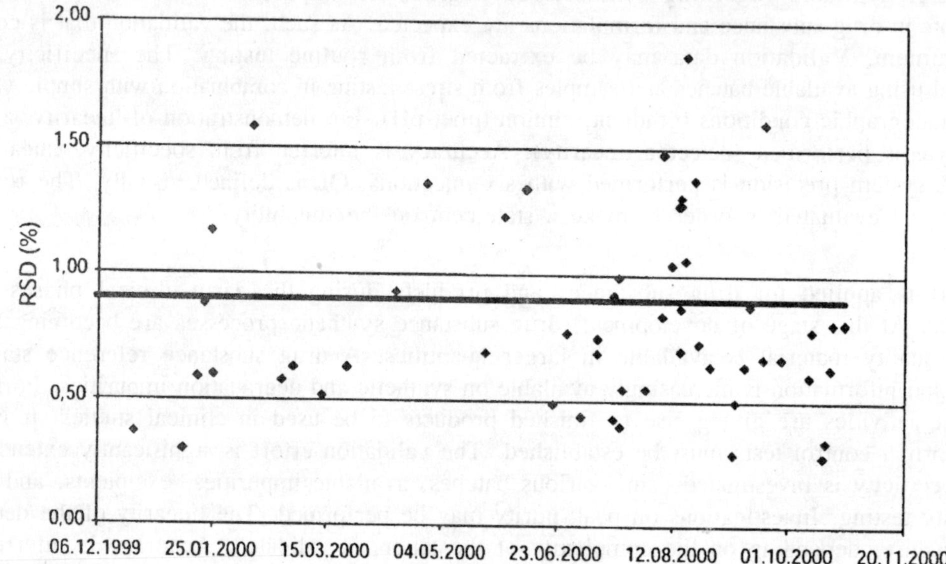

Fig. 3.9. Relative standard deviations of reference standard preparations for an LC assay procedure over a period of about 10 months.

The RSDs were calculated from the standard preparations of an assay procedure, i.e., from four injections of two separate preparations (single-point calibration). Therefore, the variability represents a combination of system precision and repeatability. It should be noted that with an average of 0.88% (representative for the true value with 58 runs over 10 months), the single results scatter regularly up to 1.6%. Two-thirds of all RSDs range between 0.5% and 1.3%. In two cases (about 3%) the RSDs exceed the SST limit of 2.0%. This was attributed to gross (weighing) errors. Quality control charts are a very effective approach to investigate not only the analytical variability, but also the accuracy. Due to the accumulation of results, additional forms of statistical analysis (statistical process control, SPC) become possible.

The continuous monitoring and the proof that the analytical procedure is in statistical control allows a reliable evaluation of the underlying process (e.g., batch manufacturing) and an early detection of trends. A control batch ("dummy") was analyzed with a single determination each time the analytical procedure was applied (over about 6 months). The target mean and the standard deviation were calculated from the first 20 determinations and normalized to 100%. All but one result are within the control limits (± three standard deviations around the mean). The group of values preceding the outlying one was obtained with the same standard solution and is shifted toward the upper control limit. For the next run, a new standard solution was prepared. The "normal" result of 99.0% indicates that the shift

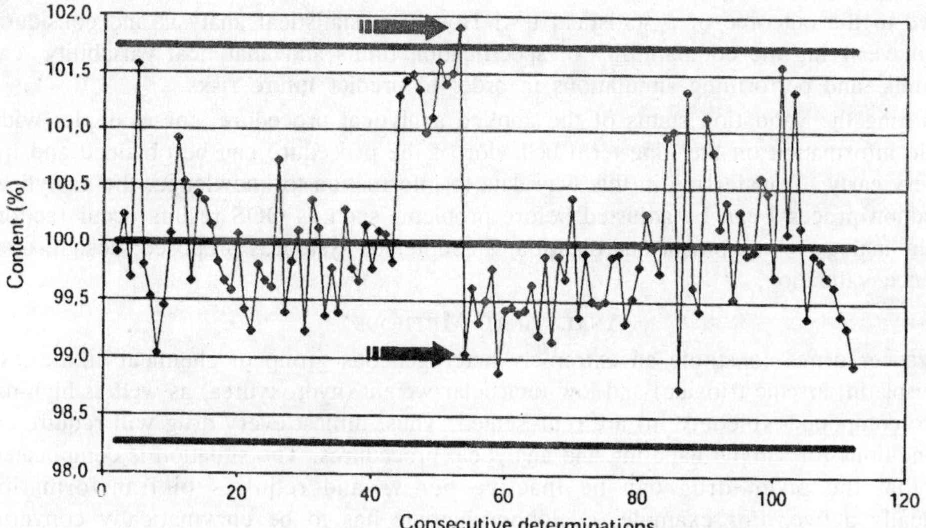

Fig. 3.10. Control chart of a single LC determination of an injection solution. The mean and the SD were calculated from the first 20 determinations. The mean is normalized to 100%.

was caused by a deviating standard preparation. The deviation from the mean is with less than 1.5% in the range of the expected analytical variability (for a single determination) and therefore difficult to detect in routine batch analyses. In contrast, such shifts and also trends can easily be detected in a control chart representation. Besides limit violations, the control chart can also inspected for "abnormal" (systematic) patterns, such as six points steadily increasing or decreasing, 14 points in a row alternating up and down, etc. This provides the chance not only to obtain reliable (long term) information on the analytical system, but also to adjust it proactively.

Such a continuous process of analytical validation can be regarded in analogy to the qualification process. With respect to the four Qs (design, installation, operational, and performance qualification), three Vs can be defined: design, operational, and performance validation. "*Design validation*" involves the method development, where the basic performance requirements are established. During the "*operational validation*," it is verified that these requirements are generally met, i.e., this part corresponds to the "*conventional*" validation. Performance validation consists of a continuous monitoring of the validation status of an analytical procedure.

Instead of an isolated and formal "checklist" activity, validation of analytical procedures should be regarded as part of an integrated quality assurance concept to guarantee the accuracy and reliability of the analytical results and therefore quality, safety, and efficacy of pharmaceuticals.

For such an integrated system, all parts (such as equipment qualification, performance of the analytical procedure, analytical variability, specification limits, etc.) must be compatible with each other to prevent (analytically caused) out-of-control or OOS results. On the basis of the validation characteristics and requirements of the ICH guidelines, each analytical procedure must be validated with respect to parameters, which are relevant to its performance. It is the responsibility of the analyst to identify these parameters and design the validation study accordingly. Acceptance criteria should be defined in the validation protocol. They can be established from previous experiences (analytical state of the art) or calculated from specification limits. For the intended use of the test procedure acceptable absolute acceptance limits are preferred. Statistical tests should be used carefully and preferably for orientation purposes. The evaluation of the validation results is the responsibility of the analyst and must not be left or reduced to the outcome of a statistical test! However, statistical analysis and consideration are very helpful in verifying the compatibility of specification limits and analytical variability, calculating acceptance limits, and performing simulations in order to predict future risks.

By monitoring the validation status of the applied analytical procedure, for example, with control charts, reliable information on the long-term behavior of the procedure can be obtained and trends can be detected very early. Transferring in this way data to information to knowledge, the analytical system (or the production process) can be adjusted before problems such as OOS results occur (action instead of reaction). In analogy to equipment qualification, a continuous system is proposed: design, operational, and performance validation.

Analytical Methods

The anticancer drugs constitute an extremely heterogeneous group of chemical entities. Inorganic compounds (cisplatin, arsenic trioxide) and low-molecular-weight (hydroxyurea) as well as high-molecular-weight organic compounds (bleomycin) are represented. Thus, almost every drug will require evaluation of optimal conditions for sample handling and analytical procedures. The situation is complicated further by the fact that the given drug can be inactive *per se* and requires biotransformation to be pharmacologically active. For example, cyclophosphamide has to be enzymatically converted to 4-hydroxycyclophosphamide in the liver and temozolamide must be degraded in vivo to the linear triazine MTIC, which exerts the antitumor activity. There are also examples where both the parent compound and the formed metabolites contribute to the cytotoxic activity, for example, chlorambucil and its main metabolite phenylacetic acid mustard. It is therefore essential to establish which substance(s) should be quantified when performing pharmacokinetic/pharmacodynamic studies and that sufficient sensitivity and selectivity are obtained by the analytical procedure used. In this section we focus on some important areas that in our opinion have not previously been sufficiently penetrated. The examples discussed will mostly come from our own research concerning alkylating agents, platinum-containing drugs, and antraquinone glycosides.

Chemical Stability in Biological Material

Alkylating agents and cisplatin

The stability of most anticancer drugs, for example, cisplatin, oxaliplatin, and busulfan, is mostly lower in biological material as compared to pure aqueous solutions. Cisplatin, for example, is stable in an acidic aqueous solution containing 0.1 *M* sodium chloride whereas the degradation half-life in human plasma is only about 0.9 h (37°C). The low stability in plasma is attributable to the fact that the compound has a high propensity to react with thiol-containing endogenous compounds, for example, albumin, glutathione, and cysteine. The stability of cisplatin in whole blood is higher than in plasma, the half-life being approx 1.43 h, most probably because cisplatin is in a chemical environment with lower nucleophilic character when partitioned to the red blood cells.

The low stability of cisplatin places stringent requirements on the handling of the blood samples. The blood is collected in prechilled tubes, stored on ice, and ultrafiltrated centripetally (20 min, 4°C) within 1 h using a 10,000 mol wt cutoff filter. Centripetal ultrafiltration allows the free fraction of cisplatin in whole blood to be determined. Less than 5% of cisplatin will be decomposed following this handling procedure.

Anticancer drugs containing the nitrogen mustard group (chlorambucil, melphalan) have for a long time been used in anticancer therapy. Recently, small peptides containing the alkylating group have been suggested to mediate a more selective delivery to cancer cells. The compounds are chemically unstable but, in contrast to the platinum-containing drugs, show an increased stability in plasma. Thus, chlorambucil has a degradation half life of 0.45 h in buffer (pH 7.4, 37°C) but is considerably more stable in the presence of albumin ($t_{1/2}$ = 15.8 h in 45 mg/mL of albumin). Chlorambucil is extensively bound to albumin, and when bound it is about 100 times more stable than in the free form. Formation of the cyclic aziridinium ion is the rate-determining step in the hydrolysis of aromatic nitrogen mustards. The rate of formation is drastically affected by the dielectric constant of the solvent, and it can be concluded that chlorambucil when bound to albumin is in a chemical environment with solvating properties quite different from those in pure aqueous solution.

Anthraquinone glycosides

The antraquinone glycosides are extensively metabolized to their corresponding 13-hydroxyderivatives by aldo-ketoreductase. This enzyme is present in most human tissues, which has to be taken into account in the bioanalysis. The formation rate of the reduced metabolites is increased with increasing lipophilic character of the drug. Incubation studies in whole blood reveal fast formation of large amounts of daunorubicinol and idarubicinol from the two most lipophilic anthraquinone glycosides commercially available. The conversion could be diminished by immediate cooling of the blood samples on ice or by treatment of the samples by an ultrasonic cell disruptor. None of the anthraquinone glycosides are metabolized in cell-free plasma.

Stability during Storage

It is of utmost importance that the stability of the compound during storage conditions is thoroughly investigated. For example, both cisplatin and oxaliplatin have a degradation halflife of approx only 2 d in plasma at –20°C, which means that 10% of the compounds have decomposed already after 8 h during this storage condition. In ultrafiltrate both substances are stable for at least 1 mo at –80°C.

The concentration of doxorubicin in spiked-frozen (–20°C) plasma samples decreased during storage. Most likely the decrease was not the result of chemical degradation of the drug but caused by changes in the plasma matrix. The amount of precipitates in the thawed samples increased with increasing storage time and also by repeated freezing and thawing of plasma samples. Probably the anthraquinone glycosides are adsorbed on the precipitate, resulting in a decrease of the extraction yield during the analytical procedure.

Selectivity

Selectivity is a measure of the extent to which an analytical procedure can determine a particular compound without interference from matrix components, metabolites, or degradation products. Irrelevant conclusions have been drawn concerning the pharmacokinetics and the fate of the platinum-containing drugs in in vitro cell systems because of the use of analytical methods with insufficient selectivity. The pharmacokinetics of oxaliplatin has almost exclusively been based on the determination of the platinum content in plasma or ultrafiltrate using flameless atomic absorption spectroscopy (FAAS) or inductively coupled plasma mass spectrometry (ICPMS). The reported terminal half-lives in humans show large variations, the shortest 31–47 h, being obtained by FAAS and the longest, 189–273 h, by the more sensitive ICPMS. Using highly selective liquid chromatography in combination with postcolumn derivatization with *N,N*-diethyldithiocarbamate in a microwave field, the kinetics was studied in patients with colorectal carcinoma. A median terminal half-life of 14 min was found. Oxaliplatin rapidly reacts with endogenous low-molecular-weight species such as cysteine and methionine and high-molecular-weight compounds such as albumin, globulin, and hemoglobin. The long terminal half-lives reported ($>$ 200 h) by measuring ultrafiltrate platinum most probably reflect the turnover rates of endogenous high-molecular-weight species representing inactive platinum conjugates.

The extensive studies of chromatographic properties of the anthraquinone glycosides using reversed phase systems showed that the chromatographic selectivity increased with decreasing concentration of organic modifier in the mobile phase. The choice of organic modifier is also of importance in pharmacokinetic studies of anthraquinone glycosides. Acetonitrile is superior to alcohols and acetone because of a higher chromatographic selectivity in separation of intact drugs and their corresponding active 13-hydroxy metabolites. Thus, a number of pharmacokinetic studies have been conducted using reversed phase liquid chromatography with this organic modifier in the mobile phase, for example, a study of the influence of the infusion time on the pharmacokinetics of doxorubicin and a comparative pharmacokinetic study of doxorubicin after intravenous and intrahepatic administration.

Limit of Quantification (LOQ)

LOQ is the lowest concentration of an analyte that can be measured with an acceptable level of precision and accuracy. The LOQ should be measured using the anticancer drug in the biological matrix and is usually the lowest point of the calibration curve. This value must of course be determined experimentally and never by extrapolation. An acceptable precision at LOQ is in general considered to be 10–20% coefficient of variation. It is essential that the analytical technique has sufficient sensitivity to establish accurately the terminal elimination half-life of the drug.

Photometric detection at 600 nm gives a high detection selectivity and sensitivity for quantification of the anthraquinone glycosides. Fluorometric detectors can preferably be used, as recent technical improvements have increased their sensitivity considerably.

Cisplatin has a low molar absorptivity but can be determined photometrically at 344 nm after postcolumn derivatization with *N,N*-diethyldithiocarbamate, giving a derivative with a molar absorptivity of 20,000 M^{-1} cm^{-1}. Busulfan, initially used in the treatment of chronic myelogenous leukemia, has today an important place in combination with bone marrow transplantation. A gas chromatographic method was developed for the analysis of busulfan in patients. The method comprises derivatization with iodide, extraction, and sample concentration in one single step. Replacing the methane sulfonate groups by iodide gives a derivative that can be determined with high sensitivity using electron capture detection as well as mass spectrometry.

Calibration Curves

Calibration curves are usually constructed by making up a series of the biological material, for example, blood or plasma, containing known amounts of the analyte and taking each sample separately through the analytical procedure. The analytical instrument generates a signal, which is plotted on the *y*-axis of a calibration graph with the standard concentrations on the *x*-axis. A straight line (or sometimes a curve) is drawn through the calibration points. Calculated regression coefficients are then used for the determination of sample concentrations.

The use of improper techniques for the determination of the regression coefficients might, however, introduce large systematic errors. Unless a proper test of accuracy is performed, these errors are difficult to detect.

Calibration curves are generally evaluated by ordinary linear (unweighted) regression. This technique might, however, be less accurate in the lower part of the calibration curves when a wide range of concentrations is to be determined, because of the regression equation to a great extent is determined by values in the high concentration range. In such cases, calibration curves sometimes are generated for different concentration ranges, that is, different regression equations are used. The choice of the various concentration ranges with corresponding regression equations is mostly arbitrary. The use of nonparametric statistical methods has become increasingly important for the evaluation of experimental data because these methods are valid even when the underlying distribution is not normal. Moreover, nonparametric regression procedures are less sensitive to outliers than least- squares regression.

Nonparametric linear regression is almost as efficient as the least-squares method when the errors are normally distributed but much more efficient when the errors are not normally distributed, especially when *n* is small. The precision of the regression parameters is expressed by nonparametric confidence intervals. Nonparametric linear regression can easily be implemented with modern computers, for example, by the use of basic programming or spreadsheet programs. Least median of squares regression is an alternative robust regression technique, minimizing the median squared residual. The median squared residual is not changed by outlying observations, and hence robust estimates of regression parameters are obtained. Extended least-squares regression, a general statistical estimation method, is a powerful tool for analysis of individual pharmacokinetic data, used to avoid the weighting problem in the data analysis.

Visual inspection of the corresponding calibration curves often gives the impression that almost identical sample concentrations are obtained irrespective of which of the previous principles for evaluation of calibrations curves has been used for quantification.

The ratio plot is an indispensable tool also for the validation of calibration curves. Calculated values of C_{est}/C_{actual} (C_{est} is the sample concentration in the standard solution determined from the regression coefficients and C_{actual} is the known concentration in the standard solution) have demonstrated that nonparametric, least median of squares regressions and extended least-squares regression are more suited for calculation of regression coefficients of calibration curves than ordinary linear regression in cases with large concentration intervals. Weighted least-squares regression might possibly increase the accuracy of estimated concentrations in the low concentration range, but the proper choice of weights is not obvious.

The high selectivity of the chromatographic system enables construction of calibration curves with two different anthraquinone glycosides as internal standards at different concentrations to cover the wide concentration ranges of doxorubicin and doxorubicinol expected in plasma samples from cancer patients. For pharmacokinetic studies two calibration curves were prepared for doxorubicin, one with a plasma concentration range of 2–200 ng/mL, using daunorubicin (30 ng/mL) as internal standard (IS) and one with a plasma concentration range of 200–1400 ng/mL, using idarubicin (400 ng/mL) as IS. A standard curve for doxorubicinol, 2–45 ng/mL, was prepared with daunorubicin (30 ng/mL) as IS. Daunorubicin and idarubicin were added as internal standards for all plasma samples from patients receiving doxorubicin giving concentrations of 30 ng/mL and 400 ng/mL, respectively.

Clinical Applicability

Cisplatin

It has generally been assumed that cisplatin is present as intact drug in plasma as a result of a high chloride concentration and is converted to the monohydrated complex (MHC) intracellularly because of the lower chloride concentration. MHC is supposed to exert the cytotoxic effect by binding to DNA. The use of liquid chromatography in combination with postcolumn derivatization with *N,N*-diethyldithiocarbamate made it possible for the first time to study the pharmacokinetics of both cisplatin and MHC in whole blood in patients. This study suggested that the kinetics of MHC was formation-rate-limited. The presence of MHC in blood is due to the fact that the pK_a for MHC is 6.56 and at physiological pH it will be present mainly in its less reactive monohydroxo form. Preparative isolation of MHC on porous graphitic carbon using an alkaline mobile phase also made it possible to evaluate its cytotoxicity in an in vitro system and to study its nephrotoxic and ototoxic activity in an animal model. Previous studies on the toxicity of MHC have used hydrolysis mixtures of cisplatin in water that contained both the parent compound, MHC, the dihydrated complex, and possibly di- and trimeric platinum containing compounds.

Ototoxicity is one dose-limiting and unpredictable side effect of cisplatin treatment that together with nephro- and neurotoxicity has attracted a large amount of interest. Administration of sulfur-containing chemoprotectors, for example, D-methionine, has shown promising results regarding protection in animal models. We have recently shown that administration of D-methionine results in lower blood concentrations of cisplatin in an animal model, most probably as a result of a chemical interaction between cisplatin and the protector. It is essential to use selective techniques when performing these types of studies because analytical techniques measuring only total platinum concentration (e.g., by atomic absorption spectroscopy) will codetermine the drug and its reaction products with the protector.

Anthraquinone glycosides

Doxorubicin, an anthraquinone glycoside, is currently one of the clinically most important antineoplastic drugs. In early clinical studies epirubicin appears to be one of the most promising new anthracycline derivatives, which is suggested to have a considerably higher therapeutic index than doxorubicin.

Weenen et al. stated that accurate comparison of the pharmacokinetics of doxorubicin and epirubicin must await evaluation of a large number of patients because of the considerable interindividual variability. However, by simultaneous administration or the two drugs combined with the use of a highly selective analytical technique, it has been possible to overcome intra- and interindividual variation and to compare their pharmacokinetics. Thus, by this method even minor differences in pharmacokinetics can be evaluated.

The plasma pharmacokinetics of doxorubicin and epirubicin have been studied after simultaneous intravenous bolus injection of equal amounts of the two drugs in patients with ovarian carcinoma and after simultaneous intrahepatic administration in patients with nonresectable and symptomatic liver cancer.

The plasma concentration of epirubicin as well as of doxorubicin after intravenous and intrahepatic administration followed a three-compartment open model. The plasma concentration of doxorubicin was in all cases higher than that of epirubicin. On average the area under the plasma concentration time curve (AUC) and the maximum plasma concentration (C_{max}) were 2.1 and 1.7 times larger for doxorubicin than for epirubicin, respectively. Epirubicin was eliminated faster than doxorubicin, the terminal half-life time being, on average, 1.5 times longer for doxorubicin.

The reduced toxicity of epirubicin in comparison with doxorubicin after intravenous administration has been suggested to be the consequence of the pharmacokinetic behavior of epirubicin, characterized by constantly lower plasma levels as compared to doxorubicin, that is, a reduction in AUC and C_{max}. The importance of the differences in the pharmacokinetics of doxorubicin and epirubicin in relation to therapeutic efficacy is unclear.

The plasma concentrations of the 13-hydroxy metabolites did not exceed 20 ng/mL. Their AUC values averaged 23% of those of the intact drugs. The clinical importance of the 13-hydroxy metabolites, that is, influence on the therapeutic efficiency and side effects, is not fully understood. Extensive formation of these metabolites has been associated with a high therapeutic response. In model systems doxorubicinol in general has cytotoxic properties similar to those of doxorubicin.

Factors influencing the pharmacokinetics of doxorubicin and epirubicin administered simultaneously in equal doses as a 24-h constant rate infusion have been investigated in children (0.73–15.3 yr) with acute lymphocytic leukemia (ALL). In this pharmacokinetic study our previously published simplified sampling procedure comprising only one blood sample taken prior to the end of the infusion, that is, at pseudo-steady state, was used.

The plasma pharmacokinetics of neither doxorubicin nor epirubicin correlated with the age of the pediatric patients. It was not possible to demonstrate a statistical difference of the dose-normalized maximum concentrations between males and females. The interpatient variations of the dose-normalized maximum concentrations of both drugs were, however, larger among females than among males.

The doxorubicin/epirubicin C_{max} ratio was 1.39. The pharmacokinetic differences in children are less pronounced than in adults. Hence, the reduction of systemic side effects obtained by substituting doxorubicin with epirubicin might be less pronounced in children than in adults. However, the pharmacokinetic differences of the two drugs in children are still of such a magnitude that substituting doxorubicin with epirubicin most likely will be of clinical importance.

A comparison of C_{max} values in the pediatric patients and in a previous study of adult breast cancer patients shows that dosing based on body surface area results in similar plasma concentrations of epirubicin in children and adults, under the assumption that identical infusion rates are used. In contrast, dosing based on body weight results in lower plasma concentrations of epirubicin in children than in adults. The interpatient variation of the dose-normalized C_{max} values of epirubicin were higher in children with ALL than in breast cancer patients, underlining the difficulties in a proper dosing of anthraquinone glycosides to children. The rather marked interpatient variation in clearance has previously been demonstrated when epirubicin was used in the 5-FU, epirubicin, and cyclophosphamide (FEC) combination.

Capillary and Venous Blood Sampling

The plasma pharmacokinetics for doxorubicin (area under plasma concentration time curve and maximum plasma concentration) show more than a 10-fold interindividual variability despite dosing based on body surface area. An individualized doxorubicin dose, based on determined plasma concentrations, would therefore most likely result in an improvement of treatment. The drug concentration in one single venous plasma sample drawn at the end of a constant infusion (2 h or longer) gives highly accurate estimates of the systemic exposure of the anthraquinone glycosides doxorubicin and epirubicin and may substitute a complete pharmacokinetic evaluation requiring at least 12 blood samples collected over a 24-h period. The clinical applicability of this method has been established. Plasma levels of anthraquinone glycosides have so far been measured using blood samples obtained by puncturing of a peripheral vein. With increased sensitivity of analytical techniques, for example, by using modern fluorometric detectors it is now possible to quantify anthraquinone glycosides in capillary samples, collected by a finger lancet puncture.

Potential concentration differences of doxorubicin in plasma from capillary and venous blood samples were evaluated in 16 patients (7 females and 9 males; median age: 37 yr, range: 1–77 yr). The quantitative analysis of doxorubicin was carried out by reversed phase liquid chromatography with fluorometric detection. The very high correlation between concentrations of doxorubicin in capillary and venous plasma samples ($r = 0.98$; $p < 0.0001$) might falsely give the impression that capillary and venous sampling sites can be used interchangeably. In contrast, the ratio plots clearly demonstrate minor but significantly higher capillary plasma concentrations, the median capillary/venous plasma concentration ratio being 1.13 (95% confidence interval: 1.06–1.20). The wide plasma concentration range of doxorubicin, because of inclusion of samples from patients treated with large variations in dose and infusion times, did not affect the relative concentrations of doxorubicin in capillary and venous samples. Multiple regression with stepwise variable selection revealed that gender was the only variable tested affecting the capillary/venous plasma concentration ratio, the concentration ratio being significantly higher in males (median: 1.18) than in females (median: 1.01). Gender differences in plasma protein binding, body composition, or blood flow might influence the amount of doxorubicin diffusing into the tissue, thereby affecting the capillary/venous concentration ratio. The observed concentration differences of doxorubicin in plasma from capillary and venous samples are, however, of minor importance only.

The practical advantage of collecting capillary blood instead of venous blood is evident, but is most pronounced in pediatric patients, who often find venous blood sampling very traumatic. In addition, deterioration of the veins caused by treatment with antineoplastic drugs often results in difficulties in obtaining venous blood samples from cancer patients. Capillary blood sampling can now be recommended for therapeutic drug monitoring and pharmacokinetic studies of doxorubicin. To minimize the dilution of the blood with the interstitial fluid, the capillary blood sampling must be conducted with free flowing blood with minimum squeezing of the finger.

A careful examination of drug concentration differences in capillary and venous blood samples is necessary prior to change of sampling site. Even though concentrations of large numbers of drugs in capillary and venous blood samples have been compared, the results are in general difficult to interpret because of unsuitable treatment of data, that is, the use of scatter diagrams. A high correlation coefficient and/or a p value < 0.05 is often considered sufficient for conclusions of interchangeable sampling sites. Hence, it was concluded that methotrexate venous blood sampling can be substituted by capillary blood sampling, as a scatterplot of the concentration data showed a correlation coefficient of 0.934. A closer examination of the data showed that the capillary/venous concentration ratio ranged from 0.2 to 3.1, a fact that may have serious consequences when basing the leucovorin rescue on measured methotrexate concentrations.

Many of the anticancer drugs are demanding from an analytical point of view, for example, chemical instability, low blood/plasma concentrations, and sometimes also the need to quantify several chemically closely related compounds. To obtain optimal results in pharmacokinetic/pharmacodynamic studies and therapeutic drug monitoring, a close interaction among analytical chemists, pharmacokinetic expertise, clinicians, nurses, and experts working in other disciplines is mandatory.

4

Control of Bioanalytical Methods

Validation and control of bioanalytical methods as practiced in U.S. Food and Drug Administration (FDA)-regulated drug development studies is the approach most often used for anticancer drugs. The discipline has progressed from one that was in its infancy a decade ago to a largely mature endeavor more recently. Validation and control procedures in other areas of bioanalysis such as clinical chemistry and forensic toxicology have been largely consistent for a number of decades. The primary difference between the drug development discipline and other areas of bioanalysis is the fact that drug development requires application of consistent standards for analytical methods that are investigational rather than routine. Validation and control attempts in drug development studies carried out prior to 1990 were the result of individual policies that varied a great deal from company to company. The importance of consistent procedures for validation and control in drug development was first outlined by Shah in 1987 and specific procedures were proposed by Karnes in 1991. Since these two works on the subject, a number of reviews and research articles have been published along with two conferences that have led to the establishment of a "Guidance for Industry" on Bioanalytical Method Validation. The first conference was held in 1990 with the results published in 1992. A draft guidance was also published as a result of this conference in 1999. Following an acknowledgment that small molecules should be treated differently than large molecules, two more conferences were held in 2000 and the proceedings published in 2000 and 2001 for small and large molecules, respectively. All of this activity resulted in the final guidance that was approved by the Center for Drug Evaluation and Research (CDER) of FDA in cooperation with the Center for Veterinary Medicine (CVM) and published in May of 2001. The guidance has regulatory implications for a variety of biological matrices analyzed in human and animal clinical and preclinical studies.

The document applies to chromatographic, spectrometric, immunological, and microbiological procedures and was intended as a nonbinding general recommendation that can be adjusted depending on circumstances. The document outlines fundamental parameters for bioanalytical method validation that include accuracy, precision, selectivity, sensitivity, reproducibility, and stability. The document addresses situations in which a bioanalytical method may be modified and suggests different levels of validation to ensure that validity is maintained. The document also includes a glossary of terms. Although this document represents the current thinking of the FDA and is based on the conferences held, the procedures and criteria were primarily negotiated. They were based on an amalgam of procedures that existed within the industry prior to the conferences and are not necessarily based on the best scientific approach. This chapter endeavors to present the best scientific approaches based on the literature while considering them in the context of the FDA guidance.

There are two major divisions in the endeavor to ensure the quality of analytical results. The two divisions consist of method validation and method quality control. There are referred to as prestudy validation and during-study validation, respectively, in the draft FDA guidance but no nominal distinction is made in the final FDA guidance. Another division that is used often in describing validation and control processes is a method development or establishment phase in which the method is not yet complete but some validation results may be collected in an effort to establish optimal conditions. As such, the method development or establishment phase should be free from regulatory scrutiny for the most part since the method is dynamic at this point. The validation phase represents the stage at which a method is complete but has not yet been used for analysis of "*real samples.*" The question to be addressed at this phase is whether or not the method is good enough for an intended purpose. It could be argued that the criteria used here should be flexible so that methods used for critical purposes such as therapeutic monitoring of a narrow therapeutic index drug would require strict and tight guidelines, whereas other situations may not require such rigorous criteria. The approach of the FDA recommendations has been to apply a "one size fits all" approach without built in flexibility for a large variety of drug types and for a large number of different applications. The FDA guidance makes no distinction between the method development/establishment and validation phases. The quality control phase represents the period in which data are collected from quality control samples and exists to ensure the quality of "*real sample*" results. The question to be addressed in this phase is no longer related to how good a method is but to determining whether the method is performing according to specifications set during method validation. The procedures used for these three phases should reflect the goals to be achieved. The FDA guidance does this for the most part but fails to address some valid scientific issues related to these goals in some cases. The following sections presents approaches suggested in the guidance along with scientific justifications when appropriate. Other approaches are presented as alternatives to the guidance that may have more scientific validity or better address the individual goals of method development, validation, and quality control.

Method Development

Two important factors in achieving good performance of bioanalytical methods in the method development phase are selective recovery from sample processing and calibration with appropriate primary standards. Selective recovery for a bioanalytical method refers to the provision of an analytical response for the entire amount of analyte contained in a sample without residual interferences or matrix effects from other sample components. Although selectivity must be dealt with in method development from the standpoint of achievement of selectivity, this is largely a validation parameter and is dealt with in that section. Recovery of a bioanalytical method most appropriately refers to analyte extraction efficiency and is termed absolute recovery. Absolute recovery may be measured in a number of ways and is calculated using the general formula below:

$$\frac{\text{Extracted response}}{\text{Unextracted response}} \times 100 = \%\ \text{Recovery}$$

The extracted response is the quantitative instrumental measurement from a sample, spiked at a known concentration, into a blank matrix sample that is processed and measured. The unextracted sample may be represented by a number of response values depending on the particular situation. The simplest experiment is to measure the unextracted response from a nonmatrix solvent solution spiked at the same concentration. This provides absolute recovery, although the value may not be representative because of residual matrix effects in the extracted sample or poor reproducibility of the instrument response. Matrix effects can be compensated for by adding an appropriate amount of analyte to an extracted blank matrix and then measuring the unextracted response in the presence of the blank extract.

Instrument response variability can be lessened by addition of an internal standard to both the extracted sample following the extraction process and at the same concentration to the unextracted sample. The measured response then becomes the response ratio of the analyte to that of the internal standard. Absolute recovery can also be easily estimated if radioactive analogs of the drug are available. In this experiment, radioactivity counts prior to extraction provide the unextracted response, whereas the radioactivity counts following extraction from the same spiked sample provide the extracted response. This procedure eliminates intersample variability and the possibility of a matrix effect with an isotopically labeled analog is remote. Sufficient replication needs to be employed to provide sufficient confidence in the calculated recovery and the more variable measurements (typically the extracted samples) require greater replication than the less variable measurements (typically the unextracted samples).

There are a number of experiments that have been referred to as recovery experiments that do not provide absolute recovery or an estimate of sample processing efficiency. They include experiments evaluating the measured response ratio of a sample extracted from the intended matrix to that extracted from a nonmatrix solution. This experiment provides information on the effect of components of the matrix on the measured signal and is an important experiment to evaluate method selectivity, but should not be confused with an experiment to measure absolute recovery. Another experiment that has been reported as a recovery experiment is the ratio of the assayed concentration to that of the prepared concentration. The is an accuracy experiment and again does not address recovery as is intended in the FDA guidance. One last example of an experiment that may be reported as recovery but does not address processing efficiency is the ratio of the internal standard compensated response that has been extracted to the corresponding response unextracted, provided the internal standard is added prior to processing. This experiment will evaluate how well the internal standard is functioning, but again provides no information on sample processing efficiency. The FDA guidance defines recovery as specifically pertaining to absolute recovery experiments that indicate extraction efficiency. The guidance suggests that recovery experiments should be conducted but that recovery need not be 100%.

For chromatographic methods, another question to be addressed pertains to the use of an internal standard. As mentioned above the use of an internal standard involves adding a structural or isotopic analog to a sample prior to processing so that errors in sample processing can be corrected for by including a ratio of the response of the analyte to that of the analog. It has been noted by a few authors that the use of an internal standard is not necessary in many cases or can actually lead to a degradation of analytical results in the absence of systematic errors. Method degradation from the use of an internal standard will occur if the following is true:

$$\text{RSDb} > r\ \text{RSDa}$$

where RSDb and RSDa are the relative standard deviations of the internal standard and analyte responses, respectively, and r represents the correlation coefficient for the responses of the analyte vs the internal standard. This relationship was derived mathematically and proven with experimental data by Haefelfinger et al. Even though there are good arguments for not using an internal standard for chromatographic procedures, they are based on random and not systematic error. It is well accepted that internal standards are essential for correcting technical systematic errors such as loss of sample caused by variable phase transfers or dilutions and allow for many volume transfers to be nonquantitative, thus increasing sample throughput. Correction of errors or shifts related to partition, chemical reactivity, and detector stability will depend on the characteristics of the internal standard relative to the analyte and the closer the chemical and physical properties of the analyte and internal standard are, the greater the probability that these errors will be accurately corrected for. Internal standards that are isotopes of the analyte have become popular for this reason although a mass detector is required to discriminate between responses. The FDA guidance does not specifically require the use of an internal standard, but it is generally expected for chromatographic procedures. Care must be taken, however, not to use an internal standard that is chemically inappropriate simply to address this expectation or the quality of results could suffer.

Calibration of an analytical method is an important consideration in method development. The concentration range for calibration must be established and an appropriate model applied to the data that will allow accurate calculation of unknown sample concentrations. The lower limit of calibration is usually established through a consideration of the lower limit of quantitation (LLOQ) and the point at which the data no longer fit the calibration model determines the upper limit. Practical considerations such as the concentration range expected for samples are also employed in setting up the calibration range. The choice of a calibration model should be determined by experimental concentration vs response data, and the model that best fits the data should be used. The FDA Guidance suggests that the simplest model that adequately describes the relationship be used, thus indicating a bias toward the linear model, but use of nonlinear functions is not prohibited. Determination of the appropriate range for calibration and application of the most appropriate model requires a consideration of the quality of fit of the experimental data and is intimately related to method validation, which is covered in the following section.

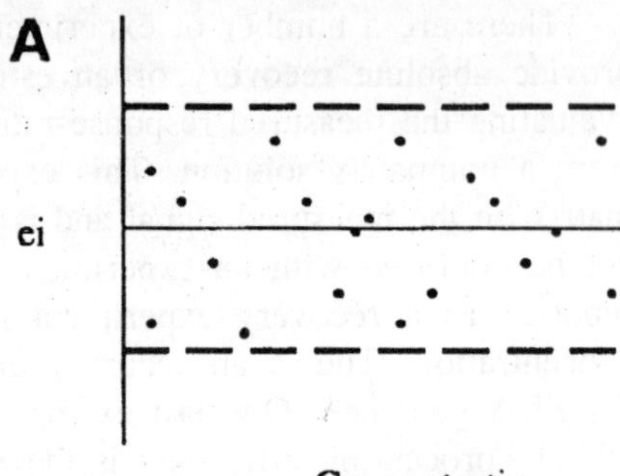

METHOD VALIDATION

Calibration

Method calibration is the crossover point between method development and method validation, as it involves both setting up procedures and also showing that they work well enough for a stated purpose. The quality of fit of the data to the selected calibration model will determine the allowable upper limit of calibration. This will be the highest concentration that will consistently provide an acceptable fit throughout the entire range of calibration. To establish the range and model for calibration it is most helpful to evaluate residual errors and to use the model that provides the lowest residual error. For example, residual error for the linear model can be calculated as follows:

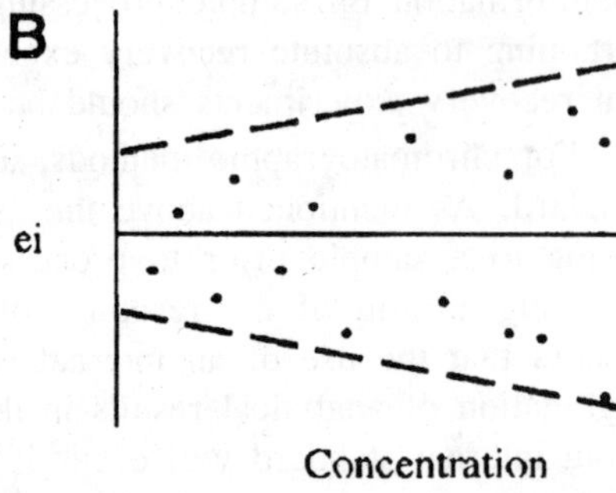

$$e_i = y_i - a - bx_i$$

where e_i represents the residual error at a given concentration, y_i and x_i are the dependent and independent variables, respectively, and a and b are the best fit intercept and slope form a linear regression of the entire calibration range. These residuals are often expressed as a concentration by "backfitting" individual calibration data. Although the FDA guidance has a bias in favor of the simplest calibration model (linear), it does not prevent use of nonlinear calibration models that may provide a better fit to the data and allow more accurate calculation of unknown values over a wider concentration range. If residual values are plotted vs concentration, a pattern as shown in Fig. 4.1A will result for homoscedastic data and the use of a nonweighted linear calibration model can be considered

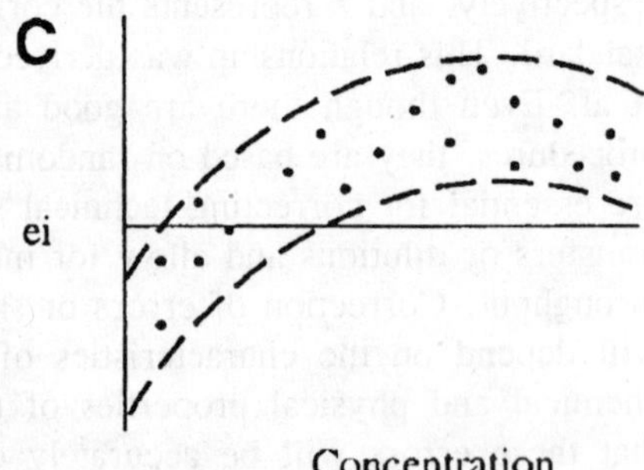

Fig. 4.1. Schematic representation of calibration residuals vs concentration.

appropriate. If the residuals demonstrate heteroscedastic data in which there is a proportional increase in the residuals as concentration increases, represented in Fig. 4.1B, a weighted linear calibration is most appropriate. Figure 1C is representative of a residuals pattern that indicates the data to be nonlinear and the linear model is therefore inappropriate. Weighted linear calibration is carried out using a normal linear regression modified to include a weighting factor as a multiplier when calculating the sum of squared residuals. The most appropriate weighting factor is the inverse of the variance at each concentration; however, because this variance has been shown to be proportional to concentration, the inverse of concentration squared or simply the inverse of concentration can be used. These weighting factors can be used on a trial basis to determine which factor provides the lowest residual error throughout the concentration range. If a pattern of residuals emerges that is similar to the heteroscedastic pattern, then a systematic departure from the model is indicated and an alternative to the linear model such as a power or a polynomial fit should be investigated. Caution should be used in attempts to force truly nonlinear data to a linear calibration model in response to the FDA bias. It can be seen that the linear calibration provides unacceptably high residuals at low concentration. These residuals are improved significantly by use of the weighted linear model. The function of the weighting factor is to increase the influence of the low concentration data on the best fit regression slope, and therefore the low concentration residuals are improved whereas the high concentration residuals are made worse. This occurs because forcing the line closer at the low concentrations acts as a fulcrum to force the inflexible linear calibration line away from the data at high concentrations. The solution to this problem is to allow some flex in the calibration curve and to use a nonlinear calibration model that will provide a better fit at both extremes of calibration for such data.

Table 4.1. Back-calculated standards mean deviation (n = 5,%)

Conc. (ng/mL)	*Power fit*	*Weighted 1/conc.*	*Unweighted*
10	5.15	5.98	18.55
20	3.40	3.40	6.06
50	1.78	1.82	1.70
100	2.23	4.04	3.26
250	0.99	0.34	0.23
500	3.26	4.31	3.32

There are many approaches to assessment of the quality of fit for analytical calibration data in addition to an evaluation of residuals. These include but are not limited to correlation coefficients, sensitivity plots, polynomial fits, log–log plots, and the *F*-test for lack of fit. Sensitivity plots, polynomial fits, and log–log plots are limited to evaluation of the linear model and are not widely used in bioanalysis. Log–log plots have been shown to provide comparable results to the *F*-test for lack of fit and residuals analysis, whereas the polynomial fit approach was found to be more conservative. For linear analytical data, calculation of the correlation coefficient involves the false statistical assumption that the independent variable in regression analysis (concentration) is errorless. The correlation coefficient is essentially a measure of the amount of variation in the dependent variable (analytical response) that is accounted for by the independent variable (concentration). It does not distinguish random from systematic error well. Also, with regard to testing the linear model, correlation coefficients have been shown to produce good correlation for data that do not conform to the linear model and have been shown to be a more liberal criteria than other approaches. For these reasons, the correlation coefficient has been deemphasized as a method of evaluation for goodness of fit and is not mentioned in the final FDA guidance.

The *F*-test for lack of fit is a statistical test of whether or not the sum of the variances attributable to lack of fit (the differences between mean and fitted values for the analytical response at each calibrator concentration) is significantly different from the sum of the variances attributable to pure error (the differences of individual calibrators from the mean at a given concentration). The *F*-test for lack of fit has been shown to provide comparable results to residuals analysis and log–log plots. Although the *F*-test for lack of fit is the most appropriate test of goodness of fit statistically and can be used to evaluate both liner and nonlinear models, replication is required to obtain statistical significance and the test may not be easily understood at all levels of bioanalytical practice. The only specific criterion for calibration goodness of fit to the model offered by the FDA guidance is a criterion applied to concentration residuals. This criterion states that all concentration residuals must be within 20% of the nominal value for the lower limit of quantitation and within 15% at all other concentrations. This criterion is easy to understand and does not require deviation from a set protocol to achieve statistical significance. A criticism of this criterion is that it is based on consensus opinion and does not possess a statistical foundation.

Selectivity

There has been confusion over the terms selectivity and specificity, and they are often used interchangeably. Specificity may be used appropriately to refer to an analytical method that provides a response for only a single analyte. The term has also been used appropriately to describe the absolute condition of selectivity. Selectivity is the more appropriate term for analytical purposes, as few if any analytical systems can be said to respond to only a single species without being affected by components of the matrix. In an analytical method in which concentration is determined as a function of response, the degree to which the response is unaffected by contributions from the matrix is referred to as the selectivity of the method. There are two independent components to selectivity referred to as matrix effects and interferences. Interferences are predeterminate errors caused most frequently in bioanalysis by a component of the matrix producing a measurable response. This causes an error in the intercept of the calibration curve, where the dotted line represents a calibration with the interference and the solid line represents the unaffected calibration curve. Interferences are best evaluated by analysis of the baseline from a blank measurement if a suitable blank exists. Interferences must be differentiated from contamination (a response from the intended analyte in the blank) by qualitative means when contamination is suspected. In biopharmaceutical analysis interferences are relatively easy to evaluate because the analyte is normally a xenobiotic and a blank is readily available for each biological source as a predose sample. Analysis of this predose sample by the method demonstrating a lack of significant response indicates good selectivity. The FDA guidance states that a lack of interferences needs to be demonstrated in six independent sources of blank matrix

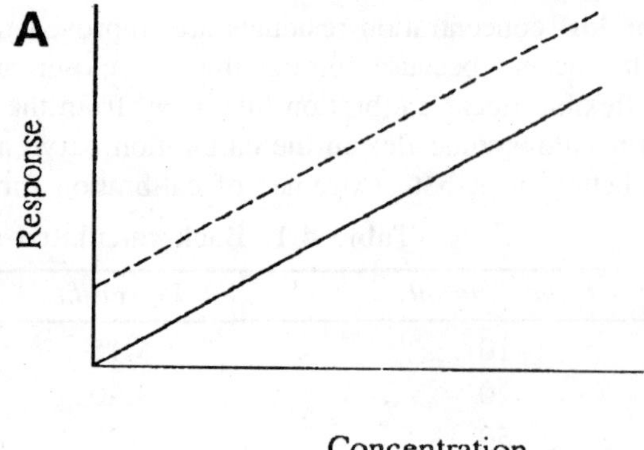

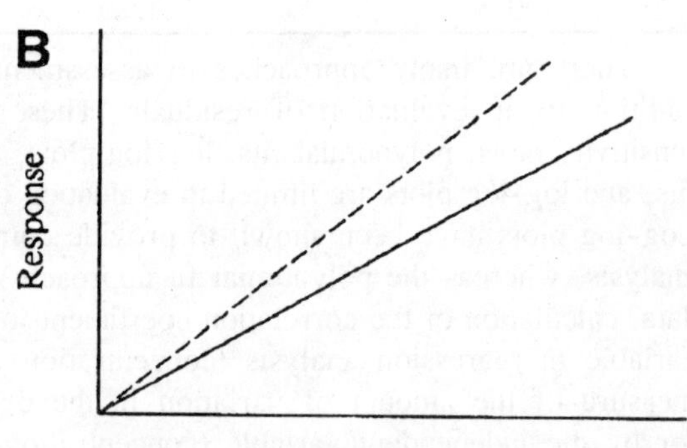

Fig. 4.2. Errors in selectivity caused by a predeterminant and constant shift in the calibration are referred to as interferences and are represented in A. Matrix effects are proportional errors of slope as shown in B.

and that there should be evidence that the substance being quantified is the intended analyte. The guidance does not specify what constitutes a lack of interference or what evidence is needed for demonstration of qualitative identification of the analyte. Commonly used criteria for chromatographic procedures include a lack of interference of $< 5\%$ or 20% of the limit of quantitation and a retention time match with a primary standard for qualitative identification.

The situations in which the predose blank matrix approach to interference evaluation does not prove adequate include instances in which interferences may appear over time because of lack of stability of the matrix or analyte, situations in which interferences are caused by metabolites of the drug that are not present in the predosed blank, and situations in which the analyte is an endogenous compound for which there is no predose sample. Stability issues are a separate concern and include a consideration of more than just the maintenance of the selectivity of the method with time under storage conditions and these will are dealt with later in this chapter. Interference from metabolites is a concern especially when using mass spectrometry (MS) as an analytical method, as the source of ions for MS is a reaction chamber where metabolites and other analogs of the analyte, most notably internal standards, can be fragmented into ions that are the same as those that originate from the analyte. This phenomenon is referred to as "cross-talk." For this reason, it is necessary for evaluation of interferences by use of primary standards of the individual metabolites or by modification of chromatographic conditions to effect a separation of the analogue from the analyte. Once the modified chromatographic conditions have been shown to produce no differences in measured response, the original chromatographic conditions may be used. This special precaution, which is important for MS, is less of a concern for other methods, as complete separation from components of the matrix is routinely carried out for these methods. No provision for this extra concern regarding interferences with MS methods is included in the FDA guidance. It is recommended practice, however, to evaluate "cross-talk" at high levels for potentially interfering internal standards and metabolites along with conducting experiments at altered retention times in dosed (ex vivo) samples.

Matrix effects are proportional errors of slope as shown in Fig. 4.2B, where the dotted line represents a calibration with the matrix effect and the solid line represents the unaffected calibration curve. Unlike interferences that are caused most often by components from the matrix that yield a response, matrix effects are generally caused by some interaction, either chemical or physical, of the analyte with some component of the matrix. An example of this is shown below for charge transfer and proton transfer reactions that occur in atmospheric pressure ionization (API) MS:

Charge transfer: $A^+ + M \rightarrow M^+ + A$

Proton transfer: $AH^+ + M \rightarrow MH^+ + A$

where A^+ and AH^+ represent charged and protonated analyte molecules, respectively, and M^+ and MH^+ represent the corresponding species for a matrix component. A and M represent the uncharged, unprotonated forms and negative charges may be involved as well as the positive charges pictured. These reactions both lead to ion suppression matrix effects that result in a decreased response for the analyte as compared to nonmatrix analysis. The proportional nature of the matrix effect error is a result of this type interaction because the effect is mediated through an interaction constant and is proportional to concentration in the simplest case.

Matrix effects can often be compensated for by duplication of the sample matrix in calibration standards. This will adjust the slope in calibration standards to match that of the sample matrix. The assumption involved is that the blank matrix used for calibration standards is sufficiently similar to that of the samples to yield accurate results. This assumption is generally valid for most bioanalytical methods that involve an extraction and chromatographic separation, as the factors that may affect extractability and separation such as pH and protein content are relatively constant in biological samples from the same origin. MS methods again require special attention because quantitation is often carried out without complete extraction and separation of the analyte from matrix components. Although the FDA guidance does not specify any test of matrix effects, it is recommended practice for MS methods. It is advisable to use an isotopically labeled internal standard if possible, to increase chromatographic retention times as a test to see if results change, and to evaluate instrument response in a variety of sources of biological matrix. A very useful experiment for validation of the lack of ion suppression or enhancement in MS is the post-column infusion experiment in which a steady infusion of the analyte is pumped into the system post-column generating a steady response from the analyte. In this configuration, blank matrix is injected precolumn and the ion suppression or enhancement appears as a negative or positive deflection of the baseline response. This negative or positive deflection in the baseline can be compared to where the analyte elutes if injected precolumn. The chromatography can then be modified so that the elution time of the analyte is not coincident with suppression or enhancement peaks.

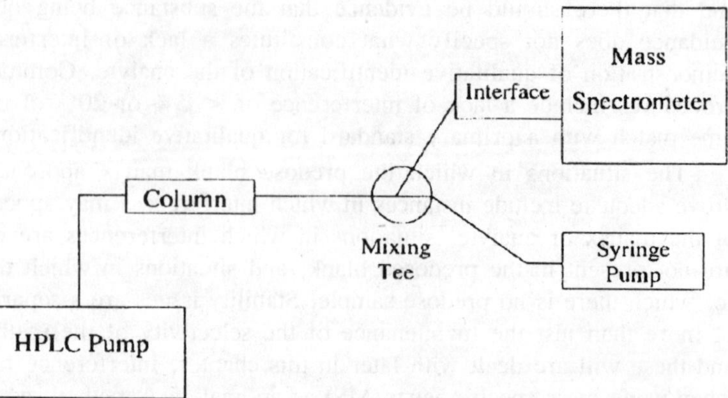

Fig. 4.3. A schematic representation of a post-column infusion hardware setup in which a steady infusion of the analyte is pumped into column elluent.

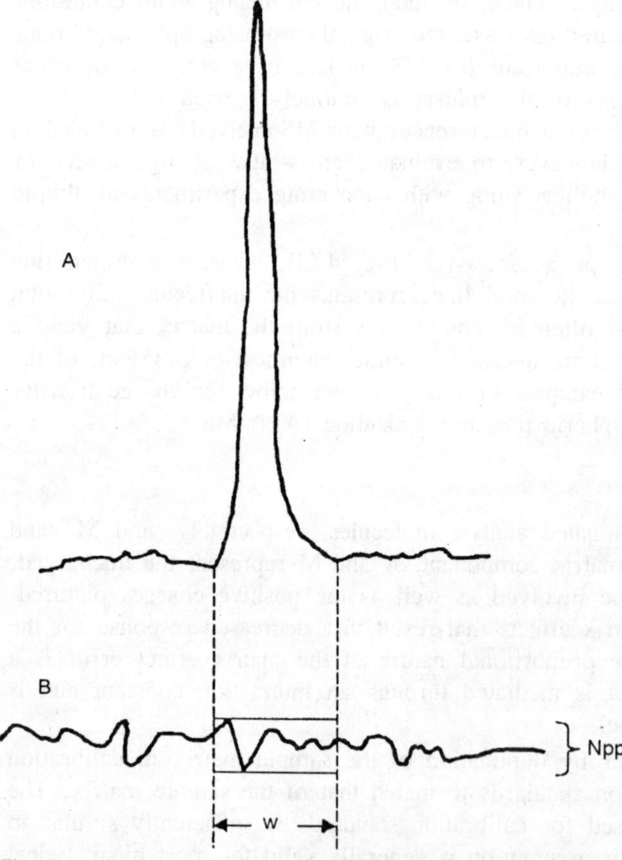

Fig. 4.4. A common way to calculate signal to noise ratios. A- represents a chromatogram of standard material and B- represents the baseline from a blank injection.

Detectability

Detectability has been one of the most broadly interpreted parameters of validation. The term detectability is used here because it more accurately reflects the parameters used for validation of the lowest concentrations to be measured. The term sensitivity is often used for this purpose. It is used in the literature to indicate the slope of the analytical calibration curve, however, and is not defined in the FDA glossary of terms, so it would seem inappropriate to use it to refer to detectability except in the most general sense. There are a number of different mathematical definitions for detectability that will yield different results and many of them are referred to by the same terminology. Most often, detectability has been defined based on blank noise measurements. Valid statistical approaches have also been based on confidence limits associated with a calibration curve. Discussion of detectability is limited to the blank noise approach here because this approach is more accepted in FDA-regulated drug development. Blank noise can be defined in a number of ways. For chromatographic methods this consists of measuring the biological analytical signal over the elution window of the peak of interest in a matrix blank sample. This is shown in Fig. 4.4, where Fig. 4.4A represents a chromatogram of standard material and Fig. 4.4B the baseline from a blank injection. The blank signal should be an average from a number of blank matrices. The most conservative estimates will be yielded by use of the peak-to-peak noise signal rather than the peak noise signal although both have been used. Root mean square (RMS) noise has also been used, although use of this noise estimate would provide a very liberal estimate of detectability relative to the others. The blank noise approach involves multiplication of some factor (K) times the standard deviation of the blank noise to yield a confidence interval. The confidence interval then allows prediction of an error probability associated with making an incorrect decision of detection for the analyte. This value is then divided by the slope of the calibration curve to yield results in concentration units as shown below:

$$K\,S_b/m = X_{LLOD}$$

where S_b represents the standard deviation of the blank noise measurement, m is the slope of the calibration curve near the limit and X_{LLOD} is the lower limit of detection. This limit represents the concentration that can be distinguished as nonzero with great probability or with low probability of actually being a blank. The K factor used determines the width of the confidence interval and thus the probability of an incorrect decision, that is, the sample being measured as above the lower limit of detection (LLOD) but one that is truly blank. Typically used values for K are 2 and 3, representing error probabilities of 95.4% and 99.7%, respectively, 3 being the most conservative and most commonly used. The LLOD calculated in this way is not useful for the purpose of setting a parameter for quantification and should be used only to compare absolute detectability potentials of analytical systems. This is the case because an analytical measurement made at the LLOD would yield a high probability of being indistinguishable from a measurement made at zero. To solve this problem, a new limit is defined as the lower limit of identification (LLOI), which uses a value for the K factor of 6 and defines the concentration at which there is a low probability of being less than the defined LLOD. The lower limit of identification has a practical meaning as the threshold for presence of an analyte in a sample. It can be said with a defined level of confidence that if the measured concentration is above the lower limit of identification, then the analyte is present in a sample. The most useful application of this is in purity testing of chemical substances and dosage forms, but the parameter has little application in quantitative bioanalysis except for situations in which a method selectivity argument is made.

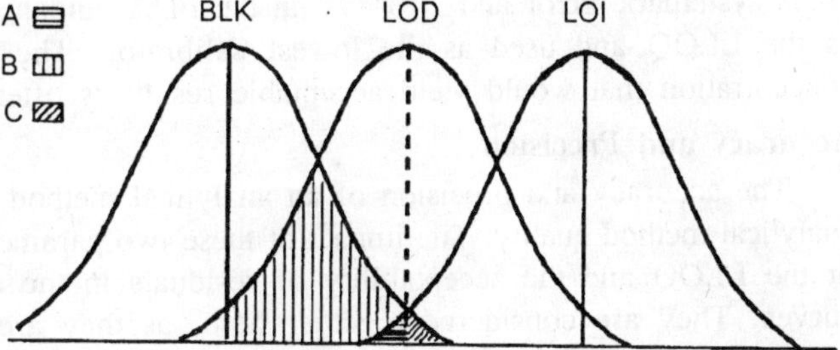

Fig. 4.5. A graphical representation of the probabilities related to various detectability parameters.

The most useful limit in quantitative bioanalysis is the LLOQ. The LLOQ represents the concentration above which accurate and precise quantification can be carried out. This limit can be traditionally estimated using the blank noise approach with a K factor of 10. This factor for K is intended to target a coefficient of variation (CV) of 10%, in the absence of systematic errors. An appropriate K factor for a desired level of precision can be arrived at through the following expression:

$$K = 1/\mathrm{CV}$$

where CV is the coefficient of variation expressed as a decimal fraction. The above expression is derived through a combination of the general lower limit of detection equation and the expression for CV. A K factor of 5 as recommended in the FDA guidance would therefore predict a CV of 20% which is the precision limit at the LLOQ allowable in the FDA guidance. The FDA guidance is therefore consistent with accepted theory although the approach does not account for the fact that this value is lower than the LLOI and is technically not present in the sample with great probability (99.7%). A slightly more conservative approach would be to use a K factor of 6 or 10 as an estimate of LLOQ.

LLOQs may be estimated with the blank noise approach but are established through actual testing of concentrations prepared at that level to ensure that precision and accuracy limits are met. The estimates provided by the blank noise approach should be used as a guide as to where to set concentrations for evaluation but should not be used as evidence for validation. The best approach to establishment of the LLOQ is to prepare several concentrations near the LLOQ estimate and to measure them in replicate. The lowest concentration to yield the desired acceptable level of accuracy and precision would therefore represent the LLOQ and should be established as the lowest concentration in the calibration curve. The greater the number of concentrations tested, the better will be the estimate for LLOQ. In practice, it is inefficient to measure a large number of low concentrations with sufficient replication to establish the LLOQ rigorously. Typically, the blank noise estimated LLOQ is used as a guide and a single LLOQ is tested. If the results of this test yield acceptable accuracy and precision (20% systematic error and 20% CV in the FDA guidance), then this single concentration is established as the LLOQ and used as the lowest calibrator. The question of whether or not there is a lower concentration that would yield acceptable results is often not addressed.

Accuracy and Precision

The accuracy and precision of an analytical method are by far the most important determinants of analytical method quality. The impact of these two parameters has already been discussed in establishment of the LLOQ and the acceptability of residuals in the evaluation of the quality of fit for calibration curves. They are considered together here, as they are often lumped together to represent the total error of a measurement and it is important to distinguish these three parameters. Accuracy and precision are interdependent in assessment of the acceptability of an analytical method. The FDA guidance defines accuracy as "the degree of closeness of the determined value to the nominal or known true value under prescribed conditions." The accuracy component of total error can be represented by the following:

$$\frac{u = \bar{x}}{u} \times 100 = \%\ \text{Accuracy deviation}$$

where u is the "true" or "nominal" value and $\bar{x}$ is the average of measured values. It is important to make sure that the average has been calculated from enough measurements to allow for an adequate reduction in the random (imprecision) error so that only the systematic (inaccuracy) error is represented. It is therefore incorrect to represent accuracy for an individual measurement. This concept is illustrated in **Fig. 7**, where the Gaussian distribution shown represents a distribution around a measured average that determines an analytical method's precision. The difference between this average and the true value is the accuracy as described mathematically above, and the sum of the two errors is referred to as total error or bias. Both accuracy and precision are traditionally evaluated through control samples prepared at various concentrations to reflect the range of expected values and should be measured independent of the calibration standards. The "*true value*" for these control samples can be established either through comparison of results to a reference method or through assigning a known concentration from spiking of weighed standards into a blank matrix.

The imprecision or random error component of total error can be estimated from calculation of the percentage relative standard deviation (RSD), which is also referred to as the coefficient of variation (CV). This value is calculated as follows:

$$\frac{sd}{\bar{x}} \times 100 = \text{RSD}$$

where *sd* represents the standard deviation of a group of multiple measurements of the same sample and $\bar{x}$ again represents the calculated average from the same group. Precision is often confused with reproducibility and repeatability, although these terms have distinctly different meanings. Reproducibility is the closeness of results measured under different conditions, such as different laboratories, and repeatability refers to the closeness of results from successive measurements of the same sample. Precision is normally assessed on a within- batch and a between-batch basis. The within-batch assessment is considered an estimate of the precision under optimal conditions without the variability associated with batch-to-batch results. It is for this reason that it is advisable to run unknown samples generated from the same subject but different legs of a clinical study in the same batch if possible. The between-batch assessment is a more realistic estimate of the precision of a method because it normally is subjected to a greater number of sources of variability.

The total error or "bias" of an analytical measurement is appropriately represented for individual measurements and it is not appropriate, therefore, to apply an accuracy criterion to a single measurement. Any criterion for individual measurements should be referred to as a total error criterion. The criterion should be broad enough to include both the random and the systematic error components of the total error. Total error for an individual measurement can be calculated as follows:

$$|x-u| + 2.58\ sd = E$$

where x represents the individual measured value and E represents the total error or bias of that individual measurement. The random error component for the example above has been considered to be the width of a confidence interval specified at 99%. The random error component of an analytical measurement is a characteristic of the method and the primary measure of the method's performance. Systematic errors are theoretically correctable errors and are related more to calibration and the purity of primary standards. It may be desirable to determine if the observed error is due to random error alone so that systematic errors can be corrected if they exist. This is accomplished through application of a *t*-test to determine whether or not the average value of a set of measurements differs significantly from that of the true or nominal value. If the difference is significant, there is some correctable systematic error.

The FDA lists accuracy and precision criteria for acceptance of a method for the purpose of bioanalytical data submissions. It is recommended that four control concentrations spanning the range of calibration should be employed, one of which is no more than three times the LLOQ and one prepared at the LLOQ. The percentage accuracy deviation and percentage RSD must be within 15% for all controls except for the LLOQ, which is expected to be within 20% RSD and accuracy. This absolute approach taken by the FDA guidance is generally appropriate for validation of analytical methods, as the question addressed in validation is whether or not the method is good enough for the intended purpose. The fixed acceptance criteria for bioanalytical methods suggest that all data be at least as good as a minimal threshold value and that all methods should conform to this threshold. It could be argued that some methods that are very precise by nature or that measure relatively high concentrations should be held to a higher standard or conversely that very challenging methods should be given more flexibility. It also follows that certain applications such as very narrow therapeutic window drugs might require tighter control whereas other applications may not. These situations may be compensated for in application of the guidelines although deviations from the fixed recommendations will no doubt require rigorous scientific justification. If it is simply not possible for a given analytical method at a needed concentration to provide results within the fixed guidelines, the most straightforward solution to the problem is to conduct sample analysis and validation in replicate. The RSD of a method can be effectively reduced by a factor of $1/\sqrt{n}$,. where represents the number of replicates assayed. In this way. the variability of both the sample measurement and the validation data will be lowered through use of an average value rather than the single individual measurement. This approach is recommended in the FDA guidance. In cases in which inaccuracy exceeds the threshold value, use of the average of replicate measurements may provide a better estimate of the true value but will not necessarily reduce inaccuracy. The systematic error may also be corrected through better calibration or standardization of the method or by limiting calibration to a smaller concentration range.

Stability Testing

Stability of an analyte in the matrix in question is an important part of the validation process. The stability of an analyte is not only a function of the chemical nature of the substance itself but also of the matrix and container in which it is stored. Instability can result from both chemical and physical processes and the most accepted way to show stability is to monitor the concentration of the analyte in question over a time period and under conditions set to reflect the handling of unknown samples. Although the FDA guidance suggests that stability should be evaluated during the sample collection process, there are few analytical laboratories that have control over this process. Stability studies that are normally carried out by analytical laboratories include:

1. Freeze/thaw stability testing in which three control samples are frozen at the storage temperature and thawed and refrozen a total of three times. The sample is then analyzed after the third cycle and the results are compared to results measured prior to the freezing cycles.
2. Short-term stability in which controls are stored at room temperature for 4–24 h (based on the expected time samples will be kept at room temperature), then analyzed and compared to results from samples not left at room temperature.
3. Long-term storage stability in which samples are stored under long-term storage conditions and analyzed after a time expected to be the longest storage time for samples. Results measured from freshly prepared controls are compared to the results from the stored samples to indicate storage stability or instability.
4. Stock solution stability in which standard solutions in the appropriate solvent and container are analyzed before and after a minimum of 6 h of storage, or the longest time expected for stock solution storage. The storage conditions should replicate that which is employed for normal conditions. The instrument responses of these samples should then be compared to those of freshly prepared solutions.
5. Prepared sample stability in which processed samples stored under the conditions needed for analysis such as on an autosampler tray are analyzed and compared to results obtained form samples not stored for the indicated period of time.

All of these stability studies involve comparison of results from stored samples to those freshly prepared or unstored. The guidance suggests that samples from dosed subjects may also be investigated for stability but stop short of requiring that this type of sample be tested. There is no acceptance criterion established in the FDA guidance, although it is suggested that a statistical approach based on confidence limits may be employed. The guidance does not prevent employment of combined stability studies, and these may make sense in terms of preserving laboratory efficiency. For example, samples could be analyzed that not only have been frozen and thawed three times but have also been kept at room temperature and left prepared on an autosampler for a designated amount of time. In this way three stability studies are combined into one and if stability is indicated, nothing further needs to be done. If instability is indicated, however, individual studies should be carried out to determine the source of the instability. In contrast to procedures for determination of accuracy and precision, the FDA guidance offers little information as to how to conduct stability studies. General principles for stability tests of drug products have been established and would apply to bioanalytical studies as well. These include the following:

1. The method used for stability testing must be shown to be stability indicating. For bioanalytical methods, this should consist of making sure that degradation products, either known or created through forced degradation, do not interfere with quantitation of the analyte.
2. The time zero reference should be a measured (not nominal) value that has been rigorously established with sufficient replication.
3. Sufficient replication of the timed stability samples needs to be carried out to provide a reliable mean measured result.
4. The entire concentration range in question should be investigated, as significant differences in rated of degradation can occur at different concentrations.
5. Blank matrix samples should be run in conjunction with stability samples to ensure the absence of interferences that may appear with time.
6. Freshly prepared and matrix matched samples should be used.

The decision as to whether or not to conclude stability or instability should be based on the precision of the method and the acceptance criterion for validation. As the FDA guideline states that a method should be accurate to within 15 %, it would follow that an acceptance criterion for stability should be similar. This would result in a straightforward fixed threshold value that would be consistent with the accuracy criterion. Accuracy is based on a comparison to the nominal value and stability studies are more appropriately based on a measured mean reference value. If a criterion of 15 % is to be applied to stability testing in a matrix, then it should be measured relative to a mean time zero reference. A more statistically valid approach would be to compare the measured stability values via a confidence interval approach. This may involve the upper limit of the confidence interval of stability measurements being not less than some lower acceptable limit (usually 90% of the reference) or that the lower limit of the confidence interval be not greater than some higher acceptable limit (usually 110% of the reference). This approach ensures that a method does not fail the stability test unless there is a high level of confidence that the sample mean is outside the acceptance range. The level of confidence or probability that the sample is actually unstable when you have concluded that it is not, is determined by the size of the confidence interval chosen. Ninety-five percent and 90 % confidence intervals have both been used for this purpose.

QUALITY CONTROL

The goal of a good quality control program is to determine whether or not a method is performing up to specifications during the process of analyzing unknown samples. This is in contrast to the goal of validation, in which it is desired to show that a method is good enough for an intended purpose. For this reason, it is necessary to view the quality control process as more of a relative criterion than an absolute one. Relative assessment of quality control data from a sample run can be efficiently carried out employing the use of quality control charts. The control chart concept involves setting up an acceptance criterion based on the mean of quality control measurements at a given concentration plus and minus some factor, related to the desired level of confidence, times the standard deviation of the quality control measurements. For example, an acceptance range of 12.06–18.34 would result from a mean of 15.2 with a standard deviation of 1.22 if the level of confidence chosen were 99% (a factor of 2.58). The mean and standard deviation are established with the control results themselves as collected or based on validation data collected prior to the sample run. They can be updated with new data as quality control runs are carried out. The precision of the method itself therefore determines the acceptance criterion, and more precise methods would generate a narrower acceptance range whereas less precise methods would generate a broader acceptance range. This is appropriate if the established goal is to monitor whether or not a method is performing as well as it should be expected to perform. A fixed criterion applied to the same data set would not allow this kind of flexibility and the fixed criteria would inherently be too wide to be effective for precise methods and would be sufficiently narrow such that less precise methods would fail at a high rate, even though the method is performing as well as expected based on validation data.

The control chart approach is the standard in areas such as forensic science, clinical chemistry, and general manufacturing. There are a large number of scientific and statistical investigations and procedures to draw from that utilize the general control chart approach. These allow decision-making such as trend and shift analysis. Westgard's rules, which are based on control charts, have been shown to be optimal in terms of maximizing error detection while minimizing false rejection of data. Although control charts do a good job of monitoring method precision and consistency, they do not alone address accuracy of control data during the time samples are analyzed, and an additional accuracy criterion should be employed to make sure the mean value for the control data is accurate to within an established reasonable limit.

Questions to be addressed when setting up an analytical run incorporating quality control samples is the number and sequence of quality control samples and the way in which acceptance criteria will be applied. It is generally accepted that control samples should be prepared at three concentrations that are representative of the concentration range of the method. The number of replicates of these three concentrations will of course determine the total number of quality control samples run, which in turn will affect the error detection and false rejection probabilities as well as the sample throughput efficiency. The number of replicates is therefore an important consideration, and this number should be established as a percentage of the total number of samples in the run to preserve consistency in these critical parameters from run to run. It is also important to keep the number of replicates at each of the three concentrations consistent to preserve a balanced statistical design and to ensure the same decision-making power at each concentration level.

Quality control samples should be sequenced within the analytical run to maximize the degree of concentration coverage over the entire run and to minimize the number of samples run between each control. The best decision-making power would be derived from a run sequence that involves all three controls being run before and after each sample. In this way each sample would be controlled at each concentration just prior to and after it is run, minimizing any time delay before a control sample is run. Few industries can allow such inefficient sample throughput, however, and a good compromise would be to alternate high, medium, and low concentration controls each separated by an equal number of samples. Acceptance of the sample data can then be done according to criteria applied to the entire run or the run can be subdivided into "brackets." Samples that are contained between each control would constitute a bracket and whether or not the samples are acceptable depends on the acceptability of only the controls that bracket the samples. The advantages of the brackets approach are that acceptable samples are taken only from between acceptable controls and portions of a run may be preserved even if a significant portion of the run is out of specification. The brackets approach does a much better job of controlling for transient errors that may appear and disappear during the course of a run. In contrast, a criterion based on rejection of an entire run would result in data being rejected even though the problem had disappeared if rejection was due to a transient problem. The advantage of a criterion applied to the entire run is that the process is simpler and easier to manage.

The FDA guidance favors a criterion applied to the entire run. The guidance further states that quality control samples should be run at three concentrations in duplicate but further stipulates that the number of quality control samples (run in multiples of the three concentrations to provide a balanced design) should be dependent on the number of samples in a run. The minimum percentage of quality controls to samples is specified as 5%. The FDA guidance offers no stipulation on the sequence of samples, calibration standards, and quality controls within an analytical run.

The primary acceptance criterion for the entire run is that at least four of six quality control samples must be within 15% of their respective nominal value although the two allowed outside this range cannot be the same concentration. This so-called 4/6/15 rule was modified from a draft version of the guidance that stipulated a 4/6/20 rule. The FDA Guidance also states that a confidence interval approach yielding comparable accuracy and precision is an appropriate alternative to the 4/6/15 rule but does not specify the level of confidence to be applied. The 4/6/15 rule is loosely based on a quality control procedure proposed by Causey et al. that used a 67% (1S) confidence interval to establish acceptance limits although their limit was 10% rather than 15% or 20% . The FDA guidance contains further stipulations on the acceptance of concentration residuals from the calibration curve and implies that validation type criteria are applied to intrarun quality control data.

The acceptance criterion proposed by Causey et al. is consistent with the criterion of 10% they proposed for validation of precision and is statistically valid. The 4/6/10 rule with a 10% acceptance criterion for the RSD (also based on 1S) is statistically valid, if applied relative to a mean measured value, as a 67% confidence interval around a mean would be predicted statistically to yield 67% of measurements within this interval. This is provided that the method demonstrated a precision of 1S (10% in this case) and there were no method errors beyond the level of error demonstrated during validation. These method errors that inflate the level of error beyond what has been determined to be acceptable during validation are what a quality control program is supposed to detect. The FDA guidance criterion of 4/6/15 would also be consistent with their validation criterion of 15% RSD if it were based on a mean measured value. The guidance states, however, that the criterion is to be applied to a "nominal" value, which is most often taken as the target value the quality control sample was prepared to be. This means that the FDA guidance criterion encompasses both random and systematic error. The validation criterion in the guidance for both random and systematic error (accuracy and precision) is 15%, and because these errors are additive, the criterion is actually a criterion for total error. The statistically valid criterion for quality control based on a nominal value would therefore be 30%, which is derived form the sum of the allowable accuracy and precision errors. The allowable random error is determined in this case by the 1S interval (67% or 4 of 6) and is 15% according to the guidance on precision validation. The allowable systematic error is 15% also as determined by the accuracy criterion and the criteria for bias should therefore be 30% to be statistically valid. The FDA guidance could also be

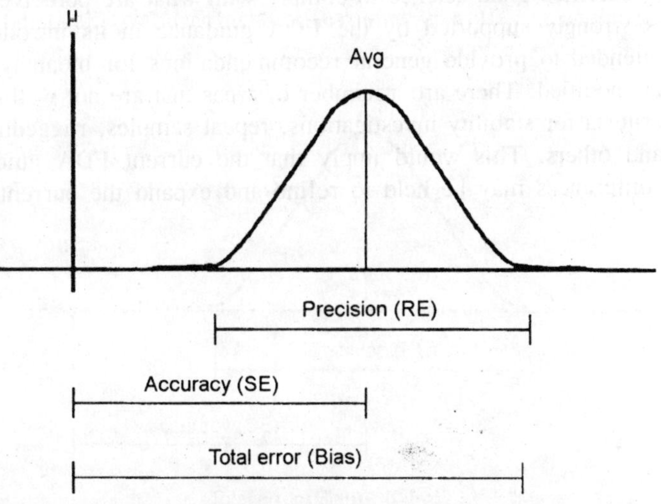

Fig. 4.6. The concept of total error. Imprecision or random error (RE) is related to the standard deviation of the set of measurements.

made statistically valid by application of the 4/6/15 rule to the mean of quality control values and with a separate accuracy criterion of 15%.

The FDA guidance approach has been compared using real bioanalytical data for 10 analytical methods and found to be in disagreement with three statistically derived approaches involving confidence intervals, Westgard' s rules, and a range chart approach. The statistically valid approaches were all relatively consistent with one another. The danger that exists for the bioanalytical scientist is that methods that pass the FDA guidance validation criteria but are borderline in terms of accuracy and precision can be expected to incur a large number of quality control failures in routine analysis. To avoid this, a reasonable practice would be to proceed with routine analysis of samples only when methods demonstrate a total error (inaccuracy plus imprecision) of no more than 15%, even though the acceptance limit for total error in validation is 30% according to the FDA guidance. It is also important to be aware that the FDA criterion is not statistically valid, and although it is the standard of practice in drug development, can be challenged successfully on a scientific basis.

A scientific and statistically valid approach to validation and quality control is important to be consistent with the standard of practice outside of the drug development discipline. The science of validation and quality control is generally well developed and easily understood for those with a background in statistics. Standard operating procedures should be developed with this in mind and a balance should be found between what is perceived to be compliance and good science. It is inappropriate to sacrifice good science to comply with what are perceived to be regulatory preferences. This concept is strongly supported by the FDA guidance in its introduction, where it states that the guidance is intended to provide general recommendations for bioanalytical method validation that can be adjusted or modified. There are a number of areas that are not well developed in the guidance such as acceptance criteria for stability investigations, repeat samples, ruggedness testing, selectivity in mass spectroscopy, and others. This would imply that the current FDA guidance is a work in progress and additional conferences may be held to refine and expand the current guidelines further.

5

Validation of Pharmaceutical Processes

Process validation is a requirement of current Good Manufacturing Practices (GMPs) for finished pharmaceuticals (21 CFR 211) and of the GMP regulations for medical devices (21 CFR 820) and therefore applies to the manufacture of both drug products and medical devices. According to the FDA Guidelines on General Principles of Process Validation, process validation is defined, "as establishing documented evidence, which provides a high degree of assurance, that a specific process will consistently produce a product meeting its predetermined specifications and quality characteristics." The process for making a drug product consists of a series of unit operations (modules) that result in the manufacture of the finished pharmaceutical. There is much confusion regarding the definition of process validation and what constitutes process validation documentation. The term validation is used here generically to cover the entire spectrum of current GMP concerns, essential most of which are; facility, equipment, component, method, and process qualification. Based upon the FDA process validation guidelines, the specific term should be reserved for the final stage(s) of the product and process development sequence.

The end of the development sequence, which should be assigned to formal (three-batch) process validation, derives from the fact that the specific exercise of process validation should never be designed to fail. Failure in carrying out the formal process validation assignment is often the result of incomplete or faulty understanding of the process capability, in other words, what the process can and cannot accomplish under a given set of operational requirements. In a well-designed validation program, most of the effort should be spent on facilities, equipment, components, methods, and process qualification. In such a program, the formalized, final three-batch validation sequence provides only the necessary process validation documentation required by the FDA to show product reproducibility and a manufacturing process in a state of control. Such a strategy is consistent with the FDA preapproval inspection program directive.

Process Validation Options

The guidelines on general principles of process validation mention three options: prospective process validation (also called *premarket validation*), retrospective process validation, and revalidation. Actually there are four, if concurrent process validation is included. Prospective validation is carried out prior to the distribution of a new product or an existing product made under a revised manufacturing process where such revisions may affect product specifications or quality characteristics. The prospective approach features critical step analysis in which the unit operations are challenged during the process qualification stage to determine those critical process variables that may affect overall process performance, using either worst-case analysis or a fractional–factorial design. During formal, three-batch, prospective validation, critical process variables should be set within their operating ranges and should not exceed their upper and lower control limits during process operation. Output responses should be well within finished-product specifications.

Retrospective validation is recognized in both current GMPs and the FDA process validation guidelines. It involves accumulated in-process production and final product testing and control (numerical) data to establish that the product and its manufacturing process are in a state of control. Valid in-process results should be consistent with the final specifications of the drug product and shall be derived from previous acceptable process average and process variability estimates where possible and determined by the application of suitable statistical procedures (quality control charting) where appropriate.

The retrospective validation option is chosen for established products whose manufacturing processes are considered to be stable and when, on the basis of economic considerations and resource limitations, prospective qualification and validation experimentation cannot be justified. Prior to undertaking either prospective or retrospective validation, the facilities, equipment, and subsystems used in connection with the manufacturing process must be qualified in conformance with cGMP requirements. Concurrent validation studies are carried out under a protocol during the course of normal production. The first three production-scale batches must be monitored as comprehensively as possible. The evaluation of the results is used in establishing the acceptance criteria and specifications of subsequent in-process control and final product testing. Some form of concurrent validation, using statistical process control techniques (quality control charting) may be employed throughout the product manufacturing life cycle.

Revalidation is required to ensure that changes in the process and/or in the process environment, whether introduced intentionally or unintentionally, do not adversely affect product specifications and quality characteristics. There should be a quality assurance program (change control) in place which requires revalidation whenever there are significant changes in formulation, equipment, process, and packaging that may impact on product and manufacturing process performance. Furthermore, when a change is made in a raw material supplier, the drug manufacturer should be made aware of subtle, potentially adverse differences in raw material characteristics that may adversely affect product and manufacturing process performance. It is recommended that every requested change be reviewed by the validation or CMC committee. Such a committee should judge if a change is significant for revalidation and decide on a course of action to be taken. The following conditions require revalidation study and documentation:

1. Change in a critical component (usually refers to active pharmaceutical ingredient, key excipients, or primary packaging);
2. Change or replacement in a critical piece of modular (capital) equipment;
3. Significant change in processing conditions that may affect subsequent unit operations and product quality;
4. Change in a facility and/or plant (usually location, site, or support systems);
5. Significant increase or decrease in batch size that affects the operation of modular equipment; and
6. Sequential batches that fail to meet product and process in-process specifications.

In some situations process performance requalification studies may be required prior to undertaking specific revalidation assignments. With the exception of sterile products manufacture, periodic revalidation is not required at the present time. The performance and state of control of the product and its manufacturing process can be adequately covered during the annual product and process review. The

FDA has issued an interim guidance document that addresses what constitutes major and minor formulation and manufacturing changes for immediate-release solid dosage forms. Such documentation and others to follow should simplify manufacturing decisions about the need to revalidate.

Validation Priorities

There is a basic concept with respect to which pharmaceutical processes should be given a higher priority over others. All pharmaceutical manufacturing processes require process validation documentation, but there is an accepted logical approach to priority selection, in the following order:

1. Sterile products and their processes
   - large volume parenterals (LVPs) infusions greater than 100 ml
   - small volume parenterals (SVPs) single and multiple dose injections
   - ophthalmics and sterile devices
2. Non-sterile products and their processes
   - low dose high potency tablets and capsules
   - drugs with inherent stability problems
   - transdermal delivery (TDD) and inhalation products
   - the rest of the oral solid dosage forms
   - oral liquids and topical products

The best approach to assessing problems with respect to a terminal sterilization method (i.e., moist heat, dry heat, radiation, and chemical methods) is to first establish the qualification, validation and stability of the pharmaceutical process prior to conducting a given sterilization procedure.

Validation Committee

In most companies, the validation or Chemistry, Manufacturing and Control (CMC) committee is charged with the responsibility of establishing and operating the complete validation program for the specific manufacturing site. In some companies the program is led by a validation manager whereas in others, quality assurance personnel have taken on expanded responsibilities in this regard. Specific process validation assignments are carried out by those with the necessary training and experience. The specifics of how the committee is organized to conduct process validation assignments is beyond the scope of this article. Other members may include Quality Control, Regularity affairs, etc.

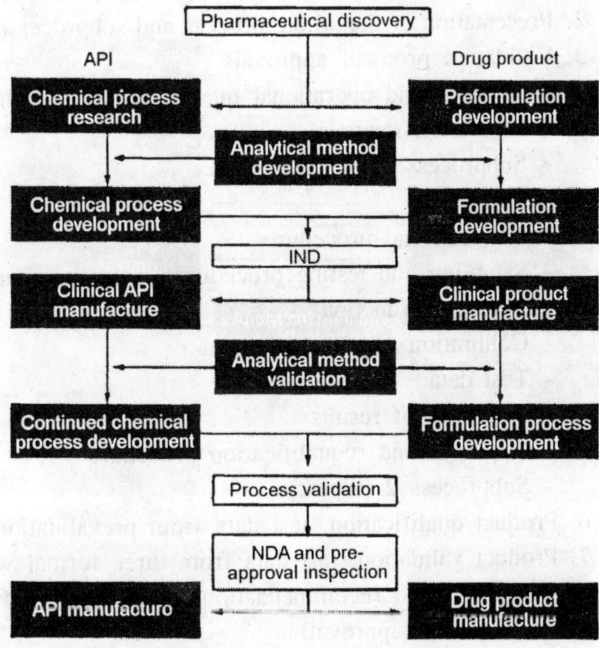

Fig. 5.1. Process validation progress chart.

Validation Master Plan

The creation of a master plan permits the development of a logical overview of the validation effort. It lays out in a logical sequence the activities or key elements or both to be performed in accordance with the approximate time schedule in a Gantt or PERT chart format. The master plan establishes the critical path through the chart against which progress can be monitored. The validation program starts with the design and development of raw materials and components, followed by the IQ/OQ of facilities, equipment, and systems through performance and process qualification stages, and terminates in the protocol-driven, three- batch, formal process validation program. Most of these activities move forward in series. However, by combining activities and elements and moving in parallel, where possible, on independent tracks with respect to active pharmaceutical ingredients (APIs) analytical methods development, facilities, equipment, support systems, and the drug product design and manufacturing process development, a great deal of time can be saved before the individual elements or grouping of activities are combined prior to the formal process validation program.

Installation Qualification (IQ)

This includes procedures and documentation to show that all important aspects of the installation of the facility, support system, or piece of modular equipment, having been properly calibrated, meet its design specifications and that the vendor's recommendations had been suitably considered.

Operational Qualification (OQ)

Following IQ, procedures and documentation show that the facility, support system, or piece of modular equipment perform as intended throughout all anticipated operating ranges under a suitable load.

Performance Qualification (PQ)

Following IQ and OQ, actual demonstrations during the course of the validation program show that the facility, support system, or piece of modular equipment perform according to a predefined protocol and achieve process reproducibility and product acceptability.

Validation Protocol and Report

The following validation protocol and format for the completed validation report have been suggested in the WHO Guidelines on Validation of Manufacturing Processes (TRS 823).

1. Purpose (for the whole validation) and prerequisites
2. Presentation of the whole process and subprocesses including flow diagram and critical step analysis
3. Validation protocol approvals
4. Installation and operational qualifications, including blueprints or drawings
5. Qualification report(s)
   - Subprocess 1
   - Purpose
   - Methods and procedures
   - Sampling and testing procedures, release criteria
   - Reporting function
   - Calibration of test equipment
   - Test data
   - Summary of results
   - Approval and requalification procedure
   - Subprocess 2 (repeat)
6. Product qualification, test data from prevalidation batches
7. Product validation, test data from three formal validation batches
8. Evaluation and recommendations (include revalidation and requalification requirements)
9. Certification (approval)
10. Summary report with conclusions

The validation protocol and report may also include copies of the product stability report or its summary as well as validation documentation on cleaning and analytical methods.

Preapproval Inspection

The FDA Preapproval Inspection Program is designed to provide a basis for determining the adequacy and accuracy of reported and factual information in New Drug Application (NDA) and Abbreviated New Drug Application (ANDA) submissions with respect to the suitability of cGMP product development, analytical laboratory, and manufacturing facilities. A preapproval inspection checklist should include the following documentation which may be required prior to the formal inspection:

1. API development and validation report(s) including impurity profile and polymorphic forms;
2. Pharmaceutical (dosage form) development report;
3. Stability and clinical batch records and history, including phase-III program;
4. Data for API and key excipients used in the manufacture of clinical and biobatches;
5. Bioequivalency report;
6. Technical transfer report (development to manufacturing/QA/QC);
7. Copy of the CMC section of the NDA including information on suppliers and vendors;
8. Copy of proposed production monograph and master batch record;
9. Equipment validation report establishing IQ and OQ;
10. Cleaning validation report;
11. Analytical methods validation and computer systems validation reports;
12. Stability report establishing expiry dating; and
13. Process validation protocol for formal three- batch validation of production-size batches.

During preapproval inspection, the FDA accepts a process-validation protocol based on the company's commitment to complete successfully three production- size validation batches prior to product launch. In some situations a prevalidation (process demonstration qualification) production-size batch is completed before the entire formal three-batch program is carried out.

Pilot Scale-up and Technology Transfer

The pilot-production program may be carried out as a shared responsibility between the development laboratories and their appropriate manufacturing counterpart or as a process demonstration by a separate, designated pilot-plant or process development department. Supporting technology transfer documentation applies to both the specific process and system being qualified and validated and the related testing standards and testing methods. The formal technology transfer is normally made from the development laboratories or the process development pilot-plant to pharmaceutical production function. In actuality, a number of technology transfer points and documents are generated as prospective validation proceeds through the various stages of product development.

Solid pharmaceutical dosage forms (tablets and capsules) are used to illustrate the various stages of product and process development. These principles and practices also apply in a general way to the development of liquid and semisolid pharmaceutical dosage forms.

Stages of Validation

Elements of the validation concept should be incorporated during each of the various stages of the product and process development continuum. These stages can be summarized as follows.

Stage Preformulation Studies: APIs plus rey excipients

Stage I Product design and development

Stage II Preparation of clinical and biobatches

Stage III Process scale-up and evaluation
Stage IV Formal process validation

Preformulation Studies: API

Preformulation testing of the specific API of interest and key excipients to be used in the product design stage, alone and in combinations with the API, should be included as a preliminary first step in the product and process development sequence. A simple check list of items worth consideration in preformulation studies with APIs and important or critical excipients is provided as follows:

API

- Key excipients
  - Fillers and diluents - Binders
  - Disintegrants
  - Glidants and lubricants Establish chemical and physical compatibility
- Minimize lot-to-lot variability in properties
- Worldwide availability from comparable suppliers
- Properties for possible evaluation
  - Color, odor, taste, solubility;
  - Particle morphology (DSC, TGA, x-ray diffraction);
  - Particle size distribution and surface area;
  - Crystal and bulk density, compaction index;
  - Angle of repose and flowability index;
  - Spectrophotometry (UV, FTIR, NMR, OR);
  - Water content, LOD, moisture uptake;
  - Microbial limits and heavy metals;
  - HPLC assay and impurity profile.

Before preformulation studies are undertaken, two-way technical communication between the manufacturers of the API (laboratory and plant) and the pharmaceutical product development laboratories must be established. It should start early and be maintained through-out the product and process development program. In addition to potency, purity, and stability considerations of the API, the product development department is especially interested in the chemical and physical form (free acid or base, salts, esters, amides, polymorphs, solvates, particle size and shape) of the API. Time spent early in the cycle in establishing these particular factors often aids and/or simplifies the subsequent product and process development program. Not every subject shown above must be tested or addressed. However, aspect, particle morphology and size, compaction and flowability, water content, spectrophotometric and chromatographic data should be studied and monitored throughout the product and process development program. Because key excipients are well established in most new product and process development programs, the same degree of preformulation scrutiny is often not required. Compatibility studies with the API, however, should be performed to study possible untoward interactions between the active ingredients and the excipients. It should be kept in mind that small or minor changes in physical and possibly chemical properties upon intimate contact in binary studies with key excipients should not automatically exclude a favored excipient without further critical testing.

Stage I: Product Design and Development

Following successful preformulation studies, the API is transferred to the formulations laboratory for preliminary product design and development studies. In most cases, the drug is mixed with an appropriate diluent or filler and glidant combination and filled into two-piece opaque hard-shell capsules for preliminary stability and subsequent phase I clinical studies versus matching placebo capsules. At or about the same time, initial studies of a prototype tablet formulation should be started. The key steps in the product design and development sequence are given below.

Stage I: Product Design: 1 × Laboratory Scale (1–10 kg)

- Hard-shell capsule (phase I clinical trials) followed by prototype tablet dosage form
  - Direct compression versus wet granulation
  - Maximize chemical and physical stability
  - Minimize product and process costs
  - Product characterization
  - Product selection
  - Process design
- Excipients are selected among the following categories:

Binder, diluents, and disintegrants including alginates, calcium phosphate, cellulose, dextrates, gelatin, povidones, starch and derivatives, sorbitol, sucrose, and derivatives. Glidants and lubricants including colloidal silicon dioxide, hydrogenated vegetable oil, mineral oil, PEG, silica gel, sodium lauryl sulfate, stearates, talc. Although the work is conducted in the research or formulations laboratory using small-scale processing equipment, it is important to gain early experience with colorant systems that have been selected for the finished tablet product; color aids in blend-uniformity evaluation.

In addition to excipient screening and selection, it is important to gauge processing parameters that are more fully explored during the scale-up phases. These processing factors include flowability, compaction and compressibility of powders and granules, content uniformity of powder and granule blends and finished tablets, moisture uptake, in vitro dissolution release profiles, and subsequent full-scale stability testing.

Products used in human clinical trials must, of course, conform to good laboratory, good clinical, and good manufacturing practice requirements.

Stage II: Process Development: Pilot Laboratory (Clinical)

After the (1X) "go" laboratory batch has been determined to be both physically and chemical stable, based upon accelerated, elevated temperature testing (1 month at 45°C or 3 month at 40°C and 80% relative humidity) the next step (stage II) is to scale the product and its process to (10X) pilot-laboratory size batch(es). This batch represents the first replicated scale-up of the designated formula. Its size usually ranges between 10 and 100 kg, 10 and 100L, or 10,000 to 100,000 units. Often these pilot-laboratory batches are used in clinical trials and bioequivalency studies. According to the FDA, the minimum requirement for a biobatch is 100,000 units.

Pilot-laboratory batches are usually prepared in small pilot equipment within a designated current GMP approved facility. The number and size of these pilot-laboratory batches may vary, depending on one or more of the following factors:

- Equipment availability
- API availability
- Cost of raw materials
- Inventory requirements for both clinical and non- clinical studies

Process development (process qualification) or process capability studies are normally started in this important stage II of the scale-up sequence. The scope of stage-II process development consists essentially of product optimization and process characterization studies.

Product optimization

- Establish formula rationale and boundary conditions for API and excipients

Process characterization

- Define unit operations, process variables, and response parameters.
  - Define critical process variables and response parameters using simple experimental designs.
  - Establish provisional control limits for critical process variables and their response parameters based on process replication.
- Maintain product stability.

  Unit operations for solid dosage-form development include:
  - Granulation
  - Drying
  - Sizing
  - Blending and mixing
  - Encapsulation andar tablet compression
  - Coating
  - Filling and packaging

Unit operations are selected for the development of a tablet (coated or non-coated) or capsule (hard shell or soft-gel) process. Unit operations that are considered to be critical are determined through analysis of the process variables and their respective measured response for each unit operation.

In order to determine critical control parameters and their unit operations, constraint analysis techniques followed by fractional factorial designs are used to challenge the tentative control limits (so-called worst-case analysis) established for the process at this intermediate stage. Time and effort spent to qualify the process at the 10X stage often simplifies the work that follows during stages III and IV.

Von Doehren et al. and Chowhan have described the various stages of solid dosage form process development as it relates to technology transfer and process validation. Their respective approaches to the topic have been integrated in this article.

Fahrner raises the following issues regarding the new role for pilot plants in product development.

1. Too much time is devoted to preliminary or applied research and not enough to the proper development of the process.
2. Often a suitable manufacturing strategy is lacking during the early phases of the program, which results in poorly planned technology transfer and an inappropriate division of responsibility with respect to the overall program.
3. Most laboratory processes are rarely scalable, since piloting is a scaled-down version of manufacturing not a scaled-up version of the laboratory batch.

Fahrner makes the case for a separate pilot facility (process development function) to bridge the communication gap between R & D and production.

Stage III: Pilot Production

The technology transfer of the product and process from the traditional product development function to a separate process development (pilot plant) function or production itself is normally carried out at the (100×) pilot-production batch stage (100–1000 kg):

- Full-scale production batch
- For possible future commercial or clinical use

- Evaluate critical process parameters; product and process are scaled to another order of magnitude (100x)
- Process optimization
  - Mixing and blending times
  - Drying times
  - Milling operations
  - Press speed, compression force
  - Encapsulation speed, tamping settings
  - Speed, air flow, spray settings, temperature
- Process qualification (prevalidation batches); determine process capability, challenge in-process control limits
- Maintain product stability

The creation of a separate pilot plant or process development unit has been favored in recent years because it is ideally suited to carry out key process qualification and/or process validation studies in a timely manner.

The objective of the pilot-production batch is to scale the product and its process by another order of magnitude (100x). For most solid dosage forms it represents a full production scale batch, in standard equipment. The technology transfer documents should include the technical information normally required for preapproval inspection:

1. Preformulation information
2. Product development report
3. Product stability report
4. Analytical methods report
5. Proposed manufacturing formula, manufacturing instruction, in-process and final product specifications at the 100x-batch size

The objectives of prevalidation trials at stage III (100x pilot production) is to qualify and optimize the process in full-scale production equipment and their facilities.

Rushing through the first (100 x) pilot-production batch in order to proceed with formal validation should be discouraged. Small problems that often arise during (100x) scale-up should be addressed immediately and not ignored. Such problems are often best addressed by returning to the laboratories (10x) for supplemental process characterization and qualification studies.

Many companies, however, proceed directly to three-batch formal validation without stage III prevalidation work and often complete formal trials prior to preapproval inspection. The downside of this alternative strategy is that finished production batches often remain in the warehouse beyond their approved expiry dating period.

When faced with a choice of strategies, there is no one ideal way of completing the pilot scale-up and validation sequence other than depending on prior experience with related products and their processes.

Stage IV: Formal Process Validation

In the normal course of events and following a successfully completed preapproval inspection, formal, three- batch process validation is carried out in accordance with the protocol approved during the preapproval inspection. The primary objective of the formal process validation exercise is to establish process reproducibility and consistency. The program is not designed to challenge upper and lower control limits (so-called worst-case analysis) of critical process variables. Such upper and lower control limit challenging is normally conducted during the stage II (10X size) process characterization, optimization, and qualification program, using suitable and reasonable experimental designs. The documentation to be established before, during, and after formal process validation is shown below. The protocols and the subsequent formal validation studies are designed to establish uniformity among the three batches with respect to granulation, blending, finished tablet, and finished capsule stages.

100 × production batches

- Complete product development program and report
- Prepare protocol for prospective process validation
- Complete preapproval inspection requirements; conduct three-batch formal process validation, establish reproducibility for mixing, blending, and compression or encapsulation operations
- Establish process documentation
  - Preformulation report
  - Analytical methods validation report
  - IQ/OQ and cleaning validation reports
  - Formula development report
  - Process feasibility report
  - Manufacturing bioequivalency report
  - Product development report
  - Process validation protocol
  - Process validation report
  - Product stability report

In that respect, the following test data and results are used to show process reproducibility and consistency among validation batches: particle or granule size distribution, bulk density, moisture content, hardness, thickness, friability, weight uniformity, potency uniformity, disintegration–dissolution profile, and product stability. Not every one of these categories have to be addressed nor followed both during in-process and final product testing. Nevertheless, testing must be sufficient to establish process reproducibility and demonstrate, with a high degree of certainly, that the product and process are in a state of control.

Whenever possible, formal validation studies should continue through packaging and labeling operations (whole or in-part), so that machinability and stability of the finished product can be established and documented in the primary container–closure system. Recently the FDA, with the cooperation of the Pharmaceutical Industry has developed a series of guidance procedures to speed approval of post approval changes with or without process scale-up changes. At the present time the SUPAC (scale-up post approval change) program covers the following product categories:

- Immediate Release (IR) solid dosage forms
- Extended Release (ER) solid dosage forms
- Delayed Release (MR) solid dosage forms
- Semisolids (SS) dosage forms
- API changes presently called BACPAC
- Packaging changes called PACPAC
- Analytical Methods changes called AMPAC
- Sterile Aqueous Solutions called SUPAC-SAS

If the program is successful, other dosage form categories will be added later.

The following changes are covered:

- Components and Composition Changes
- Manufacturing Equipment and Process Changes
- Batch Size (scale-up) Changes
- Manufacturing Site Changes

The program consists of three levels:

- Level 1 or minor changes that are made without FDA approval and reported in the Annual Report (AR).
- Level 2 or intermediate changes that may be instituted by first filing a Change Being Effected (CBE) Supplement with the FDA and waiting 30 days for a reply before instituting the change.
- Level 3 or major change in which a prior approval supplement (PAS) is filed with the FDA and approval must be obtained from the FDA before proceeding with the change.

This new program is off to a good start and is intermittently involved with the need for adequate process validation studies and documentation to support the changes requested.

CHANGE CONTROL

Procedures with respect to establishing change control should be in place before, during, and after the completion of the formal validation program. A change control system maintains a sense of functionality as the process evolves and provides the necessary documentation trail that ensures that the process continues in a validated, operational state, even when small non-critical adjustments and changes have been made. Such minor, non-critical changes in materials, methods, and machines should be reviewed by the validation commitee (development, engineering, production, and QA/QC) to ensure that process integrity and comparability have been maintained and documented before the specific change that has been requested can be approved by the head of the quality control unit. The change control system, based upon an approved standard operating procedure(s) (SOPs), takes on added importance as the vehicle or instrument through which innovation and process improvements can be made more easily and more flexibly without prior formal review on the part of the NDA and ANDA reviewing function of the FDA. If more of the supplemental procedures with respect to the chemistry and manufacturing control sections of NDAs and ANDAs could be covered through annual review documentation procedures, with appropriate safeguards, process validation will become more innovative.

OUT-OF-SPECIFICATIONS

Probably the single most important technical issue facing the pharmaceutical industry at the present time is the question: what constitutes process or batch failure in terms of an out-of-specification (OOS) assay value? The concept of product and/or process failure appears twice in the cGMPs.

According to 21 CFR Sect. 211.165(f), "Drug products failing to meet established standards or specifications and other relevant quality control criteria shall be rejected." In CFR Sect. 211.192 it is stated: Any unexplained discrepancy (including a percentage of theoretical yield exceeding the maximum or minimum percentages established in master production and control records) or the failure of a batch or any of its components to meet any of its specifications shall be thoroughly investigated [regardless] whether the batch has already been distributed. The investigation shall extend to other batches of the same drug product and other drug products that may have been associated with the specific failure or discrepancy. A written record of the investigation shall be made and shall include the conclusions and follow-up. The key to establishing product and/or process failure is to verify the accuracy, relevance, and reproducibility of deviant assay value(s), test result(s), and recorded number(s) that are reported. All companies should have SOPs in place that cover first the verification of deviant numbers in the quality control laboratories and, following that investigation and a report showing the test result to be deviant, a second set of SOPs covering follow-up actions taken as described in the following steps:

1. A written procedure for full investigation when there is not a verified laboratory error.
2. Scientific criteria for retesting and resampling during the formal investigation.
3. Description and results of the formal investigation into possible causes of the OOS result(s).
4. Results of all testing involved during the investigation.
5. A scientific basis and justification for discarding any OOS test result and accepting the batch in question.
6. Final determination of conformity to appropriate specifications and justification of the actions taken, and
7. Signature of individual(s) responsible for final decision(s) and the action(s) taken.

Even though the responsibility for batch acceptance or rejection lies with the head of the quality control unit, the help of the validation committee should prove useful in reviewing the process of OOS investigation and arriving at a recommendation for action taken.

Cleaning Validation

According to 21 CFR Sect. 211.67, Equipment Cleaning and Maintenance of cGMP regulations, equipment and utensils should be cleaned, maintained, and sanitized at appropriate intervals to prevent malfunction or contamination that would alter the safety, identity, strength, quality, or purity of the drug product. Written procedures shall be established and followed for cleaning and maintenance of equipment. These procedures shall include, but are not limited to the assignment of responsibility for cleaning and maintaining equipment; maintenance, cleaning, and sanitizing schedules where appropriate; description in sufficient detail of methods, equipment, and materials used in cleaning and maintenance operations, and the methods of disassembling and reassembling equipment as necessary to assure proper cleaning and maintenance; removal or obliteration of previous batch identification, protection of clean equipment from contamination prior to use; and inspection of equipment for cleanliness immediately before use. Records shall be kept of maintenance, cleaning, sanitizing, and inspection.

The objective of cleaning validation of equipment and utensils is to reduce the residues of one product below established limits so that the residue of the previous product does not affect the quality and safety of the subsequent product manufactured in the same equipment.

According to 21 CFR Sect. 211.63, Equipment Design, Size, and Location, of cGMP regulations, equipment used in the manufacture, processing, packing, or holding of a drug product shall be of appropriate design, adequate size, and suitably located to facilitate operations for its intended use and for its cleaning and maintenance. Some of the equipment design considerations include type of surface to be cleaned (stainless steel, glass, plastic), use of disposables or dedicated equipment and utensils (bags, filters, etc.), of stationary equipment (tanks, mixers, centrifuges, presses, etc.), of special features (clean-in-place systems, steam-in-place systems), and identifying the difficult-to-clean locations on the equipment (so-called hot spots or critical sites).

The specific cleaning procedure should define the amounts and the specific type of cleaning agents and/or solvents used. The cleaning procedure should give full details as to what is to be cleaned and how it is to be cleaned. The cleaning method should focus on worst-case conditions, such as highest-strength, least-soluble, most difficult to clean formulations. Cleaning procedures should identify the time between processing and cleaning, cleaning sequence, equipment dismantling procedure, need for visual inspection, and provisions for documentation.

The choice of a particular analytical method (HPLC, TLC, spectrophotometric, total organic carbon (TOC), pH, conductivity, gravimetric, etc.) and sampling technique chosen (direct surface by swabs and gauze, or by rinsing) depends on the residue limit to be established, based upon the sampling site, type of residue sought, and equipment configuration (critical sites vs. large surface area) considerations. The analytical and sampling methods should be challenged in terms of specificity, sensitivity, and recovery. The established residue limits must be practical, achievable, verifiable, and assure safety. The potency of selected drug and presence of degradation products, cleaning agents, perticulates and microorganisms should be taken into consideration. The following residue limits have been suggested: not more than (NMT) 10 ppm or NMT 0.001% of the dose of any product appears in the maximum daily dose of another product and no residue visible on the equipment after cleaning procedures have been performed.

PHARMACEUTICAL EXCIPIENTS

Pharmaceutical Excipients are components of finished drug products and site active components are recognized in the USP/NF. A list of key excipients for solid dosage forms is given:

1. Diluents, Fillers, and Binders:
   - Calcium phosphate, dibasic
   - Dextrates
   - Dextrin
   - Lactose (anhydrous, fast flow)
   - Mannitol
   - Starch (corn)
   - Sugar, compressible
2. Tablet Disintegrants:
   - Cellulose, microcrystalline
   - Croscarmellose sodium
   - Crospovidone
   - Sodium starch glycolate
   - Starch, pregelatinized
3. Tablet and Capsule Lubricants:
   - Magnesium stearate
   - Mineral oil, light
   - Polyethylene glycol
   - Sodium stearyl fumarate
   - Stearic acid, purified
   - Talc
   - Vegetable oil, hydrogenated
4. Other Excipients:
   - Carboxymethylcellulose sodium
   - Cellulose acetate phthalate
   - Ethylcellulose
   - Hydroxypropyl cellulose
   - Hydroxypropyl methylcellulose
   - Hydroxypropyl methylcellulose pathalate
   - Methacrylic acid copolymer

- Polysorbates
- Polyvinyl acetate phthalate
- Povidone
- Sodium lauryl sulfate

Active Pharmaceutical Ingredients (API)

A chemical is considered to be an API if it is intended for medicinal purposes. Regulatory agencies however, place greater emphasis and priority on the manufacture and validation of APIs than UPS/NF exciepients. According to Sect. 501 (a)(b) of the Food, Drug, and Cosmetic (FD&C) Act, all drugs must be manufactured, processed, packed, and held in accordance with cGMPs. No distinction is made between APIs and finished drug products. Elements common to both APIs and finished drug products include facilities and equipment qualification (IQ/OQ, and PQ), cleaning validation, validation of water supplies, microbial limits for non-sterile material, manufacture of sterile and pyrogen-free material, in-process blending and mixing, analytical methods validation, laboratory controls and in-process testing, change control procedures and revalidation, reprocessing, packaging and labeling, and stability testing.

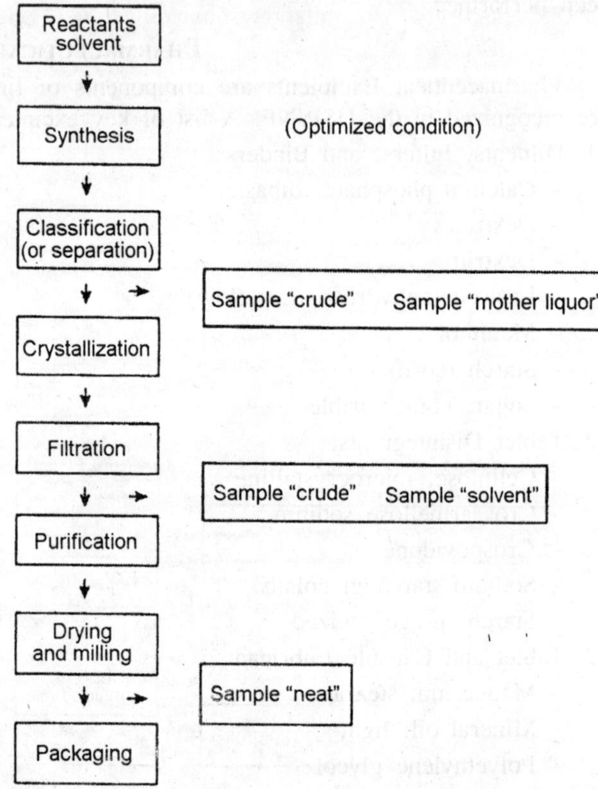

Fig. 5.2. Manufacture of active pharmaceutical ingredients (APIs).

Process

There are four primary processes used in the manufacture of APIs. They are chemical synthesis, fermentation, extraction, and purification. A flow diagram and a description of the chemistry involved are helpful in defining the process. The process description should include appropriate parameters, such as charging quantities or volumes of reactants or solvents, reaction times, temperatures, pressures, etc. Critical processing steps and critical operating parameters should be maintained to ensure batch-to-batch consistency, product yield, and quality. Where in the chain of unit operations (chemical process) does API validation start? As long as key intermediates are made in the plant, they and their reaction and processing steps should be subjected to an appropriate cGMP and process qualification- validation program. A key intermediate is defined as an intermediate in which an essential molecular characteristic, usually related to stereochemical configuration, is introduced into the final API structure (moeity).

Physical Characteristics

Besides purity (chemical potency), the physical characteristics and properties of the API are extremely important to the end user (drug product manufacturer). Characteristics such as crystal morphology, particle size and shape, bulk density, melting point, optical rotation, etc., have a profound effect upon the final drug product and its performance and stability. In addition to the reaction or extraction step, crystallization, milling, and blending unit operations must be subject to qualification and validation.

Impurity Profile

The USP permits up to 2% of ordinary non-toxic impurities. However, impurities above 0.1% should be fully characterized and quantified. Impurities may include starting materials, by-products, intermediates, degradation products, reagents, catalysts, heavy metals, electrolytes, filter aids, and residual solvents. Known toxic impurities must be held to a tighter standard, i.e., below 0.1%.

ISO quality standards series

The ISO 9000 Series was developed in 1987 by the International Organization for Standardization (ISO) in Geneva, Switzerland. It is a comprehensive set of management standards governing the operation of quality assurance to help develop and document a quality system that is useful for individual companies. The ISO 9000 Quality Management and Quality Assurance Standards, Guidelines for Selection and Use, provide basic definitions and concepts and explain how to use the rest of the series (9001, 9002, 9003, and 9004).

The ISO 9001 Quality System—Model for Quality Assurance in Design and Development provides for quality assurance in the areas of design, installation, servicing, development, and production. It is useful primarily for companies that design and develop their own products.

The ISO 9002 Quality System—Model for Quality Assurance in Production, Installation and Service applies to manufacturers, distributors, and service vendors whose products have been designed and serviced by a subcontractor. Such companies are exempt from design control requirements. Both ISO 9001 and ISO 9002 are directly applicable to cGMPs. Except for language, shades of meaning, and stresses the documents are similar. The ISO 9003 Quality Systems—Model for Quality Assurance in Inspection and Testing, designed for testing laboratories and equipment distributors only requires conformance to final inspection and testing procedures. The ISO 9004 Quality Management and Quality Systems Elements—Guidelines provide standards and guidelines for quality management planning and implementation.

6

VALIDATION OF CELL-BASED PROCESSES

Why validate? Though validation is a well-accepted and recognized cGMP requirement in today's Pharma business, this question is often posed during the product or process development (PD) activities in a start-up or even in an established company. In a nutshell, validation is not only a regulatory requirement, but it makes "good business sense." Validated processes assure production of quality product, batch after batch, and ultimately result in fewer headaches down the road in terms of fewer deviations during production, quality assurance (QA) discrepancy investigations, adverse events from the field, and regulatory observations (483s and its global equivalent) during regulatory inspections. In addition, they improve cost effectiveness in terms of preventing process failures, lot rejections, re-processing of salvageable lots, and attaining maximum plant capacity. Moreover, a sound and thorough validation strategy not only assures the production of top quality products, but also builds confidence and provides peace of mind to its customers. It also boosts the morale of the company employees and help build a sound and trustworthy relationship and track record with the regulatory agencies. The latter may come as a blessing for a company's future dealings with the regulatory agencies.

The term process validation originated in 1983 when the Food and Drug Administration (FDA) expanded the cGMP guidelines to cover demonstration of process consistency/reproducibility, but the guidelines were not finalized until 1987. These guidelines were originally intended to be adopted by all drug product and biological manufacturers, but were later extended to the medical device and diagnostic manufacturers and to the blood collection/distribution/users and blood product manufacturers. Though originally intended only for the finished drug product, these regulations have been recently extended to bulk drugs and bulk biologicals.

The original definition of the term process validation was described by the FDA as "Establishing a documented evidence which provides a high degree of assurance that a specific process will consistently produce a product meeting its predetermined specifications and quality attributes."

In practice, process validation (process performance qualification, PPQ) is more complicated than the simple definition stated above and is only one element of the overall validation process. It is a culmination of all other validation studies, such as equipment qualification (installation qualification, IQ; operational qualification, OQ; and performance qualification, PQ), computer qualification (IQ and OQ), utilities and facilities qualification (IQ, OQ, and PQ) cleaning validation (PQ), environmental qualification (PQ), and analytical qualification (PQ), all covered under a validation master plan (VMP) written for each new technology, process, or a product.

The invention of recombinant DNA technology in the late 1970s and its widespread application to eukaryotic and prokaryotic cells for developing unique medical applications/treatments resulted in the establishment of a new field known as "*Genetic Engineering*" today. These developments opened the floodgates for innovation that resulted in the establishment of many biotechnology companies worldwide. Of these, more than 50% of the biotechnology companies are working on cell culture technology for producing pharmaceutical and cellular therapies.

Due to continued innovation in this field the application of process validation concepts and guidelines are becoming increasingly complex, challenging, and difficult to understand by technical professionals, regulatory auditors, and cGMP compliance enforcers working in the pharmaceutical and biotechnology-related organizations. Since it is impossible to cover all aspects of process validation for the numerous biotechnology-derived products in this chapter, an attempt will be made only to provide a simplified version of the regulatory requirements that are needed for licensing cell culture-derived pharmaceuticals and cellular therapies. This chapter is intended to provide a bird's-eye view of the regulatory requirements for process validation to entrepreneurs before they plan for building a new manufacturing plant and expect to obtain licensure for a product or a biologic or a drug from regulatory agencies. This chapter is expected to prepare them well before they begin that challenging, eventful, exhausting, memorable, and ultimately rewarding journey.

Approach and Rationale

The innumerable amount of research and development studies conducted on a large number of medical products has enabled us to understand that the quality attributes for any given product are not an unexpected output. But, are largely dependent on the process parameters used during their production. Therefore, the control of quality attributes for any biological or pharmaceutical product is in our hands; and with the development of new technologies, quality attributes for the new products can now be built into the manufacturing process. In this respect, the process design in relation to the respective product quality attributes has become crucial for the development and licensing of the medical and pharmaceutical products.

Since the breakthrough in genetic engineering a few decades ago, numerous medical, biological, pharmaceutical, and diagnostic products and applications based on cell culture technology have been invented. They are based on microbial fermentation (*eukaryotic* and *prokaryotic*), hybridoma technology, and tissue regeneration. Even plant cell technology is being evaluated to produce medical and therapeutic products for human use. The examples of the cells used for this purpose are: bacteria (*Escherichia coli*), fungi (*Aspergillus*, *Saccharomyces*), mammalian cells (CHO, BHK, myeloma, melanoma, hybridoma, etc.), insect cells (*Drosophila*), and plant cells (tobacco, spinach, etc.). The majority of the products are secreted by the cells in the spent medium (harvest) by applying the rDNA technologies and manipulation of respective genes in the cells. The examples of recombinant products derived from these technologies are: erythropoietin (rEPO), anti-hemophilic factor (rFVIII), tissue plasminogen activator (rTPA), growth factors (EGF, TGF, PDGF, TNF, etc.), hormones (Insulin, LH, FSH, etc.), interferons (IF-1, IF-2, etc.), interleukins (IL-2, IL-4, IL-6, etc.), monoclonal antibodies (mAbs), and other enzymes and proteins (cerezyme, galactosidase, etc.). Some of the products are expressed in the inclusion bodies within cells and the cells therefore must be lysed to extract the products out (insulin, EGF, etc.). Epithelial cells, neuroblastoma, osteoblastoma and cartilage cells are being grown in laboratories and used as medical devices for a number of treatments (burns, tissue implant, tissue regeneration, etc.). A number of monoclonal antibodies are being generated from bacterial, mammalian, and plant cell technologies for the treatment of cancer, autoimmune diseases, and other immunological disorders.

A general approach to streamline validation concepts and policies has been evolving over the last number of years. These efforts have resulted in better understanding of the requirements for the validation by the industry professionals. For the purposes of clarity and better understanding this article will employ the newly emerging approach on validation concepts. Accordingly, qualification of all equipment and systems (design qualification, DQ; installation qualification, IQ; operational qualification, OQ; and performance qualification, PQ) will be referred as "*Equipment Qualification*" and not as "*Validation.*" The term "Validation"will be used only for "*Process Validation*" studies that are related with the studies (with or without active ingredient) at the small-scale (lab-scale) or full production scale (process validation, PV or PPQ).

The variety of cell culture technologies and many different approaches to use them as pharmaceutical products or medical devices makes the task of building the quality attributes in the manufacturing process very challenging. This also makes the task of process validation more difficult as generic models of process validation cannot be used, and every process validation study needs to be devised from scratch based on the technology being used. For example, the level of impurities (DNA, host cell contaminating proteins, etc.) may be substantially less in the starting material where the product is secreted out in the spent medium (harvest) as compared to the product that is expressed intracellularly such as in the inclusion bodies. Therefore, the design of the manufacturing process and the resultant process validation studies would be very different for the two approaches to isolate and purify the product(s). The possible impurities and contaminants in a cell culture-based product are: intact cells, adventitious agents [bacteria, fungi, mycoplasma, viruses, transmissible spongiform encephalitis (TSE)/ bovine spongiform encephalitis (BSE)], endogenous retroviruses, host cell nucleic acids and proteins, foreign proteins (from raw materials and microbial contaminations), endotoxins, and contaminating process chemicals. A validated process, therefore, must demonstrate effective removal, inactivation, or reduction of these impurities and contaminants to acceptable levels.

Though it is preferable to perform process validation studies at full-scale operational level, it is not always possible to perform them at manufacturing scale due to practical limitations (e.g., virus and nucleic acid reduction studies may require huge amounts of model viruses and nucleic acids). In such cases, scaled-down bench- level studies are acceptable as long as all process input parameters are kept the same as in the full-scale and the output parameters are comparable to the full-scale. Whenever this approach is used, demonstration and justification of the acceptability of the scaled-down model should be performed prior to formal process validation.

Process Development

Development of a Defined Process

We will examine below the requirements for developing a reliable and reproducible process for a cell culture derived product. The definition of a defined process may be summarized as "a process that provides a high degree of assurance that it will consistently produce a product meeting its predetermined specifications and quality attributes." This definition seems simple and doable (in the beginning phase of a project) but becomes difficult to achieve when all the details for a cell culture-based product are brought into consideration. Adequate confidence must be built by doing sufficient experimentation and development work to demonstrate that the process can consistently produce a product of pre-specified quality. Range finding (feed stream) studies should be performed for every critical and noncritical process parameter, and operational set-points must be established after completion of the range finding studies. Worst-case studies (upper and lower ranges) should be performed during the development phase, (as it is much easier to do them during development than during actual production). Alert and action levels (limits) for out-put parameters (test results and specifications) must be established with adequate justification. In-process and final product specifications (acceptance criteria) must be defined clearly with sound scientific justifications.

The success of a well executed project depends on a well written process development (PD) report with sufficient details for every aspect of the process and a well executed transfer of technology from the R&D department to the operations department. The R&D personnel not only adequately transfer the technology, but must provide training to production personnel in every aspect of the process. The role of the R&D personnel does not end here, they should actively monitor the process after successful process validation by applying the statistical tools such as statistical process control. Post-validation process data must be analyzed to ensure that the process performs within the established boundaries. Process capability (Cpk) calculations must be performed on the post-validation process data to evaluate process performance. The process data should also be analyzed by applying other statistical tests, such as Student's t-test, to determine confidence intervals on process performance. A 95% confidence interval is generally acceptable for process validation studies. Many companies, however, run their production processes at 98% confidence interval or up to ±6 SD of the validated process parameters. These analyses demonstrate whether the process is in control and build confidence for running the process on a consistent basis. The importance and relevance of good PD work that eventually pays off many fold must be emphasized here. It is generally acknowledged that many pharmaceutical and biotechnology organizations shy away from doing comprehensive PD work as they are in a rush to reach the marketplace. In our competitive world of today, timing is key for making or breaking of an organization. Often what we do not realize is that there are no short cuts and eventually (sooner or later) we have to do the required PD work. The smart approach, therefore, would be to perform all required PD work before process validation, rather than during process validation or after completion of a process validation project. In the latter case, the validation projects generally become confusing, cost a great deal of money, and delay project completion.

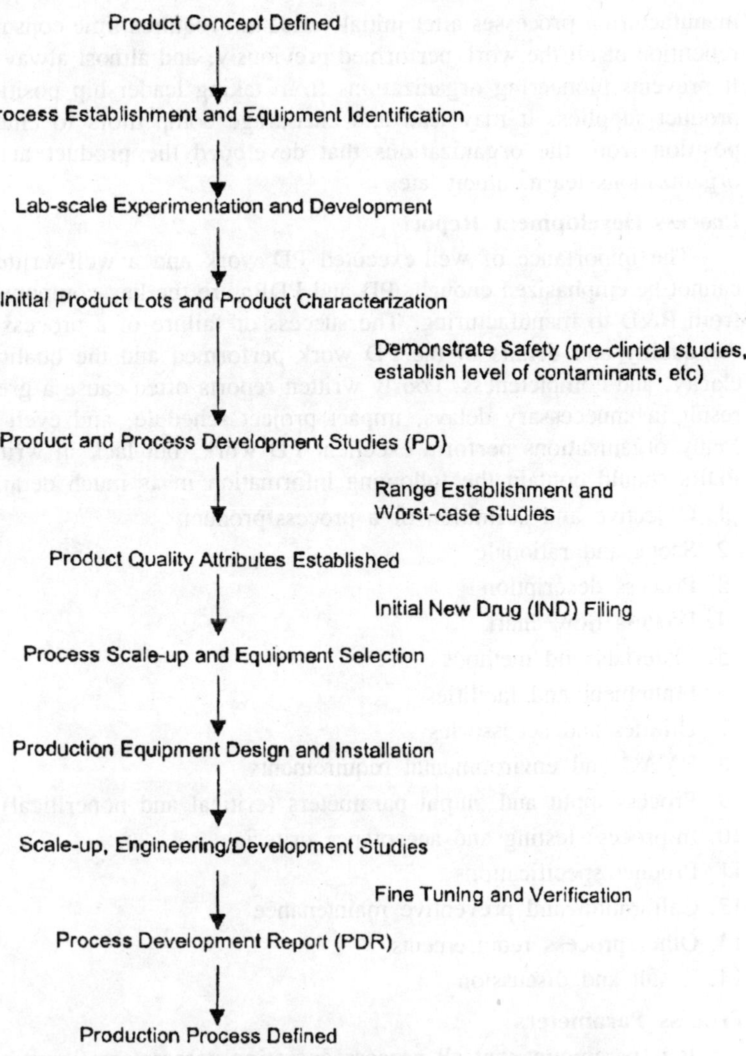

Fig. 6.1. Critical steps for developing a defined process.

A poorly developed process will typically allow only narrow ranges for operational parameters and may result in the rejection of large amounts of otherwise good in-process material produced slightly outside the narrow process ranges developed. Extension of the process ranges or scale-up of manufacturing processes after initial validation requires time consuming regulatory review and approvals, repetition of all the work performed previously, and almost always turns into a costly validation project. It prevents pioneering organizations from taking leadership positions in the marketplace due to limited product supplies. It may lead and encourage competitors to enter the field and snatch the leadership position from the organizations that developed the product at the first place. It is a lesson many organizations learn, albeit late.

Process Development Report

The importance of well-executed PD work and a well-written process development report (PDR) cannot be emphasized enough. PD and PDRs are the key components of a successful technology transfer from R&D to manufacturing. The success or failure of a process validation project greatly depends on the quality and details of the PD work performed and the quality of PDRs in terms of their content, clarity, and completeness. Poorly written reports often cause a great deal of frustration for all involved, result in unnecessary delays, impact project schedule, and even lead to ultimate failure of a project. Many organizations perform excellent PD work, but lack in writing clear and complete reports. Ideal PDRs should contain the following information in as much detail as possible:

1. Objective and definition of a process/product
2. Scope and rationale
3. Process description
4. Process flow chart
5. Materials and methods
6. Equipment and facilities
7. Utilities and accessories
8. HVAC and environmental requirements
9. Process input and output parameters (critical and noncritical)
10. In-process testing and acceptance criteria
11. Product specifications
12. Calibration and preventive maintenance
13. Other process requirements
14. Result and discussion

Process Parameters

It is paramount that all process operating parameters (input parameters) that affect product quality attributes (output parameters) are established clearly during the PD phase of a new process, product, or a technology. This is accomplished typically by performing studies at lower and upper limits of the operating ranges generally referred to as the worst-case studies, crash studies or feed-stream studies. Some studies are performed up to the edge of failure and then stepped back to the ranges where process performance is acceptable. These studies can be simulated or performed with active ingredient or product derived from starting material generated during PD phase of the project. These studies can also be performed by generating starting material by artificially setting the parameters to the upper and lower limits of the range. The process parameters are generally classified as critical process parameters and noncritical process parameters.

Critical process parameters

By definition the critical process parameters are "those operating parameters that directly influence the quality attributes of the product being produced." For example, temperature and pH in a fermenter are considered critical operating parameters as they have a direct influence on the viability of the organism and the chemical or biological activity of the product being produced. Other parameters that may be considered critical for fermentation processes are: cell viability, media conductivity, glucose concentration, oxygen and air uptake rates, and cell density in the production vessel or device.

Noncritical process parameters

The noncritical process parameters are "those operating parameters that have no direct influence on the quality attributes of the product being produced." For example, cell age and media flow rates in a fermenter are considered as noncritical operating parameters as they have no direct influence on the viability of the organism or the activity of the product being produced. Other parameters that may be considered noncritical for fermentation processes are: cell density in the inoculum, cell productivity, agitation rate, perfusion rate, and cell osmolality in the production vessel or device.

Cell Culture and Fermentation Process

A number of different approaches have been used to exploit cell culture technology and develop pharmaceutical products and medical devices, for example expression of the molecule of interest by cells through genetic manipulation or the use of cells as such for treating certain medical conditions. Of these, the technology based on product expression through genetic manipulation is most common. Commercial fermentation processes and bioreactor technologies have been developed in the last several decades to state of the art production of pharmaceutical agents of interest. The introduction of rEPO, rTPA, rFVIII, rInsulin, rHGH, rPDGF, etc. to treat many medical problems would have not been developed without these advances in the technologies. We will discuss below the steps involved in the development of a commercial cell culture process in the light of process validation. Of special interest here is the establishment of critical and noncritical process parameters that will be verified during the process validation phase.

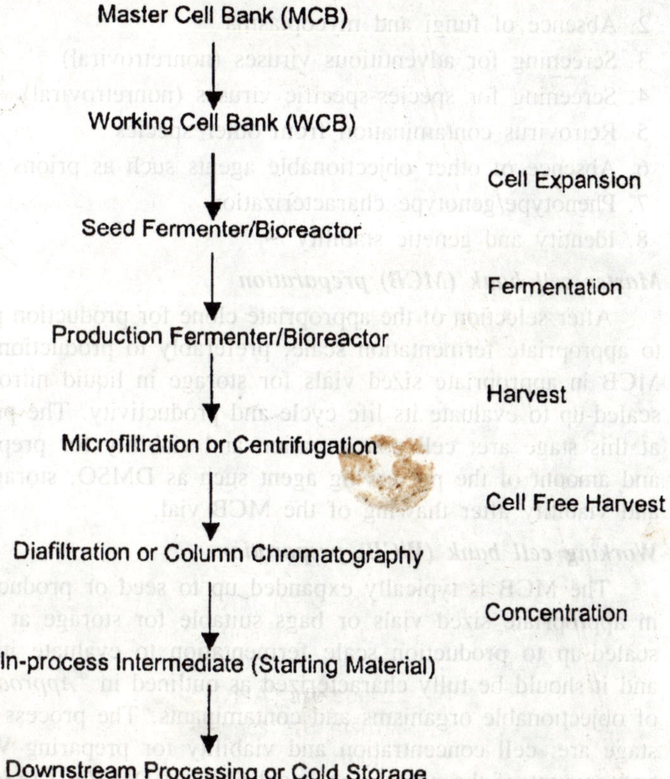

Fig. 6.2. Typical fermentation process flow diagram.

Cell line development

Once a clone has been selected for commercial development it is crucial that the nutritional requirements for the cell line must be defined. The cell line may need to be adapted for growth in certain cases, such as the expression and production of a product in a serum-enriched or serum-free media. The following nutritional requirements in terms of their concentration (% or molarity) or amounts (g/L or PPM or PPB as appropriate), and growth conditions must be established:

1. Chemically defined growth medium
2. Need for protein/serum/plasma or a protein-free media

3. Requirements for vitamins or fatty acids
4. Requirements of any special chemicals
5. Requirements of growth factors or hormones, etc.
6. Optimizatipon and maintenance of appropriate pH and ionic strength
7. Requirements of oxygen, carbon dioxide or other gases
8. Optimizatipon and maintenance of appropriate temperature
9. Frequency of media changeover
10. Frequency of harvesting of the cell line or product

Cell line characterization

The cell line must be fully characterized for the absence of objectionable organisms or contaminants as follows:

1. Absence of bacteria or spores
2. Absence of fungi and mycoplasma
3. Screening for adventitious viruses (nonretroviral)
4. Screening for species-specific viruses (nonretroviral)
5. Retrovirus contamination from other species
6. Absence of other objectionable agents such as prions and TSE/BSE
7. Phenotype/genotype characterization
8. Identity and genetic stability

Master cell bank (MCB) preparation

After selection of the appropriate clone for production purposes, the clonal cells should be expanded to appropriate fermentation scale, preferably to production scale fermentation, and used to prepare an MCB in appropriate sized vials for storage in liquid nitrogen. After preparation, the MCB should be scaled-up to evaluate its life cycle and productivity. The process parameters that need to be established at this stage are: cell concentration and viability for preparing MCB, cell volume in the vial, purity and amount of the preserving agent such as DMSO, storage temperature, and acceptable cell recovery and viability after thawing of the MCB vial.

Working cell bank (WCB) preparation

The MCB is typically expanded up to seed or production scale fermentation to prepare the WCB in appropriate sized vials or bags suitable for storage at –70°C or colder. The WCB should also be scaled-up to production scale fermentation to evaluate its productivity and other growth conditions, and it should be fully characterized as outlined in "*Approach and Rationale*" to ascertain that it is free of objectionable organisms and contaminants. The process parameters that should be established at this stage are: cell concentration and viability for preparing WCB, cell volume in the vial or bag, purity and amount of the preserving agent such as DMSO, storage time and temperature, and acceptable cell recovery and viability after thawing of the WCB vial or bag.

Cell expansion and seed preparation

Procedures (SOPs, BPRs, etc.) should be prepared that describe in detail all the steps for the expansion of cells starting from WCB through preparation of the seed for inoculation of the final-scale production device (fermenter, bioreactor, bag or bottle or vessel). The cell expansion procedure may require only a few steps or may have a number of steps before a seed is ready for inoculation of the production device. In addition, the seed may be used immediately to inoculate a production vessel or it may be stored further until use. Therefore, it is important to evaluate the process and identify the critical and noncritical process parameters for each process independently. The examples of the process parameters that may be established at this stage are: thawing time and temperature, volume of media and size of flask or bottle for initial cell growth, time and temperature for initial cell growth, media pH, conductivity, temperature, glucose concentration, oxygen and air uptake rates, cell viability and cell recovery at different stages, cell density for scale-up to the final seed vessel (bottle or bag or fermenter or bioreactor), cell density and cell viability in the seed to be used for inoculation of the production device (bottle or bag or vessel or fermenter or bioreactor), and storage time and temperature for the seed (inoculum).

Production scale fermentation

Fermentation at the production scale may be carried out in a vessel (fermenter or bioreactor), bottle, or a bag depending on the product type. The product may be the cells themselves, for which efficient cell growth may be critical, or the product may be a biochemical entity (enzyme, protein, hormone, etc.) expressed either in the cells intracellularly retained in the inclusion body or secreted out of the cell in the spent medium. In the latter case, the stability of the molecule in the spent medium should be explored as storage time and temperature for the harvest will be critical for the stability of the product. The process parameters required to be established for the fermentation are: cell viability and cell density in the inoculum, media pH, conductivity, temperature, glucose concentration, oxygen and air uptake rates, cell productivity, cell life span, agitation rate, perfusion rate, cell density, cell viability, and cell osmolality in the production vessel or device.

Continuous fermentation (perfusion)

Continuous fermentation, where the product is generally secreted in the spent medium, is the most efficient and commonly employed technology for the production of biopharmaceuticals today. The main concept of this technology is to keep the cells alive as long as they produce a quality product. The number of days the cells are kept in a fermenter (fermenter days) varies depending on the cell type and established time period (weeks or months) for producing a quality product. In this approach the cells are expanded to desired optimum concentration and induced to adhere to coated (with proteins such as collagen) or noncoated acrylic beads where they can survive for many months as long as their nutritional needs are met. Fresh medium is introduced (per- fused) and spent medium (harvest) is removed from the fermenter on a continuous basis. A number of cell sedimentation devices (conical, incline or plate settlers) are used to separate the cells from harvest. The cells are returned to the fermenter and the harvest is collected in a harvest tank or bag. The fermenters used in this technology are typically smaller in size (50–2500 L), as continuous perfusion of media allows sufficient volume of harvest collected on a daily basis.

Since the equipment used is more complex and the fermenter cycle is typically long (months), the validation effort is more rigorous for this technology. Establishment of acceptable fermenter days requires full cell characterization at the beginning (early), middle, and end (late) of fermentation to demonstrate that the cell characteristics do not change over time. In addition, product quality attributes are evaluated for the product derived from early, middle, and late stages of fermentation. These activities are performed and established during PD phase and confirmed during formal process validation (PPQ).

Batch fermentation

This nonperfusion technology is employed for products that are either secreted in the spent medium or expressed intracellularly. The cells or the harvest is collected for the isolation and purification of the product depending on the expression of the product in the cells or in the spent medium. The fermenter cycle is generally short (days) for batch fermentation process than for continuous fermentation process (weeks or months). This technology is most efficient for products that are expressed intracellularly where cell mass expansion is critical for productivity. It is less efficient for cell secreted products as the cost of operation is high. The fermenters used in this technology are typically larger in size (500–25,000 L), as it is a batch operation that allows collection of cells or harvest only once per fermenter cycle. Since this technology does not use cell sedimentation devices and fermenter cycle is short (days), the validation effort for batch fermentation process is less rigorous.

Cell mass expansion

This technology is similar to batch fermentation process except the main objective of the fermentation is to expand cell mass. It is used mainly for the products that are expressed intracellularly or where the cells themselves are used for medical treatment (as a medical device), and the cell mass is critical for productivity. The fermenter cycle is short (days) for this technology than for continuous fermentation process (weeks or months). The fermenter sizes used in this technology vary depending on the requirements of the cell mass. Since the equipment used is simpler and the fermenter cycle is short (days), the validation effort for this fermentation process is less rigorous.

Though validation of fermentation process may be simpler for medical devices using biologically active cells, process validation for their formulation, storage, and delivery are more complex. Since mammalian cells are more fragile than protein molecules, their storage without impacting their quality attributes are more challenging. Demonstration of biological activity retention for a heterologus cell-based product during production, distribution, and storage is a daunting task. Cell characterization studies may have to be performed more rigorously after formulation, storage, and end of shelf life of these devices. In addition, the level of impurities and contaminants would also require rigorous investigation during these stages. Moreover, an assurance that the biological activity and safety do not impair and adverse reactions do not increase during these stages also needs to be demonstrated.

New approaches and future of cell-based therapies

The manipulation of cell culture technologies to generate unique therapies and medical treatments has just begun. Further development of these technologies would be essential for their impromptu use in new ways to treat diseases. Mammalian cells are being evaluated for grafting, transplantation, tissue regeneration, and organ culture. Stem cells are being developed into numerous cell-based treatments/cure for many diseases such as cancer, HIV, Alzheimer's, Parkinson's, etc. Gene therapy is expected to be the ultimate cure for many diseases in the 21st. century. This field is expected to grow exponentially in the next 25 years and bring numerous challenges for cell culture scientists. A number of microbial hosts (bacteria, plasmids, viruses, etc.) are being evaluated as carriers or vehicle for gene therapy products. For a successful gene therapy product it is crucial that it is free of any side effects, is long lasting, and is fully effective. To accomplish these goals the gene therapy products would have to be pure, free from undesirable components, easy to use, effectively targeted to desirable site, effective transformation and expression of desired genes, complete correction or deletion of defective genes, and they must prove to increase longevity. Cell culture scientists would definitely address all these issues and develop appropriate technologies to attain desired results. However, imagination for validation of all these diverse technologies and processes is mind-boggling today. New approaches to validate these technologies, production equipment, and production processes would have to be developed to meet yet to be established regulatory requirements.

Product isolation, separation, and concentration

The procedures for the isolation of the product, its separation from impurities and contaminants, and its concentration by different technologies, depending on the product type, are performed after the fermentation process is complete. The cell separation techniques such as centrifugation or microfiltration may be applied to concentrate cells for product recovery or remove cells from the harvest that contains the product. The parameters that may be critical for process validation for this process are: cell concentration and viability in the fermenter effluent (spent media with or without cells), storage time and temperature for the effluent, centrifugation speed or microfiltration rate for cell separation, cell separation time and temperature, and storage time and temperature for the concentrated in-process intermediate (IPI, starting material).

In-process intermediate (IPI) or product preparation and stabilization

The IPI may be the cell suspension or cell extract or concentrated harvest fluid depending on the product type. Some of the processes require stabilization of the IPI for storage prior to further processing of the product. In these cases a formulating agent may be added to the concentrated IPI prior to its storage in the cold. The parameters that should be considered for process validation here are: the purity and concentration of formulating agent, mixing of the formulating agent with the IPI, freezing time and temperature for the formulated IPI, and storage time and temperature for the formulated IPI.

For medical device applications, the IPI (cell suspension/tissue) may be the final product that may require cleaning and removal of impurities, formulation for stabilization, and preparation of the product for clinical use. In such cases, the parameters that need to be established for process validation are: amount of contaminants (DNA, proteins, etc.) in the final product, cell/tissue morphology, genetic characterization of the cells/tissue, amount of formulating agent, storage time and temperature, and shelf life of the product.

Downstream Process Development

The pharmaceutical or therapeutic proteins expressed in cells are further purified from the IPI generated during the fermentation. The purification steps may involve microfiltration/diafiltration, salt or solvent fractionation, and column chromatography (ion exchange, hydrophobic interaction, affinity, gel filtration, etc.). The examples of critical process parameters that should be established here are: pH, conductivity, salt or solvent residues, membrane life cycle, column operation parameters (equilibration, load, wash, elution, regeneration, storage, cleaning, life-cycle, etc.), impurities and contaminant clearance (DNA, microbes, viruses, proteins, etc.), and hold times and temperature for in-process material and equipment. There is a whole battery of process parameters that should be established for process validation for these operations.

Bulk Formulation, Stabilization, and Final Packaging

The purified in-process material (bulk) is typically formulated for stabilization and either stored until further processing or filled and/or freeze-dried depending on the mode of application for the product. These operations are generally performed in the clean room environments (class 100) that require detailed and cumbersome PQ studies. At this stage, the product is characterized in detail and every lot of the product is evaluated against pre-established specifications and quality attributes. These include: product amount (units or weight), purity, strength, pH, ionic strength, amount of trace metals, amount of impurities and contaminants (DNA, proteins, microbial load, endotoxins, etc.), amount of residual reagents (solvents, polymers, chemicals, etc.), amount of formulating agents (excipients, sugars, etc.), sterility, storage time and temperature, and product shelf life. The process parameters governing these quality attributes should be considered as critical parameters during process validation studies. The filled or lyophilized product vials are inspected for container closure integrity and labeled appropriately. The product coming from validation runs is placed on stability to demonstrate that the product is stable during its entire shelf life. In addition, shipping studies are performed to demonstrate that the packaging is shatter-proof and the product is stable during shipping. All appropriate process parameters covering these quality aspects of the process should be established and verified during the process validation studies.

Process Validation

Process validation projects are complex and cover a great deal of details. The process validation begins with the receipt of a PD report from the R&D arm of an organization, and ends with the approval of a process validation report and applicable SOPs/BPRs by the QA arm of the organization. A well-written PD report with adequate details of the developed process greatly facilitates process validation. In addition, efficiency and success of a process validation depends heavily on the extent and quality of PD work and/or engineering runs performed on associated equipment. Prior to formal process validation, processes should be run rigorously on associated equipment to gain valuable experience. The experience gained is well worth as it saves time and resources during the formal validation stage by efficiently resolving any unforeseen problems, discrepancies or deviations. In no event, the engineering runs or PD studies be left for performance during the formal process validation stage (PPQ phase). Successful completion of a process validation study requires good coordination among the responsible departments such as production/manufacturing, quality control, QA, engineering, R&D, regulatory affairs, etc. We will discuss below the types of processes that are generally covered under process validation projects (PV or PPQ).

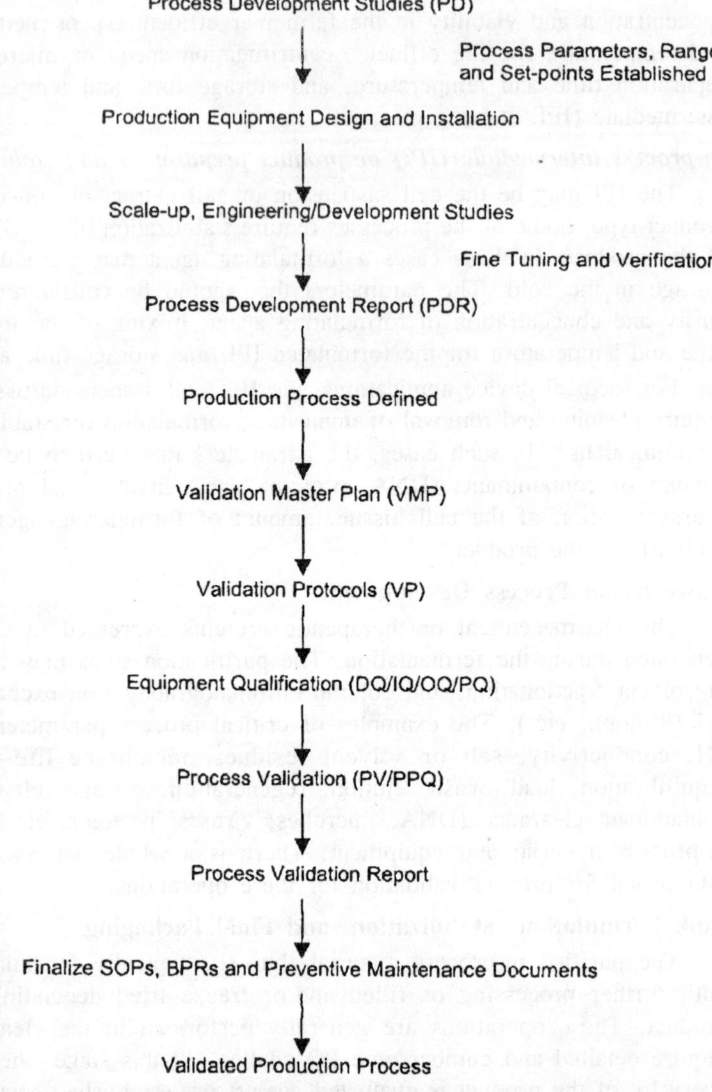

Fig. 6.3. Critical steps leading to process validation.

1. Manufacturing procedures for fermentation, product isolation, purification, formulation, sterilization, filling, and freeze drying of products
2. Microfiltration, ultrafiltration, and sterile filtration
3. Cleaning procedures for equipment and processes (clean-in-place, CIP)
4. Lifecycle determinations for chromatographic resins, membranes and filters
5. Impurity/contaminant clearance (DNA, viruses, host cell proteins, etc.) studies
6. Impurity/contaminant inactivation (virus, endotoxins, TSE/BSE, etc.) studies
7. Sterilization and steam-in-place (SIP) systems

8. Critical utilities such as water for injection (WFI). (PPQ is performed to demonstrate process reproducibility/consistency and product quality)
9. Environmental qualification for facilities (EQ). (EQ is a combination of air handling, equipment/facility cleaning, sanitation, gowning, and environmental monitoring)
10. Re-processing of process intermediates, bulk, and final product
11. Revalidation of processes due to major change control requests (CCRs)

Unlike equipment re-qualification, revalidation of a production process is currently not a mandatory cGMP requirement, but must be considered after implementation of a large number of CCRs or as soon as a process shift is noticed. The purpose of the process revalidation should still be to demonstrate that the implementation of CCRs or an observed shift in the process has not affected quality attributes of the final product. Even if no major changes were implemented or process has not shifted, process revalidation should still be considered to demonstrate that the process is running within controlled limits, at some appropriate time intervals after original process validation (after 100/ 500/1000 lots or 2/5/10 years, as appropriate).

Life Cycle of Process Validation

Process validation is a continuous process, it does not end after the sign-off of the original process validation report. It is not uncommon for companies to initiate change control requests within days or weeks after the completion of the original process validation. Many companies have made major process changes within one year of the original process validation.

Since cell culture and fermentation processes are continually evolving, changes are being made to manufacturing processes on a regular basis by many companies. In fact, a number of second-generation products are derived from the same cell lines, except the cell lines have been adapted to produce the product in a protein-free (serum/plasma) media.

Though such changes improve the product quality and safety tremendously, the process validation task is nevertheless the same. Such changes often lead to the construction of a new manufacturing plant and complete re-validation of the production process. Therefore, the life cycle of a manufacturing process after original validation is mainly dependent on the volume of change control activity.

Though regulatory agencies have not made a guideline yet for process re-validations, they have been advising drug/biological manufacturers for some time to evaluate the need for process re-validation at some regular intervals. Many companies do not feel the need for process re-validations based on the activities that are covered under their change control management programs. However, it may be prudent to perform process re-validation after a major process change or after a number of small changes to assess the cumulative effect of many change control requests. One possible mechanism may be to perform process re-validations after every 100/200/500/1000 production runs or, 2/5/10 years or sooner, as justified by the evaluation of the historical process input and output parameters, specifications, set-points, action limits, or other observations that suggest that the validated process may have shifted.

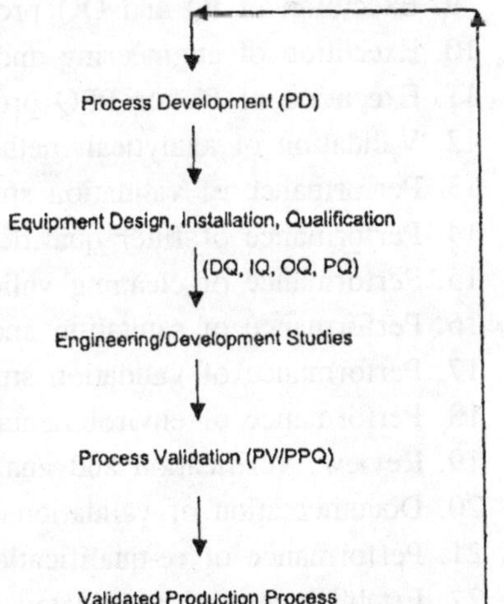

Fig. 6.4. Life cycle of process validation.

Validation of the Manufacturing Processes and Associated Equipment Qualification

Validation SOPs

Establishment of sound validation SOPs and strict adherence to them is crucial for the success of any validation project in a cell culture-derived drug/biological manufacturing organization. These SOPs are typically written by validation professionals and are approved by the responsible groups (e.g., operations, engineering, validation, research, PD, QC, QA, and regulatory affairs) that have a stake in the validation projects. The SOPs should be established for the required validation functions, as listed below:

1. Site or facility validation policy and management
2. Validation master plan and final report
3. Validation requirements for DQ, IQ, OQ, PQ, PD, PPQ, EQ, and RQ validation protocols
4. Design of worst-case studies for OQ, PD, and PPQ protocols
5. Determination of acceptance criteria for validation protocols
6. Design of prospective or concurrent validation studies, and retrospective data analysis
7. Write a validation protocol and a validation final report
8. Revision of a validation plan, protocol or a final report
9. Execution of IQ and OQ protocols
10. Execution of engineering and PD protocols (studies)
11. Execution of PV or PPQ protocols (studies)
12. Validation of analytical methods, assays, and procedures
13. Performance of validation studies on clearance and/or inactivation of impurities contaminants
14. Performance of filter qualifications and sterile filtration validations
15. Performance of cleaning validation studies on equipment, accessories, and processes
16. Performance of sanitation and sterilization validation studies
17. Performance of validation studies on automated systems (computers, DCS, and PLCs)
18. Performance of environmental qualification (EQ) studies
19. Review, verification and analysis of validation data and documents
20. Documentation of validation discrepancies and deviations
21. Performance of re-qualification (RQ) studies on validated equipment, systems and processes
22. Establishment of a validated lifecycle (for cells, resins, filters, membranes, etc.)
23. Requirements for maintaining a equipment or a process in a validated state
24. Display of validation status (labels) for validated equipment and systems
25. Training and certification program for personnel involved in validation projects

In addition to these, many other SOPs may be established for performing specific validation functions depending on the need of the equipment, system or process (e.g., determination of equipment surface finish, calibration of instruments and thermocouples, determination of agitation rates, determination of HETP and Af on chromatography columns). The required SOPs are typically identified and established by qualified validation professionals depending on the need of an organization.

Validation Master Plan

It is paramount that a detailed VMP should be written before implementation of any new or unlicensed process for the production of a cell culture derived drug/biological product. The VMP provides details of an organization's plans for carrying out all validation activities on production equipment, systems, and processes. The plan should provide details of equipment, facilities, utilities, raw materials, storage times and temperatures, environmental requirements, production processes, critical and noncritical process parameters, process set points, SOPs and BPRs, in-process and final product sampling, analytical assays and methods, QC testing, in-process testing and acceptance criteria, and product release specifications. The VMPs should be approved by all responsible stakeholders or senior management of a company (operations/manufacturing, QA, QC, engineering, PD, and regulatory affairs), and should contain the following information at a minimum:

1. Objective
2. Scope and rationale
3. Process and product design
4. Description of manufacturing facility
5. Equipment description and qualification (DQ/IQ/OQ/PQ)
6. Process description and qualification (PQ/PPQ)
7. Description of utilities and supplies
8. Description of automated systems
9. Equipment cleaning (CIP/COP) and sanitation (SIP)
10. HVAC and EQ
11. Process parameters and set points
12. In-process testing and product specifications
13. Analytical methods and procedures
14. Manufacturing procedures and batch records
15. Responsibilities
16. Execution plan and schedule
17. Documentation and training
18. Modification and change control
19. Preventive maintenance
20. References
21. Attachments
22. Facility diagram
23. Process flow diagram
24. List of validation protocols
25. List of PDRs
26. List of engineering reports
27. Project schedule and Gantt charts
28. Other pertinent documents

Equipment Qualification

A great deal of information is available in the literature, web sites of the regulatory agencies (FDA, EMEA, ICH), professional societies (PDA, ISPE, AAPS, etc.), various seminars and symposia, and from professional consultants for the qualification of process equipment. The key components of equipment qualifications are covered in the following validation studies:

1. Design qualification (DQ)
2. Installation qualification (IQ)
3. Operational qualification (OQ)
4. Performance qualification (PQ)

Equipment qualification studies should be performed for all process equipment (fermenters/bioreactors, chromatography, microfiltration/ultrafiltration systems, tanks and vessels, autoclaves, CIP and SIP systems, freeze dryers, etc.), utility equipment (WFI, clean steam, solvent delivery, etc.), supply equipment and accesories (gases, filters, raw materials, etc.), automated systems (computers, DCS, PLCs, etc.), and critical facility equipment (HVAC, warehouse, storage chambers, shipping containers, etc.).

Equipment Engineering Runs and Process Development Studies

After completion of the DQ, IQ, OQ and PQ studies on the equipment, it is prudent to perform equipment engineering runs and PD studies (pre process validation studies, also known as trial runs) to ascertain that the developed process is scalable to the production scale. These studies confirm that the process can perform effectively within the ranges established at the small-scale or previously developed scale. These studies also help in ensuring that the formal process validation studies would not run into major discrepancies, deviations, or failures. They also provide an opportunity to fix any problems that may have been ignored previously. Furthermore, they provide a chance to develop or fine tune acceptance criteria and specifications for the formal process validation studies down the road.

These studies are performed under approved PD protocols. Typically three runs are performed at the production scale by following the SOPs and BPRs written for the process. All sampling and testing is performed as in the process validation studies except that some tests may not be required (have no chance of failure due to scale of operation). PD final reports are prepared after review and analysis of all results and associated data. Appropriate conclusions are drawn and recommendations for formal process validation studies are made in the final reports. The examples of these studies are equipment load studies (autoclaves, depyrogenation ovens, viral inactivation tanks, pasteurization, column chromatography, cleaning validations, etc.), mock runs (process runs without active ingredient), partial load studies (part load with active ingredient and remaining load with an excipient), and full process runs with active ingredient. In conclusion, these studies provide peace of mind that the formal process validation would be un-eventful or would be completed with minimum difficulties.

Process Validation Protocols (PV or PPQ) and Final Reports

Process validation protocols are written to demonstrate that the production processes are reproducible, are in control, and consistently produce a product of predefined specifications and quality attributes. The protocols are also used to demonstrate impurity/contaminant clearance, validation of operating ranges, equipment cleaning, and establishment of lifecycles for chromatographic resins, filters, and membranes. It is indisputable that well written process validation protocols are instrumental for efficiency and success of process validation studies. The protocols should contain details of the production process and equipment to be used, SOPs and BPRs to be used, critical and noncritical process parameters, process set-points and action limits, sampling and QC testing, analytical methods and assays to be used, and in-process and final product specifications. The process validation protocols should be designed to incorporate worst-case studies based on the acceptable level of risk for the process and the product. It is important that all pre-requisites (e.g., DQ/IQ/OQ/PQ on equipment or a system, approved SOPs/BPRs, instrument calibration, and personnel training) are completed before execution of a process validation protocol.

After execution of the validation protocols and completion of all testing, validation final reports should be written with complete details of protocol execution (BPRs and sample tables), test results, discrepancies and deviations, modifications or change control requests, passage/failures against acceptance criteria, statistical data analysis, preventive measures and maintenance, validated critical and noncritical process parameters, process set-points and action/alert limits, supporting data, and conclusions. The validation protocols (and final reports after completion of the study, see below) should be reviewed and/or approved by all responsible parties such as manufacturing, PD, engineering, quality control, QA, validation, and regulatory affairs (optional), as appropriate, prior to its execution. A typical outline of a process validation protocol and final report (validation package) are given below:

1. Approval signatures page
2. Objective
3. Scope and rationale
4. Process description
5. Acceptance criteria
6. Responsibilities
7. References
8. Prerequisites
9. Validation procedures or test functions
10. Result, data analysis and discussion
11. Validated critical and noncritical process parameters
12. List of SOPs and BPRs
13. List of supporting data and documentation
14. List of discrepancies and deviations
15. Conclusion

The validation final reports must contain all results obtained during the execution of a process validation protocol. All deviations should be described along with justifications for their acceptance. The results must be evaluated against the pre-established acceptance criteria, product specifications, and quality attributes. The data should also be evaluated statistically and confidence intervals for the data should be calculated to demonstrate process robustness. Process capability (Cpk) calculations should also be performed to demonstrate process reproducibility.

The final report should draw a scientifically sound conclusion based on the results obtained during the study. Ranges and set-points for all validated critical and non-critical process parameters should be established. In addition, alert and action limits for validated process parameters should also be established wherever applicable. Moreover, a plan to monitor process parameters during production should be devised, and the historical data should be evaluated statistically at pre-established time periods (yearly or after every 100 lots or other suitable interval). Process capability (CpK) calculations should also be repeated on historical data to demonstrate process reproducibility. The in-process action and alert limits and product specifications should be re-evaluated and tightened, wherever possible, after complete data analysis at pre-established time periods.

Raw Materials

The quality of raw materials plays a major role in attaining quality attributes for the final product and indirectly affects success or failure of process validation. The critical raw materials for a cell-derived product during fermentation are: basal media, purified water or WFI, salts and buffering agents, oxygen and carbon dioxide, amino acids, vitamins, glucose, serum or plasma proteins (animal or human), and other nutrients such as hormones or growth factors. It is essential to establish specifications for all raw materials used in the production process, and ensure that quality attributes of all incoming raw material lots are met against the established specifications. Any changes made to the specifications for raw materials should be evaluated through change control management and process validation(s) performed wherever necessary. In addition, FIFO (first in first out) procedures should be established for approved/released incoming raw material lots.

Facilities

All equipment installed in a facility must be qualified (DQ, IQ, OQ and PQ, wherever applicable). The typical facility related equipment includes HVAC, cold/freezer freezer rooms, cooling towers and heat exchangers, chemical/solvent tanks and distribution system, and waste treatment and disposal systems. The facility cleaning procedures are established based on the requirements for each classification (class 100, 1000, 10,000, and 100,000; or grade A, B, C, or D), and must be validated under the facility EQ. Emergency power systems should also be qualified (DQ, IQ, and OQ) to demonstrate that uninterrupted power supply is available to critical production equipment (cold rooms, freezers, freeze dryers, etc.).

Utilities

The critical utility systems must be qualified (DQ, IQ, OQ, and PQ). The examples of utilities that are used in a typical cell culture based production facility are potable water, purified water, WFI, plant steam and clean steam systems, gas distribution systems, CIP and SIP systems, and electricity supply systems.

Production Equipment

Besides equipment qualification (DQ, IQ, OQ, and PQ), typical production equipment used in a cell culture-based facility must be validated (PPQ). The production equipment includes media and buffer preparation equipment, media filtration equipment, media storage tanks, media and buffer distribution system, seed fermenters or bioreactors, production-scale fermenters or bioreactors, aseptic transfer equipment, cell settlers, heat exchangers, pumps and agitation systems, gas sparging equipment, harvest tanks, microfiltration and ultrafiltration systems, centrifuges, and initial capture and concentration equipment. These validation studies may be performed separately or may be combined in the process validation study for a new process, product or technology.

Instruments

Though all instruments associated with equipment systems are generally covered in the equipment qualification, any stand-alone instrument must be qualified separately. In addition, all instruments must be calibrated at the time of their qualification and must remain on a regular calibration schedule after their qualification. The established calibration schedule must be justified and scientifically sound. All test instruments used to measure a specific parameter during validation must also be calibrated.

Analytical Equipment, Instruments, and Methods

All analytical equipment and instruments must be qualified (DQ, IQ, OQ, and PQ), and associated methods, procedures or assays must be validated (PPQ). During this phase of validation, the procedures must be evaluated for precision, accuracy, repeatability, and variability. The results must be evaluated statistically to demonstrate confidence intervals for each sampling condition. The instrument to instrument, operator to operator, and intra- or inter-assay variabilities must be established.

Distributed Control Systems (DCS) and Programmable Logic Controllers (PLCs)

All automated systems (computers, DCS and PLCs) must be qualified (DQ, IQ, OQ, and PQ), and associated software must be tested for its intended function, use, and its lifecycle. The validation aspects of these systems are verified and confirmed during the process validation phase of the validation activity.

Cleaning and Disinfecting

The cleaning of the equipment including the CIP systems must be qualified (DQ, IQ, OQ, and PQ), and the procedures must be validated (PD, PV, and PPQ). The cleaning validation studies must demonstrate that the process residues and cleaning agent residues are removed to the acceptable levels after the cleaning. The acceptable levels for the residues must be established by actual scientific data or sound scientific knowledge. Appropriately validated assays to test the residues must be used. In addition, all cleaning and disinfecting agents must be qualified or approved for use. The cleaning requirements for each step of the process must be established per appropriate guidelines established by regulatory agencies.

Since the final rinse in cleaning processes for biological products is performed by WFI, many companies use the quality attributes of WFI as acceptance criteria for rinse samples. In addition to rinse sampling, cleaning agent residues and process residues (protein, fatty acids, nucleic acids, raw material components, etc.) are tested by surface swabbing and evaluated against pre-established acceptance criteria. The typical assays used for cleaning validations are pH, conductivity, TOC, microbial load, endotoxin, protein assays=analysis, and other assays for specific residues. A cleaning monitoring program should be established to maintain the equipment in a validated state.

Standard Operating Procedures (SOPs) and Batch Production Records (BPRs)

The appropriate SOPs and BPRs must be drafted, reviewed, and approved prior to beginning of process validation studies. These procedures may be modified, if needed, with appropriate justifications during validation as long as the last validation runs (three or more) are performed after making the modifications and all validation acceptance criteria are met. The modifications to the procedures during validation should be made through the change control system of the organization. It is important that all changes made during validation are fully incorporated in the SOPs and BPRs prior to approval of the final validation package.

Personnel and Training

The success of a process validation project depends solely on two things—first an effective and detailed technology transfer program, and second an effective and detailed training program for the new processes or technologies. Therefore, it is crucial that the organizations establish a very effective and practical technology transfer function, and an effective and practical training program for the operations personnel. The initial training is typically provided by the R&D arm of the organization (or whoever developed the process and has the most knowledge or experience). The training program and procedures must be well documented and must follow cGMP guidelines.

Documentation

The regulatory agencies have stated in no uncertain terms that the lack of documentation (even if the work was performed) would be interpreted as if no work was performed. Therefore, the importance of documentation cannot be emphasized enough. The following documents need to be in place for the purposes of process validation:

1. An approved validation master plan/report, if applicable.
2. An approved validation protocol/report/final package.
3. Original or copies of all approved specifications or acceptance criteria.
4. Original or copies of all PD reports.
5. Original or copies of all approved process validation parameter documents.
6. Original copies of all prerequisite sheets completed during validation.
7. Original copies of all validation attachments/execution documents.
8. Original or copies of all SOPs/BPRs employed during validation execution.
9. Original or copies of all QC test reports.
10. Original or copies of all other test reports.
11. Original or copies of all raw data, or location of all archived raw data.

12. Original or copies of all supporting data related to validation.
13. Original or copies of all change control requests implemented during validation.
14. Original or copies of all deviation reports encountered during validation.
15. Original or copies of all corrective action reports, if applicable.
16. Original or copies of all SOPs/BPRs/documents revised during or as a result of validation.
17. Original or copies of all other documents related to validation.

Preventive Maintenance

Maintenance of validation post-licensure is as important as original validation, as it transforms into cGMP compliance after licensure of the production process. To maintain a process in the validated state, it is crucial that procedures for preventive maintenance (PM) be established prior to original validation, modified as appropriate during validation, and are followed thoroughly and timely after validation. In addition, the processes should be monitored regularly with respect to process parameters observed during production.

The historical process parameters data should be evaluated at some fixed intervals (annually or sooner if needed) with respect to validated parameters and be tightened or loosened (in principle) as appropriate and justified by the data based on sound scientific principles and policies. The historical data must be evaluated by applying appropriate statistical methods and calculation for process capability (Cpk). The procedures for the following activities should be established as needed:

1. Evaluation of production equipment, parts, and accessories.
2. Calibration program for all instruments used in production and testing.
3. Equipment re-qualification and process re-validation program.
4. Preventive maintenance program for equipment, facilities, and processes.
5. Change control program.
6. Evaluation of validated process parameters.

Change Control

A change control system must be instituted to document all changes made to validated production processes (32). The change control activity begins after the installation of the equipment systems and continues throughout the lifecycle of the process or product. The change control requests (CCRs) should be initiated prior to making the change, except in emergency situations, and must be reviewed and approved by all involved groups. The impact on validated systems and processes must be assessed and any identified validation work must be completed before closing the CCR. If the change is minor, little or no validation work may be required, however if the change is major, full revalidation may be required. The US FDA published a guideline in July 1997 that requires notification of all changes to the agency depending on the extent of the change in the following manner:

Major changes require submission and approval of a supplement prior to the distribution of the affected product. Moderate changes require submission of a supplement at least 30 days (CBE30) prior to the distribution of the affected product. Minor changes do not require any submission prior to the distribution of the affected product, but must be documented in the annual report.

Manufacturing Plant Qualification

The manufacturing plant qualification and licensing requires additional validation, testing, and documentation besides equipment qualification, utilities=facilities qualification, process validation, and establishment of PM and change control programs. Successful completion of the following items is key to the licensure of a manufacturing plant for a cell culture-derived pharmaceutical or therapeutic or diagnostic product:

Plant Design and Construction

The manufacturing plant must be designed and constructed per appropriate local, state and federal regulations and bylaws. The plant must be built by keeping the product and personnel flow in mind. In general, the product flow should be unidirectional. All required essential utilities (power, water, waste disposal, sewer, etc.) and facilities (warehouse, receiving, shipping, etc.) must be planned for and built into the manufacturing plant. Location and installation of all production equipment, process utilities, facilities, and support systems must be designed and procured per requirement of the production process.

Validation Master Plan

A VMP must be written, approved by the management, executed, and revised/updated as needed starting with the site selection and plant construction and ending with the licensure of the manufacturing plant.

Equipment Installation

The production equipment, utilities/facilities equipment, and all support system equipment as designed for the process must be procured from quality manufacturers and installed per manufacturer's recommendations in the manufacturing plant. All essential utilities (power, water, disposal, etc.) and supplies (gases, solvents, etc.) must be available prior to the installation of equipment systems. Equipment check-outs (ECOs) must be performed to evaluate safe and normal operation of the equipment prior to equipment qualification. It is also essential that the equipment life cycle be established at this phase to ensure that the equipment performs as designed during the entire life of the equipment.

Equipment Qualification

Please refer to Equipment Engineering runs and Process Development Studies, and Process Validation Protocols and Final Reports Sections for details on equipment qualification. It is crucial that ECOs and dry runs (trial/engineering runs) are performed during the equipment qualification phase to ensure that the equipment operates within the ranges as designed for the process and certified by the manufacturer.

Equipment Performance Qualification

These studies are performed during the qualification phase of the equipment to ensure that the equipment delivers the desired output for the manufacturing process such as flow rates, temperature, pH, conductivity, agitation rates, sparging rates, cell retention, bioburden reduction, endotoxin removal, depyrogenation, sterile filtration, sterilization, etc. Equipment loading studies (autoclave loads, vial washer loads, depyrogenation loads, stopper processing loads, chemical inactivation tank loads, etc.) are performed during this phase to ensure that the equipment loads are processed appropriately to meet all quality attributes desired in the qualified loads. It is essential to evaluate which of the equipment needs to be placed on equipment re-qualification program to ensure that equipment delivers desired quality attributes in the processed loads during the entire life of the equipment.

Heat, Ventilation, and Air Conditioning (HVAC)

The qualification of HVAC system (DQ, IQ, OQ, and PQ) for the manufacturing plant must be completed during the validation phase. This includes qualification of the air handlers, HEPA filters, distribution piping, and associated equipment. The PQ on the HVAC system must demonstrate that the adequate air flow and particle levels (viable and nonviable) are achieved per specification (Federal Standard 209E or European ISO Standard or equivalent) for the different manufacturing environments.

Cleaning and Sanitation

Effective equipment and facility cleaning and sanitation procedures play a major role in maintaining equipment in a validated state and maintaining its life cycle, and by doing so, assures maintenance of product quality attributes. Cleaning and sanitation procedures should be developed that can effectively clean equipment product contact surfaces, working and processing areas, work surfaces, floor and wall surfaces, and drainage and disposal systems. The cleaning=sanitation procedures must be validated by using appropriate acceptance criteria. The specifications or acceptance criteria for cleaning and sanitation should be established on a case by case basis by consideration of the manufacturing process, processing time, and in-process materials used. Hold times for process equipment after cleaning must be established and demonstrated (qualified). PD studies should be performed to evaluate effectiveness of the cleaning agents and procedures and establishment of acceptance criteria before PPQ studies are performed. The typical tests used to demonstrate cleaning of equipment product contact surfaces are visual examination, microbial load, endotoxin level, pH, conductivity, level of residual process impurities, level of residual cleaning agents, TOC, and any other appropriate test for a residue. The typical tests used to demonstrate effective sanitation procedures are visual examination, levels of viable particles, level of nonviable particles, and absence of objectionable organisms. The following cleaning and sanitation procedures should be established at a minimum:

1. Procedures for cleaning inner and outer surfaces of equipment.
2. Procedures for cleaning of chromatography columns, filters and membranes
3. Recipes and methods for CIP/COP systems.
4. Manual cleaning procedures.
5. Cleaning/sanitation procedures for work surfaces, floors, and walls.
6. Cleaning/sanitation procedures for drains and disposal systems.
7. Cleaning/sanitation procedures for utilities (WFI, gases, steam, etc.)

Gowning and Personal Safety

Appropriate and protective gowning is essential for preventing the product from getting contaminated by human interaction and also to safeguard humans from any undesirable effects due to exposure of finished products, in-process materials, process chemicals, and supplies or accessories used during production. The personal safety devices used are lab coats or gowns, eye/hearing protection devices, gloves, face shields, and chemical or solvent handling devices. Clear procedures should be written for effective use of gowning and personal safety devices.

Environmental Qualification

In addition to qualification of HVAC, equipment/facility cleaning, and gowning; an EQ should be performed to demonstrate clean manufacturing environment as a combination of an effective HVAC system, effective equipment cleaning procedures, effective gowning procedures, and effective facility cleaning procedures at dynamic and at rest conditions. The acceptance criteria for the EQ for class 100,000, 10,000, 1000, and 100 (grade A, B, C, and D by European Standard) are different and are derived from Federal Standard 209E and other US and European regulations. The typical documentation and testing performed during EQ are as follows:

1. Number and gowning status of the operators present during dynamic conditions.
2. Number and gowning status of the operators present during rest conditions.
3. Swab testing of operator's gowns for presence of viable and nonviable particles.
4. Verification of air flow changes/hour and air flow rates during testing.
5. Testing of viable and nonviable particles in the air. Testing of viable and nonviable particles in swab samples from work surfaces, floor surfaces, and walls.
6. Verification of all cleaning performed during the testing period.
7. Presence/absence of objectionable organisms in the environment.

8. Discrepancy investigations and implementation of corrective actions.
9. Establishment of an environmental monitoring program.

Preventive procedures to check the presence of insects, pests, reptiles, and rodents should also be employed.

Capacity Evaluation

Though not a regulatory requirement yet, regulatory agencies sometimes request that a production capacity evaluation be performed for each manufacturing facility that requires licensure. Capacity evaluation should be performed by verifying the capacity of the equipment, utilities, supplies, facilities, raw materials, in-process materials, and final product production. The following items should be evaluated for the capacity assessment of the manufacturing facility:

1. Capacity for manufacturing areas in terms of space and production for equipment such as seed and production fermenters, media/buffer tanks, harvest tanks, filtration/microfiltration, ultrafiltration/ diafiltration, chromatography columns and skids, in-process material and bulk storage tanks, filling machines, lyophilizers, vial washers and processors, stopper washer and processors, cold rooms and freezer rooms, refrigerators and freezers, warehouse capacity, storage of raw materials and process intermediates, and storage of quarantine and released product.
2. Capacity for processing/storage of potable water, purified water, WFI, plant steam, clean steam, CIP, SIP, cooling towers, heat exchangers, gases, etc.
3. Capacity or production/storage of critical raw materials such as plasma, serum, hormones, peptides or proteins, affinity-matrix for columns, etc. used in the production.
4. Capacity in terms of processing supplies such as autoclave loads, depyrogenation oven loads, vial/ stopper processor loads, filters, etc.
5. Capacity in terms of cleaning of equipment and turnaround time.
6. Capacity for maintaining appropriate manufacturing environment
7. Capacity in terms of personnel for working space, production schedule training, document archival, etc. performed in an orderly and a normal way.

A capacity report should be prepared and approved by responsible departments after evaluation of the above listed and any other requirements for capacity. The capacity report should clearly demonstrate the plant capacity in terms of product produced per day/week/month/year based on the capacity of each equipment, process, schedules, and trained personnel.

Access and Security

The manufacturing areas should be accessible only to qualified and authorized personnel. Adequate security procedures should be established to demonstrate that the manufacturing facility is secure and not accessible to unauthorized people. Regulatory agencies have been paying special attention to this issue lately due to recent product counterfeiting incidents in generic drug companies.

Building Licensure

A BLA is submitted to the FDA or its equivalent EMEA or other global regulatory agencies, after completion of the above listed and other required activities and documentation, for licensure of the manufacturing facility. A pre-approval inspection (PAI) is often performed by the regulatory agencies to verify that the information submitted to them is accurate and complete. The FDA and other global regulatory agencies have indicated recently that they may make PAI optional, if the previous compliance or system based inspections of the applying company have been satisfactory. Upon successful inspection or verification of the information submitted, a BLA may be approved by the regulatory agencies permitting shipping of the approved product produced from the manufacturing facility to its customers.

In summary, process validation for a new cell culture derived-product, process, technology, or a new manufacturing facility should be carried out with a lot of careful planning and brainstorming along with a pinch of passion and dedication to details. Often process validation projects end up in tremendous delays and exorbitant costs due to poor planning, unrealistic goals and schedules, and inexperience of the assigned staff. It is a very expensive activity and should be carried out with good planning and caution. Validation activities take time on their own and often cannot be sped up no matter how many resources are poured into it. Albeit challenging and tough, it is an unforgettable journey that more often than not results in a joyful regulatory approval of a new product, process, technology, or a new manufacturing facility. Once taken successfully, one craves for this journey again and again and again.

7

DISTRIBUTION MANAGEMENT VALIDATION

As a provider of supply chain services to the pharmaceutical, medical device, consumer (OTC) and hospital services industries, Exel (from now on referred to as the organization) recognizes the requirement to validate systems used to ensure regulatory compliance, a high level of assurance to clients and to continually improve on services provided. Although the organization identified this as a global requirement that could potentially apply to food, cosmetics, and perishables, over time it was decided to establish the processes in one geographical area, Europe, and roll this out globally as shared best practice. This meant that the initial development of the organization's validation expertise is based on our European healthcare operations. As a supply chain service provider, the emphasis within the regulatory compliance arena had been more focused towards complying with current good distribution practice (cGDP), whereas the majority of the focus from our customers had been on the other cGxP critical processes, including cGMP, cGLP, and cGCP. There was increasing overlap as the organization expanded services into areas such as clinical trials logistics, repackaging and rework of returned goods which are essentially GMP regulated processes.

The fact that the organization's healthcare sector provides services to a large number of clients means they are potentially subject to a broader level of inspection by a wider audience of audit teams than a standard manufacturer. These consist of client QA teams in many different industry segments, as well as country regulatory authority such as FDA inspectors. This results in a considerable variance in type and depth of audit and inspection, dependent upon the local country, market, or segment regulatory requirements. The challenge of ensuring that the organization complies with these differing requirements has historically been addressed through the sector-wide implementation of cGDP. However it was recognized that there was a need to embrace the GAMP 4 guidelines, as an international standard covering all healthcare areas, to reflect the increased reliance on IT systems to manage and control cGxP stocks.

The service-based nature of our healthcare operation compared to our customers' manufacturing-based products, has meant that when interpreting whether a system or operation has GxP impact, it is not as straightforward as we would like. An example of this ambiguity is a new building access control system for installation in a new pharmaceutical validated warehousing facility. In a manufacturing operation, the access control system would have clear GxP impact, since uncontrolled access to the manufacturing process would have obvious consequences for the guaranteed efficacy and quality of the products produced. The case is not as clear in the storage environment. Since the manufacture is complete, the opportunity to directly compromise the product is limited to flaws in the warehouse management process which could affect, for example, shelf life or batch identity. These can be said to be under control through the validation of the warehouse management or inventory systems. Of course, it can still be argued that the access control system has GxP impact because unauthorized access could result in direct tampering with the products and influence product efficacy. In this case therefore the access control system was included in the final validation master plan ensuring we erred on the side of caution. The organization sought to build upon our existing project processes and pro-cedures, in order to map them to the GAMP 4 guidelines. This meant that the revised processes would be a development of existing processes, which reduced the level of retraining and disruption to the existing implementation and support methodology.

Revisions were viewed much more positively as strengthening the established methods, rather than introducing a new approach. Instances of these improved processes are the improvements in the organization's system specification techniques, where increased clarity and control in project scope now results in clear tracking of project scope creep. This helped to eliminate a common source of problems for project teams. As a result the final protocols use existing project implementation terminology and terms such as IQ, OQ, PQ, which are primarily pharmaceutical industry terms, and the 'V' Model, which was not widely used. However, for clarity at audit and inspection, this terminology is referred to when relevant, e.g., in the process mapping documentation and quality manual. Other examples where alternative models can be used to implement validated systems are the capability maturity model (CMM) and the project activity model (PAM).

A dedicated validation team was established using internal resources and leveraging external consultancy firms. The recognition that systems validation is an important area for the organization has meant that there has been very high level sponsorship for this project from our global president for the sector. The validation team has been working in conjunction with operational site teams, our suppliers, and customers (blue chip pharmaceutical and medical device manufacturers) to establish a standard protocol within a dedicated quality manual, which is now complete. This quality manual contains all the procedures to be followed by the project, the site support and the validation teams when producing documentation for new system implementations. These procedures also cover legacy system validations and the maintenance of existing validated systems. They also contain all the process maps, which link all the procedures and explain how the validation protocol functions in terms of the inputs and outputs of each process step. The quality manual also contains a breakdown of the process steps using the IDEF0 process-modelling tool, an integration definition tool, developed by the U.S. Air Force and released by the National Institute of Standards and Technology as a standard function model in 1993. The organization found IDEF0 useful, not only in mapping out the process steps involved, but also in educating project and site teams. Consequently, at each step the inputs, outputs, restraining controls, and mechanisms are explained, and team members can clearly see the process transition from one step to the next. In our experience, communicating the functional purpose of a system in clear graphical terms is probably the greatest strength of this technique.

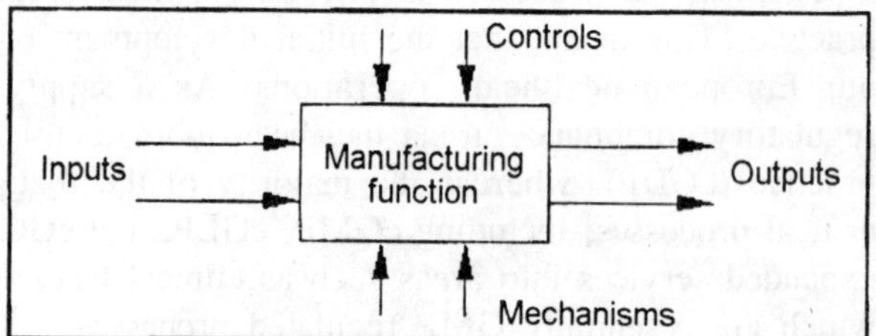

Fig. 7.1. Example taken from Exel's healthcare quality manual.

Developing the Protocol

The team made a conscious decision not to directly follow the "V" model, outlined in detail in the GAMP 4 guidelines. Although the "V" model is a sound and entirely logical process model, it was accepted early on that disruption to the teams who were implementing and running our computer systems should be minimal. Consequently the decision was taken to utilize existing project methodology, already of a high standard. This enabled the teams to refer to terminology already well understood within the business. During successive brainstorming sessions with various members of the project delivery teams the existing project lifecycle were mapped to the key phases. Using the process flows of the GAMP 4 guide, the team analyzed the existing life cycle in terms of the key validation phases and process steps. As a result, the implementation lifecycle was broken down into four distinct project phases:

1. Planning and specification.
2. Design.
3. Construction and testing.
4. Final testing and operation.

Each phase was then broken down (as illustrated in the figures) to represent the activities and documents required by the project and validation teams, the software houses and the organization's quality assurance team in order to produce a fully validated system.

The swimming lanes highlight the ownership of each document or process step. This schematic illustrates how the business development team finalize the requirements for the system solution (e.g., a new warehouse management system) to be implemented. In tandem, the project team will create implementation and project plans, along with a project definition document (PDD) as a general reference for project information. These three high-level project documents will all be inputs into the first project document that is reviewed by the validation team, the high level business processes (HLBP) (in some cases the HLBP document may be included as part of the user requirements specification.). The planning documents also feed into the first documents produced by the validation team, the validation master plan (VMP) and the individual validation plans (VP).

The distinction between the VMP and VP is key to the way that the organization approaches validation of its systems. The VMP will lay out the general approach to validation of all systems as part of an overall project implementation or site activity whereas the VP will describe in detail the activities to be undertaken in validating a particular instance of a system for a particular client. The organization will therefore not say that it has validated one particular system but instead, in most cases, will state that it has validated a system as it is used by a specific customer. This is because of the differences in configuration, network requirements, and hardware that occur between multiple users of the same system. This approach is a direct consequence of operating sites on a multiuser basis in order to make best use of key areas of expertise across a number of clients. Operating multi-user facilities is another key factor in the approach that the organization has taken to computer system validation. Where a manufacturer validates a computer system used for a specific task, the organization, as the logistics partner for several manufacturers, will be operating a system that contains data sets for all the manufacturers using the same set of programs.

Although not explicitly using the "V" model, many of the principles are derived from it. Ensuring that every activity or step laid out in the VP is referred to in the final Validation Report guarantees that each activity is verified.

For a new supplier, a supplier assessment is conducted to gauge quality processes and procedures in place before detailed project and validation planning documents are put together. This occurs at a later stage. This is a key step in the validation process for the organization. One reason for the importance attached to the assessment is that Exel's healthcare sector division does not design any of its software solutions itself. Consequently any system that is to be validated will be designed and constructed by a third-party supplier. The supplier assessment therefore has to thoroughly ensure that the process of code design, construction and testing is sound. The procedure or template for carrying out a supplier assessment reflects these needs.

Following the production of the VMP, VP, and HLBP by the validation and project teams respectively, the project team then constructs its user requirements specification, following a set procedure or template. This URS is reviewed and signed off internally and by client before it is submitted to the supplier (subject to a successful supplier assessment). The supplier will then respond to the URS by providing a formal functional specification document, which is fully referenced to the URS and details how each requirement is to be satisfied. One key output of the GAMP 4 guide is a quality plan. During initial validation exercises the validation team did produce a quality plan with the QA staff in conjunction with the VMP. However, as the process evolved, the quality plans for each system were so similar in content that the decision was taken to produce a single high-level quality plan. This could be applied to any system implementation. It states the commitment to quality in certain defined areas and describes how the organization would achieve its aims in the area of quality through the quality manual.

The validation team also establish an ongoing risk, threat, and issue log which tracks all issues considered to have a potentially detrimental impact on the ultimate validation of the system. Once these documents have been produced, all the deliverables for the planning and specification stage are in place and the first formal validation review can take place. Following a set procedure the validation team will meet with the project team and a representative of the QA team to review each document against the procedures laid out in the quality manual. During this review each document will be checked for adherence to the quality plan, consistency and completeness, and against all the checklisted points of the review procedure. At this point the review members can make a decision, based on the review checklist, as to whether to accept the documents in their current state and proceed to the design phase or to recommend necessary amendments before progressing. A formal report detailing the results of the review process forms an input into the final validation report.

Upon successful review of the planning and specification stage, the system implementation then moves into the "design" phase. Having established the key specification documents, the project team now create a new series of documents, which detail the configuration of the system. Existing and well-established procedures are followed to produce specifications for hardware, network and software configurations. (The latter only applies where there will be interfaces between different software modules.) There will also be a master data definition document outlining which static data needs to be set up on the system prior to full testing and operation. An example of such data are the locations of defined pick faces or customer and supplier address details. This is a document that is not included in the GAMP guidance. However, the characteristics of the multiuser environment not only necessitate this, but mean that it becomes a key specification. As the validation and project teams handle individual instances of the same system with data sets for each client, the static data, which needs to be configured prior to live operations for a client, becomes a vital area when maintaining close control over the system for each client. Similar issues can be seen in the software configuration specification required for modular computer systems. Other documents produced by the project team during this phase are the disaster recovery and business continuity plan. The testing specification document defines the approach to testing from the philosophy to the structure of the scripts, their acceptance criteria and the testing scripts themselves.

The project team will also at this stage compile a traceability matrix linking all the key system documentation and the functional areas within them. This allows an external reader such as an inspector, to follow any functional requirement, from the initial specification or business process document through to the eventual testing of that function in the delivered system. This matrix is updated throughout the system's life by the site support teams reflecting any changes resulting from change requests. These are recorded and retain full traceability for the URS, the FS, and the testing scripts. Using such a matrix has also been an incidental benefit of implementing GAMP methodology, since tracking areas of functionality through documentation had occasionally been a problem area. This is now much improved in terms of speed and reliability.

Again, when the deliverables are in place, the validation, project, and quality team members will carry out a formal review of the project phase before deciding whether to proceed to the construction and testing phase. Moving into the third project implementation phase, the initial versions of the software were installed. The testing strategy laid out previously in the testing specification can now be implemented. The schematic for this project phase lays out all the possible areas of testing, and also bridges the terminology gap between GAMP and the existing project terminology. The IQ, OQ, and PQ steps are identified without creating extra process steps for the testing teams. The testing specification is included in this phase as well as the previous one. Here it is used as a reference to ensure that the test scripts have been produced according to the testing plan. If the business processes are to be expanded then they should be included in this section. The other key deliverable here is the structured training material that is produced to support users of the finally implemented system. This may include project training material. As before, once all the deliverables are in place, a formal review will determine whether the project team can progress to the final phase of the implementation.

The final project phase involves completing the system testing (as per the testing specification) so cutover testing documentation is included. All of the change control documentation is also collated for future reference. This involves making sure that all the specification and testing documents, as well as the traceability matrix, are current prior to the handover from the project to the site support team. This will also be documented, following a predefined procedure or template. Upon completion, the final review can take place. Once all the project deliverables have been satisfactorily completed, then the final validation report can be written. This report will be written by the validation team, reflecting the results of all the activities planned, in light of the original validation plan. Once the validation team is satisfied that the system has been implemented in line with all the processes and procedures as set out in the quality manual and all risk and issue logs are closed out, then a validation certificate will be issued and the systems or validation register is updated. This will then reflect that the system implemented in this particular instance is considered validated and inspection ready.

Maintaining the Validated State

One of the biggest misconceptions that we encountered within the organization was that once we had implemented a validated system all the work is done! Using MS Visio Process models and IDEF0 charts we also constructed detailed mechanisms for maintaining the validated state, which were held within the quality manual. The emphasis here is on the work to be done by the site support team who provide live support to the individual clients once the system has been implemented. Typically there will be one analyst or super user per client who will have support from the validation team in maintaining the validated state. This time the starting point is the systems or validation register, which shows the validation status of each system, and reflects the work required to achieve and maintain this status. The work flow for the site team begins by following the operational plan as laid out in the quality manual. This details how the system must be maintained in terms of:

1. Training.
2. Problem management,.
3. Service level agreements (SLA).
4. System backups.
5. Business continuity planning.
6. Performance monitoring.

7. System security.
8. System retirement.

It is through adherence to the operational plan, associated procedures, and regular document reviews that the validation team assure adequate system maintenance.

Legacy System Review

The retrospective process therefore forms the third plank of this approach to validating all systems with GxP implications (e.g., after new systems and maintaining the validated state). This is still very much based on the processes already discussed. However the emphasis here is on ensuring that the key deliverables are already in place. This involves carrying out "*gap analysis*" and then performing any necessary remedial work. In this sense the organization's approach as a distributor does not differ significantly from a manufacturer, although the deliverables do, of course. As in a prospective implementation, validation plans are created. Once all the documents have been collated then a series of validation reviews will determine if the system meets the required standards prior to production of a final report, and update of the systems or validation register.

Electronic Records and Signatures

The area of electronic records and signatures is no easier for those working to cGDP than it is for those working to cGMP, cGCP, or cGLP. Also the recent withdrawal of guidelines and recent interpretations of the CFR 21 Part 11 legislation makes this a very difficult area in which to achieve full compliance.

Approach

The organization has incorporated the ER/ES requirements within the overall validation approach. There is no separate plan to achieve Part 11 compliance per system. There is a policy document that states how to achieve compliance published within the quality manual, detailing the requirements of each section of the regulation and sets out how compliance is achieved. Emphasis has been placed on the following areas:

1. Policies.
2. Protection of records.
3. Security (system and logical).
4. Sequential checks.
5. Training.
6. Documentation.

The approach achieves compliance through a combination of internal policies and procedures and the organization's software suppliers' technical controls. The three main areas considered necessary to achieve compliance are graphically represented in the Venn diagram.

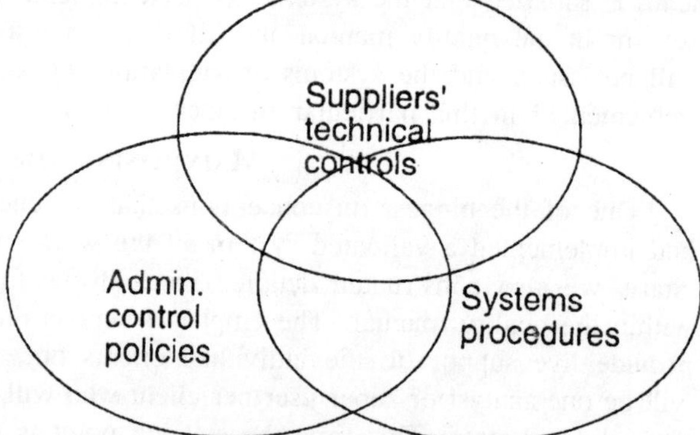

Fig. 7.2. Venn diagram representation of areas necessary to achieve compliance.

Specific Validation Work

The quality manual was first launched in the final quarter of 2002 as the validation and project team members used the new processes and procedures to retrospectively validate the core versions of the key healthcare warehousing solutions. These are the warehouse management system (WMS), task management system and the integration solution that links the WMS with our clients own ERP and

MRP systems. This exercise was termed the validation of generic versions of the systems. Identification of core functionality through the high-level business processes was followed by the creation of a URS, supplied to our software suppliers in conjunction with supplier audits. As previously illustrated this assessment is vital to ensure the software design quality, achieved through rigorously challenging the potential supplier's design methods. We experienced some issues with our suppliers because they supply systems that are not used exclusively in a healthcare environment. They also wanted to know afterwards if they were then "*GAMP compliant.*" (The answer was that there is no such thing as being "*GAMP compliant*," however vendors could be technically compliant with the guidance but this is heavily dependant on the administrative and procedural controls applied by their customers) Another benefit of doing the work was that we were able to improve, or suggest potential improvements, for some of their procedures with regard to future software development. We have also found that audited and potential suppliers with previous experience of applying the GAMP principles were much further ahead in areas such as QMS, continuous improvement, code design and review, in comparison to their uninitiated counterparts.

We were then able to follow through the rest of the validation processes, holding formal reviews at predefined stages of the implementation lifecycle to ensure that the key documents had been produced to satisfactory standards and in line with the established procedures, for example, the user requirements specification, the functional specification and the testing specification and attendant scripts. This culminated in the production of final validation reports for each of the systems, which summarized the results of each of the validation reviews and the creation of a systems or validation register, updated with the results as well as any actions, which remained outstanding. Since the completion of the generic validation project the validation protocol has been fully deployed to validate specific instances of the WMS and several other systems such as those used for clinical trials logistics and temperature monitoring.

Regulatory Environment

The regulatory environment has changed while the validation protocol has been developed, the merger between the MCA and the MDA to form the MHRA in the UK demonstrates how it is vital to constantly review the environment that we as a business operate in. Regular housekeeping tasks now include reviewing the main regulatory communications channels for white papers and new draft guidance documents. This is increasingly done in partnership with our colleagues in the U.S. and APAC regions. More specifically, recent guidance issued by the FDA, following on from the ISPE's white paper has led to a different, narrower interpretation of the scope and application of 21 CFR Part 11. This has meant that we have reviewed our approach to the issues of electronic records and signatures, and revised the documentation within the quality manual where necessary to do so.

Moving Forward

The validation protocol is rolled out as a standard implementation methodology for all healthcare systems projects as a matter of policy and has become a well-established and ingrained operating mode amongst all members of the organization's healthcare community. The European validation team has also begun to develop a common approach based on the work done for the generic exercise in the U.S. and the Asia Pacific regions (the latter taking into account the requirements of the Australian regulatory body, the TGA, which borrows from the MCA and PICS literature). The global arena offers us further validation challenges as the organization deals with several major pharmaceutical companies in different areas. A consequence of this is that care must be taken when dealing with a client who may have a validated warehouse management system in its U.K. operation and therefore assumes that an instance of a different or even the same system in Australia or the U.S.A. is also validated. This may be especially true if global system brands are used. This issue is particularly relevant when discussing global branding of computer systems.

Tackling and Solving Problems

There has been some organizational resistance by parts of the business community who have viewed validation as a commercial option rather than a necessity. It was viewed as adding to the paper workload and being an "IT" cost rather than adding any value, so a lot of education and communication has been required. This communication has taken the form of internal presentations at different levels of the business and production of information packs for project, site support, and business development teams. The validation team has tried to remove the perception that validation is something which the IT community come and do to the operations and encourage the philosophy that the organization builds validation into our way of doing things such that it becomes part of good project and support practice.

There has also been a presumption that operations more concerned with medical devices have a lesser regulatory onus than for pharmaceuticals. The recent merger of the MCA and MDA to form the MHRA in the U.K., and the inevitable harmonization of regulatory requirements, is evidence that this will no longer be the case. Again, by building the validation protocol into standard project practice this problem is gradually being eliminated. Misconceptions in some European locations have included varying interpretations of the stringency of country regulations when compared to the U.K. and U.S. Also a different perception existed in some countries of what validation involves. The organization has addressed this issue at the highest level by building validated systems into our healthcare sector brand through an insistence that all new system implementations will be validated. Another misconception has been by the third party software suppliers that has ISO900x accreditation can act as a substitute for following GAMP! The challenge here was enforcement of any noncompliance since we do not have any direct power to enforce changes without resorting to the commercial arrangement. Through our existing excellent supplier relationships we have worked together to reach a point where we are happy that our suppliers fulfil their obligations to us and our requirements.

There was also a feeling early on that only the warehouse management systems required validation, little regard was given to other software or even process control systems. Subsequently Exel's healthcare sector having recently built a new UK pharmaceutical export warehouse facility has extended validation to the building itself as part of the process of gaining MCA license approval, including the temperature monitoring system, the access control system, and the chilled goods storage areas. As has already been seen, perceptions like this would be a one-off exercise that the IT community would perform. However, as part of the education and communication process, emphasis has been placed on the importance of maintaining the validated state following initial implementation and this is a message that has gradually been accepted by the business and is now owned by the various support functions. Members of the validation team are now often present at early stage meetings or presentations to potential clients or where we are trying to extend the scope of our business with existing customers. Senior management have recognized that many pharmaceutical and medical devices manufacturers will not consider us as a third party logistics partner if we cannot offer validated systems to them. It is now recognized as an important tool by which we can differentiate itself from its peer group and provide us with a distinct competitive advantage.

8

STEAM STERILIZATION

The science that underpins steam sterilization is well known and has been long established. It is the preferred method of sterilization in the pharmaceutical industry; it is used for sterilization of aqueous products in a wide variety of presentations, for sterilization of equipment and porous materials required in aseptic manufacture, in microbiology laboratories for sterilizing media and other materials, and for sterilization of "massive" systems of vessels and pipework [steam-in-place (SIP) systems]. Numerous rules and guidelines have been published on the topic, yet steam sterilization and particularly biovalidation of steam sterilization is still a subject for controversy and debate. The purpose of this article is to reexamine the biovalidation of steam sterilization, to clarify what is needed and why it is needed, and to distinguish the scientific need from the regulatory need in areas where they may appear to differ.

PRINCIPLES

Micro-organisms are inactivated when metabolically irreversible deleterious intracellular reactions occur. At high temperatures and in the presence of moisture, as in steam sterilization, the energy input from the steam inactivates micro-organisms by denaturation of intracellular proteins. Although these reactions are complex at a biochemical level, their kinetics approximate to reactions of the first order. Thus, the kinetics of inactivation of populations of pure cultures of micro-organisms take the typical exponential form of reactions of the first order. What this means in experimental practice is that there is a linear relationship when numbers of microorganisms held at high temperatures are plotted on a logarithmic scale against time plotted on an arithmetic scale. There are two highly significant points to be drawn from the kinetics of inactivation of micro-organisms.

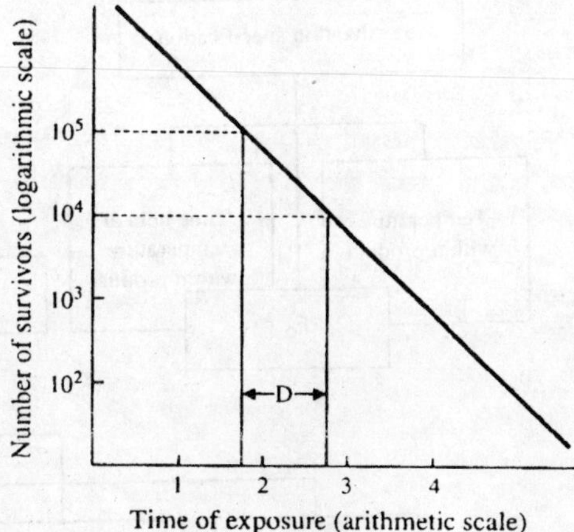

Fig. 8.1. Exponential inactivation of micro-organisms.

First, logarithmic scales never reach zero. This means that there can never be any specifications for temperature and time which can guarantee that all micro-organisms contaminating items are going to be inactivated. However, the consequences to patients of micro-organisms surviving in allegedly sterile pharmaceutical preparations can easily be fatal. Thus, sterilization processes must be specified to ensure that the probability of micro-organisms surviving in treated items is low enough to ensure patient safety. The accepted low probability indicated in the pharmacopeias is that there should be not more than one chance in one million of viable micro-organisms surviving on a treated item. This is called a probability of non-sterility of 10^{-6} or a sterility assurance level (SAL) of 10^{-6}. Second, the inactivation curve takes a regular form. This means that steam sterilization is a predictable process as long as some information is available (or can be safely assumed) about the numbers and thermal resistances of the micro-organisms contaminating items before treatment. This is important because there is no practical way to test for the achievement of SALs of 10^{-6}. The sterility or non- sterility of items cannot sensibly be confirmed in a treated item except by sacrificing the item. The pharmacopeial *test for sterility* is a sacrificial test with statistical limitations which have been so extensively criticized over so many decades that they should now be well understood. For instance, the sample of 20 items which is generally required in the test would allow a batch containing non-sterile items at a frequency of 1:100 to be passed on four out of every five occasions. This falls a long way short of being able to detect deviations from a standard of not more than one non-sterile item in one million.

Justification of the reliable achievement of SALs of 10^{-6} for particular pharmaceutical items treated according to particular specifications of temperature and time in particular sterilizers is predicated on the regularity and predictability of steam sterilization processes. The means of justification are through scientifically based development of sterilization specifications and sterilizer parameters, and through subsequent validation of the specified processes.

Development of Sterilization Specifications and Sterilizer Parameters

The development of sterilization specifications differs from the development of sterilizer parameters. Both differ from validation.

Pharmaceutical Products and Materials for Aseptic Manufacture–Sterilization Specifications

For pharmaceutical products and materials used in connection with aseptic manufacture, sterilization specifications apply to conditions of temperature and time, or F_0, or combinations of F_0, temperature and time to which the contaminating micro-organisms themselves must be exposed over the "hold" period of the sterilization process. In practice, this means actually within aqueous products, on the surfaces of rubber stoppers or metal machine parts, or within the folds of cartridge filters, etc.

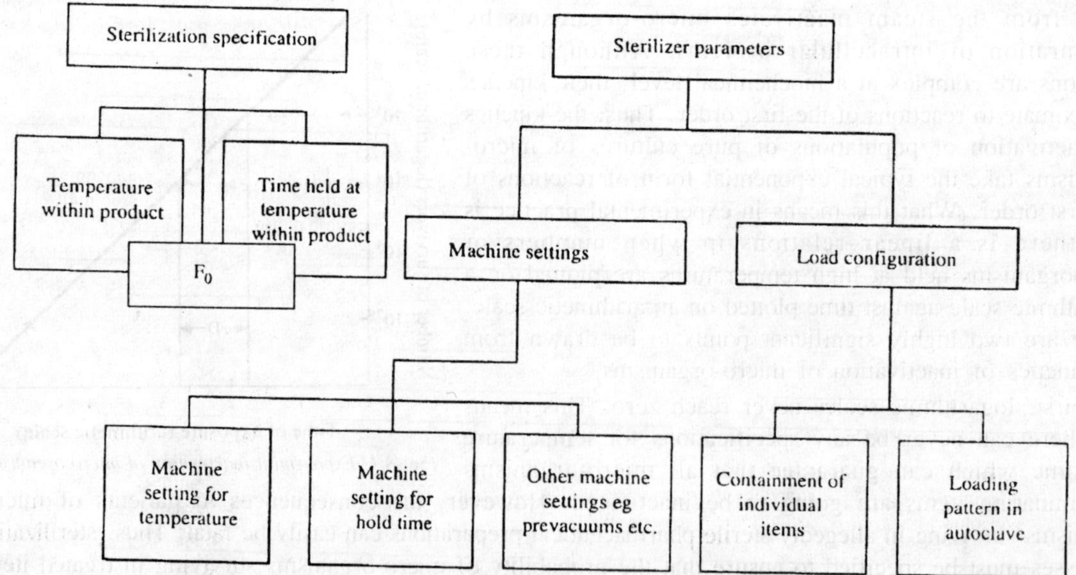

Fig. 8.2. Sterilization specifications and sterilizer parameters.

The sterilizer parameters are the practical criteria that must be specified to ensure that the sterilization specification is delivered to all parts of the load. They always include specifications for temperature and time, but it is important to recognize the distinction between sterilizer parameters applying to the machine settings on the autoclave console, and sterilization specifications applying to actual conditions within the load. Essential sterilizer parameters also include other specifications, e.g., for load configuration, number and depth of prevacuums, cooling characteristics, etc. Sterilization specifications are product specific. Sterilizer parameters are specific to combinations of product, presentation, and autoclave. Sterilization specifications may be determined from theoretical considerations or from laboratory data and are within reason transferable from presentation to presentation, e.g., from 1 ml ampules to 5 ml vials to 50 ml bags. The sterilizer parameters required to deliver the sterilization specification to these presentations differ within the same autoclave and from one autoclave to another according to differences in load configurations, chamber size, steam entry points, control systems, etc. Sterilizer parameters are not transferable and must be developed empirically for each autoclave.

Sterilization specifications should be easy to develop. The pharmacopeias allow sterilization specifications to be developed from a basis of no actual data concerning the numbers and thermal resistances of micro-organisms actually contaminating the items to be sterilized. Although this statement may appear initially to be barren of scientific reason, this is in fact not the case. What the pharmacopeias provide are either a recommended overkill specification (*PhEur*) or principles for specification development (USP) that incorporate amounts of thermal lethality well in excess of that which could ever be practically required to obtain SALs of 10^{-6}—for this reason they are called *"overkill"* specifications. In the *European Pharmacopoeia* (*PhEur*), a specification of 121°C for 15 min is given as the reference condition for overkill sterilization of aqueous preparations. The *United States Pharmacopeia* (USP) defines a lethality input of 12D. These specifications merit some examination in detail. It is worth considering the thermal resistances of micro-organisms found in pharmaceutical manufacturing environments. It is extremely rare for anyone to have isolated thermally resistant bacteria with D_{121}-values (in water) of greater than 0.3 min. The author of this paper has experience of having determined a D_{121}-value (in water) of 0.8 min for an environmental isolate of Bacillus coagulans, but this was several decades ago and was done with what would now be considered fairly primitive equipment. It is therefore probably quite reasonable to assume a worst case D_{121}-value of 1 min. Given this "worst case," the *PhEur* overkill specification of 121°C would deliver 15 decimal reductions which are equivalent to assuring a 10^{-6} SAL for contaminating populations per item of up to 10^{9} micro-organisms each with a D_{121}-value of 1 min. The USP specification of 12D under the same assumption ensures an SAL of 10^{-6} for populations of up to 10^{6} micro-organisms per item.

Thus, the pharmacopeial overkill specifications provide considerable degrees of assurance that SALs of 10^{-6} will be achieved. However, these high theoretical levels of overkill are contingent upon D-values in water being reflected by D-values in or on product. Most pharmaceutical products depress the thermal resistance of micro-organisms relative to their D-values in water, but this is not universally true. Some other materials (e.g., rubber) are known to increase the thermal resistance of micro-organisms (this may as likely be due to physical characteristics of heat transference as to biochemical protection). These product effects on thermal resistance can only be determined empirically, and are usually done in the laboratory using thermally resistant bacterial endospores, often spores of *Bacillus stearothermophilus*. The use of *B. stearothermophilus* for this purpose and their frequent use as biological indicators (BIs) in biovalidation have contributed to a belief that steam sterilization must be defined in terms of being able to kill this micro-organism. It is not; spores of *B. stearothermophilus* are used with steam sterilization because of the convenience of their high resistance to steam sterilization and the unique and distinctive conditions required for their recovery and growth. Indeed, some major companies use *Clostridium sporogenes* or other species of Bacillus as reference or indicator organisms for this purpose. The use of "overkill" specifications is not mandatory. In some instances, there may be pharmaceutical products which are unable to withstand the temperatures or energy inputs of overkill specifications. In these cases, specifications can be developed by calculating SALs of 10^{-6} from data characterizing the number of micro-organisms actually contaminating items before sterilization treatment, or from data characterizing the actual numbers and thermal resistances of the contaminating micro-organisms. The question is this—Is this exercise worth doing or would it be better and simpler to opt for aseptic manufacture of such heat-sensitive products?

Let us consider the number of micro-organisms contaminating pharmaceutical products prior to sterilization. What are the highest and the lowest numbers which could be expected? For sterile parenteral products, the highest tolerable number of micro-organisms would be expected to be on the order of 10^2. This is because 10^3 or more per item is likely to begin to incur a risk of pyrogenicity. The lowest number which could be inferred from even an extensive number of zero counts would be one micro-organism. Achievement of a 10^{-6} SAL from an initial bioburden of 10^2 would require eight log reductions. Applying these eight log reductions to an assumed worst case thermal resistance of D_{121}-value in water of 1 min gives a sterilization specification of 121°C for 8 min. Achievement of a 10^{-6} SAL from an initial bioburden of 1 would require six log reductions. Applying these six log reductions to an assumed worst case thermal resistance of D_{121}-value in water of 1 min gives a sterilization specification of 121°C for 6 min.

The determination of thermal resistances is technically complex and requires special equipment (BIER Vessels). Since it is unlikely that *Bacillus* spp. can be excluded from any survey of microbiological contamination, it is reasonable to assume that spores with D_{121}-values on the order of 0.3 min will be isolated. Using this figure, SALs of 10^{-6} can be calculated at 121°C for 2.4 min for bioburdens of 10^2, and at 121°C for 1.8 min for bioburdens of one micro-organism per item. It is apparent that very brief sterilization specifications (on the order of 2–3 min holding time at 121°C) are obtainable when the microbiological contamination is completely characterized in terms of numbers and thermal resistances. In practice, such limits on hold times could be difficult to control precisely, are probably insignificant in terms of thermal lethality compared with heat-up and cool-down times, and could prove difficult to "sell" to regulators. Without complete thermal characterization of thermal resistances, specifications calculable by the "bioburden" approach are hardly significantly shorter than *"overkill"* specifications. Thus, it probably makes practical sense in most cases to choose only between overkill cycles for thermally resistant products and aseptic manufacture for heat-sensitive products.

Some products may be heat sensitive only above a threshold temperature; for those that can withstand temperatures in the range of 110–118°C but cannot withstand 121°C it is possible to apply the F_0 concept to the principles above and derive equivalent sterilization specifications. These specifications are summarized for 116°C. As can be seen, if there is a requirement to sterilize at (say) 116°C, there are considerable time savings to be obtained by characterization of the contaminating micro-organisms.

Pharmaceutical Products and Materials for Aseptic Manufacture—Sterilizer Parameters

Sterilizer parameters are specific to combinations of product, presentation, and autoclave. They must be established empirically. Heat penetration studies done prior to the performance qualification phase of validation serve the purpose of determining the loading patterns, prevacuums, and temperature and pressure settings, etc. which ensure that the sterilization specification is delivered to the product and that it is delivered uniformly throughout the load.

For instance, a particular proposed loading pattern may never allow for uniform conditions (within specified limits) to be achieved throughout the load. In this case the pattern would have to be changed. Or, in a particular autoclave it may be necessary to set the temperature at 122°C for 121°C to be achieved within the load. Air removal is particularly important in porous and equipment loads, but is usually of little importance in the sterilization of aqueous pharmaceutical products. Air removal can be important to the specification of new autoclaves—those which are to be designated only for aqueous product sterilization have no need for the pumps and ancillary equipment required to pull deep vacuums. The involvement of steam in the sterilization of different types of product is an important consideration in understanding and controlling autoclaves. For aqueous products, steam is solely a means of raising the product to the specified sterilizing temperature; the steam does not come into contact with the contaminating micro-organisms. The transfer of heat energy (lethality) to the contaminating microorganisms is from the product itself. To all intents and purposes any suitable form of energy source could be used to raise the temperature of the product.

For instance, if ampules of aqueous products were to be sterilized in a hot air oven, the mechanisms of microbial inactivation would still be by coagulation of intracellular proteins. However, heat transfer from hot air is much slower than heat transfer from steam, which is why this is not seen as a practical process. Microwave irradiation could be an alternative means of sterilizing aqueous pharmaceutical products utilizing the same antimicrobial mechanisms as steam; certainly there is evidence that microwave killing patterns are mainly due to heat transfer with very little direct energy being absorbed from the microwaves. For porous and equipment loads, the steam comes into direct contact with the contaminating microorganisms on the materials being sterilized and there is no intermediary in the transfer of heat. The energy content of steam is defined by its latent heat. If the steam is pure in the sense that it contains neither entrained gas nor moisture, an amount of energy defined by its latent heat at the pressure of the steam will be transferred to the micro-organisms by condensation on their surfaces.

There are many potential pitfalls in equipment and porous load sterilization, mainly concerned with air or other non-condensable gas. First, the purity of the steam is important; if it is carrying moisture, or non-condensable gas, it will not contain the same amount of energy as pure steam and its lethality will be less than that predicted for pure steam. Second, any residual air around the contaminating micro-organisms may insulate them from contact with the steam and thus reduce the amount of energy (lethality) transferred. In this type of sterilization, steam quality becomes very important and so also do the materials and manner in which the products are contained in steam-permeable wrapping or perforated trays, etc., within the autoclave, and the number and depth of evacuations of the autoclave prior to the temperature- hold phases. Thermal monitoring alone gives little information on the adequacy of the measures put in place to control these complex factors, and it is therefore generally thought essential that some empirical studies be done with BIs as part of process development to ensure that the thermal lethality being imparted by the steam is not being impeded. These development studies may be rolled into bio-validation.

Sterilization of Microbiological Media in the Laboratory

The various suppliers of microbiological media include recommendations for sterilization in their catalog under "Directions for Use," for instance, "sterilize by autoclaving at 121°C for 15–18 min." The question that must be asked is—What do these specifications mean? Are they intended to apply within the media as are the sterilization specifications for pharmaceutical products and materials for aseptic manufacture? Or are they sterilizer parameters? There may be some indication in some of the older suppliers' manuals which expand their recommendations along the lines of "sterilize by autoclaving at 15 psi (121°C) for 15–18 min." Since pressures of 15 psi are not achievable within media, it is clear that the intention was that the recommendations be applied to sterilizer parameters. In most cases, it is probably immaterial how these recommendations are interpreted. For media, "over-cooking" is bad because of deleterious effects on growth-support characteristics, and "undercooking" is generally self-disclosing through evident contamination.

SIP Systems

Systems that are sterilized in-place are often immensely complex. The initial challenges to their sterilization are the removal of air and the elevation of the temperature of the pipework to prevent heat losses and condensation. As such, most work in the development of sterilization specifications for SIP systems is concerned with the heat-up phase. Appropriate questions are: Is the sterilization temperature achieved throughout the system? Where is the slowest location to achieve temperature? Where should the control probe be located? Often vast amounts of thermal lethality calculated as F_0-values are delivered in these prehold stages of SIP. However, because these temperatures are being achieved in the presence of steam–air mixtures, it is not correct to assume that the biological lethality during the heat-up phase of SIP systems is equivalent to that achieved with pure steam.

The time for which the system must be held at temperature (the sterilization specification) is often relegated to a minor consideration compared with this earlier development work. Typically, it is decided arbitrarily to use, 121°C for 15, 20, or 30 min, with no real scientific basis. Perhaps, a basis parallel to that of the pharmacopeial overkill specifications could be developed. For instance, if the actual maximum number of microorganisms within an SIP system is assumed to be 10^{12} (since this would amount to a few grams of biomass it certainly should be maximal), then 18 log reductions would be required to ensure not more than one chance in a million of a survivor. An overkill cycle of 121°C for 20 min could be proposed by adding two log reductions as a safety factor and assuming each microorganism to have a D_{121}-value of 1 min.

Bio-validation

The performance qualification (PQ) phase of validation follows the development of the sterilization specifications and of the sterilizer parameters which will deliver them. The purpose of PQ in steam sterilization of pharmaceutical products, equipment, laboratory media, and SIP systems is to confirm that the sterilization specification consistently achieves its intended purpose. The process is run using the parameters derived from process development on (usually) three separate occasions and tested for compliance with a variety of predetermined acceptance criteria. As a subset of PQ, the purpose of bio-validation is to confirm that the lethality expected from the process does not significantly deviate from what is expected. Biovalidation is a "test'' of consistency. If the acceptance criteria are not achieved, there may be need for more process development.

In consideration of the extent, thoroughness, and history of the research evidence that micro-organisms are inactivated in a regular fashion in response to temperature and time, it is periodically suggested that biovalidation should not be necessary where there is evidence of adequate heat penetration. In practice, however, the expected lethality may not always be achieved. Most frequently, such deviations from ideality occur in equipment and porous load sterilization because of inadequate air removal. Where deviations from ideality occur for aqueous pharmaceutical products, they most likely arise from inadequate knowledge of how the product affects the thermal resistances of micro-organisms, but this is best determined in the laboratory at an earlier stage of process development, not at the bio-validation "milestone'' later in the critical path of product introduction.

Acceptance criteria for bio-validation of steam sterilization processes are usually (but not invariably) defined along the following lines:

1. *n* BIs will be placed in the load at locations defined in a drawing.
2. Each BI will contain at least 10^6 viable spores of *B. stearothermophilus*.
3. The load will be exposed to a defined autoclave treatment (the validation cycle).
4. Bio-validation will be considered satisfactory if no viable spores are recovered from the BIs after *x* days of incubation at 55–60°C.

Because this approach is the common practice, there is a widely held belief within the pharmaceutical QA community that the ability to inactivate 10^6 spores of *B. stearothermophilus* is a synonym for achieving an SAL of 10^{-6}. It is not. It is true, however, that inactivation of 10^6 spores of *B. stearothermophilus* with the pharmacopeially approved minimum D-value of 1.5 min in 10–100 replicates guarantees achievement of better than 10^{-6} SALs for worst case bioburdens. However, the converse, i.e., failing to inactivate 10^6 spores of *B. stearothermophilus*, does not necessarily mean that a 10^{-6} SAL has not been achieved.

Another area of confusion is that the USP definition of an overkill specification— "a lethality input of 12D" —can be demonstrated directly in bio-validation. It should be understood that the maximum number of log inactivations of any bacterial population is technically limited to about 9 or 10 D-values. The maximum number of micro-organisms that can be handled as a BI is about 10^7-10^8, the sensitivity of recovery of micro-organisms is restricted to more than 10^{-2}. An indirect demonstration of 12 log inactivations of a micro-organism with a D-value of 1 min can be achieved by showing inactivation of 10–100 replicate BIs each carrying 10^6 spores with D-values of 1.5 min, or by inactivation of 10–100 replicate BIs each carrying 10^4 spores with D-values of 2 min. Direct demonstration of 12D is technically impossible. In bio-validation, the spore of B. stearothermophilus is akin to an end-point analytical reagent. For instance, when litmus changes from blue to red at pH levels below 7, it shows only that the pH is not higher than 7. By killing all of 10–100 replicate BIs with 10^6 spores having D-value 1.5 min, all that is proven is that the thermal lethality delivered is not less than an F0 of 12 min. The PhEur overkill sterilization specification of 121°C for 15 min should meet this requirement easily, and so should any other longer specification at 121°C, or any specification for longer times at lower temperatures taking into account of the F_0 concept.

Numbers and Locations of BIs for Bio-Validation

It is usual for bio-validation to be done with an arbitrary number of BIs between 10 and 100. Both limits are based on practical considerations. The lower number of BIs is defined in terms of ensuring that bio-validation addresses sufficient parts of the load for confidence that items in all parts of the autoclave are receiving the required lethality.

Normal practice is to define this number in terms of placing at least as many BIs as the number of thermal probes used for thermal qualification. It is sensible to place one BI alongside each thermal probe in order to be able to relate thermal data to biological data. In addition to this, some BIs should be placed in other non- probed locations in consideration of the possibility that the leads to the thermal probes may be acting as conduits for air removal or steam penetration, and thus provide falsely high levels of lethality.

More often than not the number of BIs used is about 20–30. Larger numbers up to 100 may be necessary to address very large autoclaves or in thermal mapping studies, but in validation there is little extra statistical confidence to be gained by doing so. In most microbiology QA laboratories, 20–30 BIs can be handled conveniently. Periodically in the bio-validation of sterilization of porous or equipment "*minimum*" loads, it is not practical to locate 20 or 30 BIs. For instance, a minimum load may be one cartridge filter, one mop head, or one machine manifold. In such cases, it is important to avoid too much distortion of the statistics of biovalidation. At least five BIs are recommended no matter how difficult it may be to place them.

Choice of BIs

Spores of *B. stearothermophilus* are most commonly used for bio-validation of steam sterilization processes. This is not to say that it is mandatory to use B. stearohermophilus nor that it is used exclusively. Other micro-organisms, e.g., sporogenes, are used by some companies and accepted by the regulatory agencies. Use of B. subtilis spores with resistances to steam sterilization in the higher range of that found in natural bioburden has, in recent years, been criticized by European regulatory agencies. The principles underlying the choice of microorganism used as BIs are quite well known:

1. The micro-organisms must have high resistance to the sterilization treatment which they are being used to validate. This does not mean that they must be the most resistant micro-organism known to man. *B. stearothermophilus* has D_{121}-values of 1–4 min according to conditions of culture and the substrate upon which they are mounted. This is higher than most spores of *Bacillus* spp., which tend to have D_{121}-values below 0.5 min.
2. The micro-organisms must have stable resistances to the sterilization treatment which they are being used to validate. There are data from commercial suppliers of BIs to show that spores of *B. stearothermophilus* survive and retain stable resistances over long periods of crudely controlled storage.
3. The micro-organisms must be easily culturable and preferably be easily identifiable in culture. Very few micro-organisms share with *B. stearothermophilus* the ability to grow in simple culture media at 55–60°C.

It is customary to use 10^6 (in practical terms 10^5–10^7) spores per BI. This number is based on custom, practice, and convenience rather than on science. Larger numbers than this are difficult to handle in culture and result in large errors in counting. Smaller numbers reduce the sensitivity of the test. Unfortunately, the widespread use of 10^6 spores for bio-validation has (as described before) led to a confusion between 10^{-6} SALs and 6 log reductions of *B. stearothermophilus*. More complex decisions surround the choice of substrate within which spores are suspended or on which they are mounted for use as BIs. The decision tree may be used to help choose the spore substrate used in bio-validation of aqueous pharmaceutical products. To use this decision tree, it is essential to have some knowledge of the effects of product on the resistance of spores; as mentioned before, this requires special equipment and experience. In all circumstances water is the preferred substrate for bio-validation of aqueous pharmaceutical products. Where water would give deceptive results, it should not be used.

1. If the D_{121}-value of *B. stearothermophilus* is higher in the product than it would be in water (i.e., the product makes the spores more resistant to steam sterilization), then bio-validation must be done with the spores suspended in product. Otherwise falsely favorable results may occur.
2. If the D_{121}-value in product of *B. stearothermophilus* is equal to or less than its

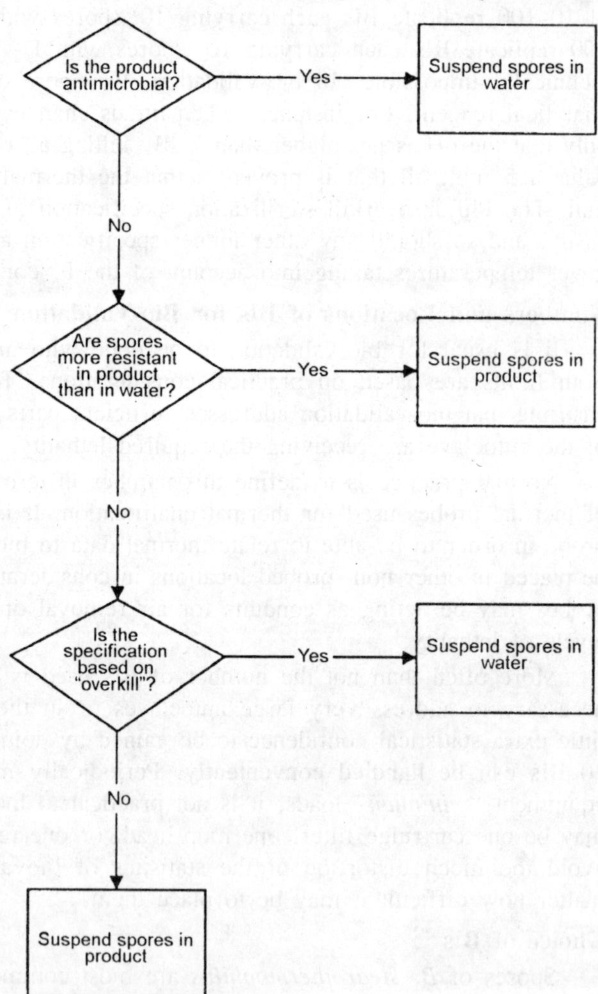

Fig. 8.3. Recommended substrates for BIs used in biovalidation of aqueous fluid loads.

D_{121}-value in water, and the sterilization specification is based on overkill, then bio-validation must be done with spores suspended in water. However, if the sterilization specification has been "*tailored*" specifically to the resistance of micro-organisms in the product, then bio-validation must be done with the spores suspended in product. Otherwise falsely unfavorable results may occur.

Under no circumstances must spores be suspended in product if that product is sporicidal. For other materials (for instance, equipment and supplies for aseptic manufacture) where the mechanisms of inactivation rely on direct contact between the steam and the item being sterilized and therefore where air removal is matter of importance, the choice of substrate for BIs generally lies between using commercially available paper spore strips and the material itself. The decision tree in 4 may be helpful. Regulatory pressure is currently toward use of inoculated product, but commercially available spore strips are more convenient. "Tailor-made" inoculated product requires substantial amounts of microbiological expertise. The decision tree may be helpful in selecting which approach is best in particular circumstances. Use of commercially available BIs transfers much of the responsibility for assuring quality in manufacture to the supplier. Regardless of this, their quality must be controlled on receipt and prior to use in bio-validation. There is no reason why any microbiology laboratory should not verify the numbers of spores per commercial BI. On the other hand, the determination of resistance requires special equipment and expertise and is probably best accepted on the basis of the supplier's certification. If this is done, the user of the BIs is responsible for knowing what the certified measures of resistance mean, how they were determined (on the strips, in aqueous suspension, or in or on something else), and that they were determined correctly and in compliance with applicable standards and legislation.

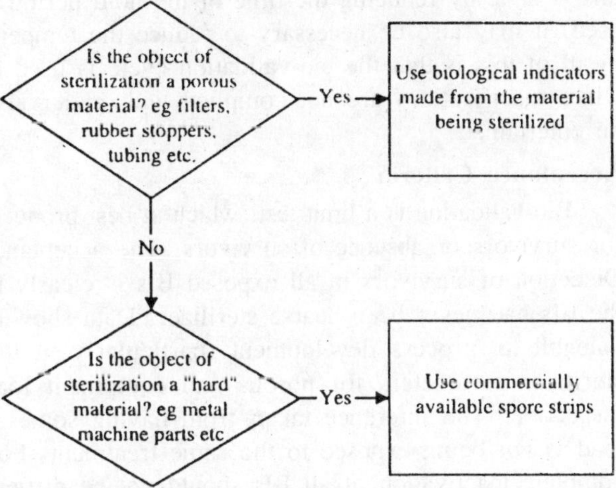

Fig. 8.4. Recommended substrates for BIs used in biovalidation of porous loads.

Validation Cycle

Bio-validation is usually done against a sterilization specification which delivers less lethality than the lower limit of lethality allowed by the sterilization specification defined for the material being sterilized. It is clearly intellectually flawed to choose to validate something different to that which is ever to be used in practice. So what is the reasoning behind this practice?

Sterilization specifications in the "hold" period are presented in terms of temperature and time with upper and lower tolerances set around them. The lower specification limits are critical to sterilization.

Time is generally easily controllable to quite high levels of accuracy and precision: A steam valve allows steam to enter the autoclave until the hold temperature is reached; the valve is then closed and the process is controlled by a timer which, at the end of the specified hold period, sends a control signal to activate the exhaust valves and cooling sequences. The hold time is usually specified in terms of whole minutes—well within the accuracy and precision of all but the most inappropriate of timers.

Temperature is less easy to control precisely. The temperature in the hold period in autoclaves is generally maintained by modulating valves which open to allow steam entry when the temperature (or pressure, because these valves are more often than not controlled through pressure transducers) begins to drop toward the critical lower limit of the specification. It is generally not possible to control an autoclave to run through a complete hold period at the lower limit of its temperature specification. However, even quite apparently trivial errors in temperature above or below the limit can make significant differences in the amount of lethality delivered. For instance, at a nominal temperature of 121°C, an error of 1 K can increase or decrease the amount of lethality by 25%.

Bio-validation cycles are therefore designed to ensure that no more lethality is delivered than that specified by the lower limits of lethality of the sterilization specification used in routine practice. Ideally this is done by reducing the time of the hold period, but sometimes, when quite short cycles are being used, it may also be necessary to reduce the temperature set point on the autoclave as well. The risk in all of this is that the bio-validation cycle is used as a justification for the release of sterilized items when specifications are not complied with under atypical production conditions. This idea should not be entertained.

Acceptance Criteria

Bio-validation is a limit test, which at best produces quantal data. Each BI should be tested separately for survivors or absence of survivors. The acceptance criterion should be that there are no survivors. Detection of survivors in all exposed BIs is clearly unacceptable; such a result would be obtainable if the BIs had never been near a sterilizer. Data showing survival on some but not all of the BIs may be valuable in process development (particularly in the development of sterilization specifications and sterilizer parameters for porous and equipment loads), but would likely raise issues at regulatory inspection. The inference taken from having some survival could be that each item in the autoclave load is not being exposed to the same treatment. For initial validation of a newly developed process, complete inactivation of all BIs should not be difficult to achieve.

The range of D_{121}-values acceptable to USP for spores of *B. stearothermophilus* allowed as BIs for use in steam sterilization is 1.5–3.0 min. An overkill sterilization or bio-validation specification delivering an F_0 of 15 min would deliver 10 log inactivations or, if there were 10^6 spores per BI, one chance in one million of finding a survivor on any one BI, one chance in one thousand of finding a survivor in 10 BIs, one chance in one hundred of finding a survivor in 100 BIs, and so on. In other words, there are pretty long odds against failing the acceptance criteria. However, spores of *B. stearothermophilus* may have D_{121}-values of 3 min. In such a case there would be practically no chance of meeting the acceptance criteria of killing 10^6 spores with an F_0 of 15 min. What are the implications of this?

On the face of it, the implication is that this sterilization specification/sterilizer parameters combination is invalid. However, remember that this same sterilization specification/sterilizer parameter combination would have been valid if the BIs used had D_{121}-values of 1.5 min. In practical terms the pharmacopeial specification for thermal resistance in BIs has been set naively. Many companies purchasing spores of *B. stearothermophilus*, either for preparing BIs or as commercial strips, order against their own specifications which include upper D_{121}-value limits (in water) of around 2 or 2.5 min. The author of this paper has published recommendations for determining biovalidation cycles appropriate to challenge numbers and D_{121}-values of the spores available, but in the long run it is far more convenient and easier to justify compliance to regulatory agencies when there is bio-validation to show that 10^6 spores have been inactivated in 10–100 replicates.

Requalification

Periodically it is wise to repeat bio-validation. Changes do occur in autoclaves and no change control procedure, no matter how rigorously implemented, is infallible. The purpose of requalification is to determine if any unforeseen change has arisen to affect the sterility assurance provided to the items being sterilized. It is important for requalification that the numbers, resistances, and substrates for the BIs are closely similar to those used in the initial validation. For the same reasons as resistance variation within BIs as discussed before, it is possible if these factors are not well controlled to emerge from requalification with either a false confidence in the security of the process (use of BIs which are less resistant than those used in initial validation), or with the incorrect opinion that the process has failed (use of BIs which are more resistant than those used in initial validation).

Biological requalification is usually done following significant process changes or on an annual frequency. The establishment of a frequency should, in principle, be based on business risk: in fact, however, with well- designed and controlled autoclaves, the risk to the business of extending the interval beyond 1 yr is probably more one of incurring regulatory criticism at inspection than of releasing non-sterile products to market.

Bio-Validation of Laboratory Autoclaves Used for Sterilizing Microbiological Media

It is not difficult to argue that the effectiveness of sterilizing microbiological media is self-disclosing and should not therefore merit bio-validation. The pertinence of bio-validation to the qualification of laboratory autoclaves is more to do with having confidence in the sterility of media before or after it is used in the laboratory (and risk false positive results if the media is not sterile), or take it into (say) aseptic manufacturing areas for environmental monitoring (and if it is non-sterile contaminate areas and products which may otherwise have been secure). Many regulatory bodies see bio-validation of laboratory autoclaves as mandatory.

Bio-Validation of Steam-in-Place (SIP) Systems

SIP systems range from very small systems (say, a mixing tank) where all parts may reach temperature within 2 or 3 min, to absolutely massive arrangements of vessels, valves, and pipework in which the expulsion of air, the drainage of condensate, and the attainment of the sterilization specification temperature at the "*slowest point*" can take 20 or 30 min. Bio-validation is essential. The placement of BIs is largely a matter of judgment. Certainly the "slowest point" to reach the sterilization specification temperature must be challenged. Certainly vent filters and low points where condensate could accumulate must be challenged. Thereafter, it is a regulatory expectation that there should be sufficient BIs placed to give coverage to the whole system, which in effect may mean placing BIs in locations which, due to the heat-up time of the system, have been exposed to the sterilization specification temperature for two, three, or four times longer than the "*slowest point*." Undue confidence should not be taken from favorable results from these locations.

9

Aseptic Processing

Aseptic processing is a widely used methodology in the health care industry for the preparation of sterile materials. The term aseptic processing as it is applied in the pharmaceutical industry refers to the assembly of sterilized components and product in a specialized clean environment. The clean environment may be a conventional human scale classified clean rooms or an environment engineered to further reduce the likelihood of contamination by reducing (or as much as is possible eliminating) direct human contact with the product and components being assembled "aseptically." The idea of sterile products manufactured aseptically is inherently contradictory, a demonstrably sterile product cannot be produced aseptically using even the most advanced technology available today. Nevertheless, on any given day millions of putatively sterile dosage form units are produced using aseptic techniques that in the literal sense are inadequate to achieve sterility. A sterile product is one that is free from all living organisms, whether in a vegetative or spore state. This is an absolute condition, something cannot be partially or nearly sterile, the presence of a single viable organism represents a failure of the product, and the systems (environment, equipment, and procedures) used to produce it. Asepsis, that state in which all aseptically filled sterile products are manufactured, cannot be established as "*sterile*." Asepsis is commonly defined as a condition in which living pathogenic organisms are absent.

Putting aside the classical definitions, one must consider the real difficulty in establishing an aseptic environment, let alone a sterile one. The practitioner is left with a insurmountable task, to somehow create an environment free of any organisms, but also one (with the exception of isolators) in which personnel must be present to perform critical functions. The problem is further compounded if it recalled that personnel are considered the single greatest source of microbial contamination in aseptic processing. Recent experiments have shown that personnel clothed in new, sterile clean room garments slough viable contamination at a rate of roughly one viable particulate to 10,000 non-viable particles. During slow deliberate movements with the best possible clothing, operators will slough particulate and viable organisms. Therefore, the probability of human borne microbial contamination being released in the conventional clean room is one over the course of any reasonably long operational shift. With this fact in mind, how then is one to accomplish a truly sterile or even aseptic environment? Especially when we must consider that many organisms that are normally non-pathogenic, can under certain circumstances become opportunistically pathogenic. Among those circumstances are a debilitated condition of general health in the patient, or, as is increasingly common, immunological insufficiency due to age or pre-existing condition. Other than the obvious considerations of proper facility design, sterilization validation, and sanitization procedures, the focus of attention must be on the personnel and the activities which they must perform. These actions are broadly termed, aseptic technique, and like any other human activity they can be accomplished in a variety of ways. In order to better understand aseptic technique, some general guidance and examples of good and bad technique can be used to delineate what should and should not be permitted.

The fundamental concept behind every aseptic processing activity is that non-sterile objects must never touch sterile objects. This is often accomplished by the establishment of a "sterile field" in which the core activities are performed. All of the surfaces of the gowned human operator must be always considered non-sterile. Non-sterile objects including the operators hands must never be placed between the source of the air and a sterile object. The operators' hands and arms must always be kept at a level beneath that of open product containers. Sterile components should under no circumstances be touched directly with gloved hands, a sterilized tool should always used for this purpose. Since gloved hands and arms will enter the sterile field they must never touch walls, floors, doors, etc. Strenuous lifting and moving of tanks, trolleys, etc. must not be done by operators assigned to work within or near the sterile field, because the more strenuous the activity the higher the level of particle generation, and at least some of the particulate released by the operator will surely by viable microorganisms. Some of the techniques to avoid include: reaching over exposed sterile objects to make adjustments beyond them; correcting a stopper feed problem with a gloved hand; touching face, eye shield, or any other non-sterile object with gloves; taking an air sample directly over open containers; continuously standing inside flexible partitions that mark the boundary of the sterile field; breaking up clumps of components with gloved hands. Each of these actions exposes the sterile objects to undue risk of contamination from the personnel. Certainly there are more ways to contaminate the "sterile field" than we can imagine. For this reason, the procedures used in and around the "sterile field" must be carefully defined and followed closely by all personnel. These procedures should follow the general principles outlined above and are evaluated in a media fill simulation and performed in an identical fashion during aseptic processing. It is beneficial to define in writing how each procedure is to be performed and train the operators in these exact procedures.

Worst Case

No discussion of aseptic processing validation can be considered complete without some mention of "worst case." As initially defined by the FDA, worst case included consideration of numbers of personnel, temperature, relative humidity, and other aspects. This aspect has been adopted with some degree of modification by industry which has included some, but certainly not all of the FDA guidance. Some of the more common worst case situations which industry employs include: number of personnel, maximum hold time for containers and other items prior to filling, number and type of interventions performed. It is important to note that the determination of worst case conditions in a aseptic processing has been largely intuitive and highly subjective. Quantitative risk analysis is rarely if ever undertaken to establish and categorize actual modes of failure. Thus, worst case conditions for tests are established largely by precedence rather than actual data. The most significant worst case condition that is employed is the use of a microbiological growth media itself. Because the majority of aseptic formulations have either a preservative system and some products are inherently inhibitory or non-supportive of microbial growth, the media represents a substantially more favorable environment for the survival of microorganisms. The protocol prepared for the aseptic processing validation effort should delineate where worst case type considerations have been incorporated into the experimental plan. Throughout this document, recommendations will be made to worst case assumptions where choices in the definition of the validation effort must be made.

Prerequisites

The validation of aseptic processing should be preceded by the formal validation of the various systems, which contribute to the sterility assurance of the materials to be produced. In essence that mandates that the facility, HVAC system, sterilization procedures for the product contact surfaces, equipment, components and product, sanitization/disinfection procedures for the suite, and personnel gowning. Merely listing the activities, which must be completed, serves to indicate the magnitude of the effort required to prepare for the aseptic processing validation effort. It is sometimes tempting to begin the validation of aseptic processing while these tasks are still underway, especially when one considers that it is universally accepted that the primary source of microbial contamination in an aseptic process are those activities which are performed by gowned personnel.

Table 9.1. Most likely sources of microbial contamination in aseptic processing

1. Personnel borne contaminants
2. Human error
3. Non-routine operations during aseptic process
4. Assembly of sterile equipment prior to use
5. Mechanical failure
6. Inadequate or improper sanitization
7. Transfer of materials within APA
8. Routine operations during aseptic process
9. Airborne contaminants
10. Surface contaminants
11. Failure of sterilizing filter
12. Failure of HEPA filter
13. Inadequate or improper sterilization

It should be evident that virtually all of the items that top the list are either performed by or corrected by the human operator. The impact of the remaining factors is widely acknowledged to be of secondary consideration. Yet proceeding with the validation of aseptic processing before completing the validation of the supportive processes and systems raises the risk of failure unnecessarily and makes failure resolution well nigh impossible. Obviously, given the significance of human borne contamination as a risk factor, training and qualification of operators is a significant prerequisite to aseptic process validation. However, in an effort to move validation along quickly many firms do not emphasize training or even take short cuts with personnel education. Fortunately the various validations, which are required, are well documented in the literature and the practitioner should have no difficulty finding information on their execution.

Regulatory and Historical Perspectives

Aseptic processing activities are evaluated through process simulations in which a microbiological growth medium is utilized in the process in lieu of the product. The media is incubated after completion of the process to evaluate the procedures utilized. When utilized to evaluate aseptic filling, it is more narrowly defined as "a means of validating the aseptic assembly process that involves the use of a microbiological growth nutrient medium to simulate sterile product filling operations." This technique was first applied in the late 1940s by Rhode, and incorporated into a World Health Organization guideline in the mid 1970s. In the late 1980s, the PDA developed one of the first guides to the execution of media fills for the evaluation of aseptic processing. Several years afterwards the U.S. Food and Drug Administration defined its aseptic processing requirements for the first time. Additional guidance has been developed by other regulatory and pharmacopeial sources, which have defined the required activities. The PDA latest guidance documents provide perhaps the most comprehensive source of information on process simulation tests. The desire to evaluate aseptic processing activities other than sterile drug filling has made for some adaptation of the classical media fill test, and for this reason the term process simulation test has come into vogue to embrace a wider range of aseptic processing activities. Process simulation tests can be defined as a means for "evaluating an aseptic process employing methods that closely approximate those used for sterile materials using an appropriate placebo material." As mentioned previously, central to the evaluation of an aseptic process is the inclusion of the required interventions which must be performed. Any process simulation that does not properly evaluate employee aseptic technique and does not fully consider the process human interface is technically invalid.

Mechanics of Media Fill (Process Simulation) Execution

The conduct of aseptic processing validation ordinarily requires the use of a microbiological growth medium in lieu of the product. The PDA/PhRMA joint task force of Validation of Sterile Bulk Processes has outlined some process simulation methodologies which do not require the use of media (see later discussion on this subject), but aside from bulk applications process simulation testing has become essentially synonymous with media fill.

Media Sterilization

The execution of a media fill begins with the sterilization of the liquid media. This can be accomplished using either bulk sterilization of the liquid media in a large (glass or stainless steel) container or by filtration with a sterilizing grade filter. The choice of sterilization method is based on considerations of the volume of media required, growth promotion requirements, and filtration rate for the media. Provided that the media is introduced into the process at or before the point in which the production process being simulated becomes sterile, the choice of sterilization method is open. Whether the media be sterilized by filtration or by steam in bulk, there is no benefit to be gained from requiring that the sterilization method used be identical to that for the production materials. It is often suggested that a media fill test can be used to verify formulation bioburden control and process filter validation; however, this is not the case because as already pointed out the growth promoting and physical characteristics of media are far different from those of nearly all pharmaceutical preparations. Sterilization validation is established independent of the process simulation, and is the appropriate activity in which to confirm the appropriateness of the methods employed.

Manufacturing Activities

Once the sterile medium is in place the simulation can begin in which the aseptic processing steps are executed through the conclusion of the process. In many cases the simulation entails the filling of the product into its final container and explains its more commonly used name—media filling. To conclude however that media filling is all that is required in the validation of aseptic processing ignores the many possible human interventions which can take place during the manufacturing and prefilling activities. Many sterile dosage forms require the execution of a significant number of complex aseptic manipulations after the materials become sterile. Suspensions, creams, ointments, implants, and liposome formulations are among the more common examples of processes where aseptic processing involves activities other than filling of containers. In the more ordinary production of sterile solutions there are manufacturing activities such as sampling and integrity testing of filters which can potentially expose sterile materials to contamination. Thus, a process simulation must include all of these prefilling activities in order to mimic the actions routinely performed in production of sterile materials.

Understanding these additional requirements makes it evident why process simulation has come into vogue as a more appropriate description for this activity as opposed to more restrictive media filling. Evaluation of aseptic manufacturing activities can be achieved independently of the filling process using a variety of methods. If performed as part of an integrated activity with filling, the evaluation of the filled containers serves as verification of both aseptic manufacturing and filling practices. The bulk production of sterile drug products such as antibiotics, corticosteroids, insulin, and certain biotechnology products requires that a number of processes be carried out under aseptic conditions. These processes can be evaluated in a manner adapted from those employed for aseptic filling processes. A joint PDA/PhRMA task force has developed the definitive guidance document on this subject.

Aseptic Filling

Media is filled into sterile containers using methods identical to those required for production of the sterile product. This activity has been the subject of numerous papers and several surveys of industry practice. Attention must be paid to the specifics of the aseptic filling process itself. The range of sterile dosage forms, which can be produced, encompasses variations in container type, container size, formulation, lot size, filling speed, and other aspects which should be embraced in the design of the validation program. Each of these must be given careful consideration in the definition of the program requirements and a sound rationale for the selection of the test conditions included in the validation protocol. Presented later are brief discussions of some of the issues to be addressed and some recommendations for execution. While the focus of these points is on activities during the simulated filling of containers, many of these are relevant to both the manufacturing of sterile bulk materials and the compounding of bulk sterile formulations.

Product-Related Considerations

Type of container

Sterile products are aseptically filled into a variety of containers including glass and plastic bottles, metal and plastic tubes, ampules, and plastic bags. The variety of these containers is matched by the variety of methods required to prepare them for use in the aseptic filling process. Where a filling line is used to fill different types of containers, the differences in sterilization and handling suggest that each type should be assessed independently of the others. Attempting to identify a worst case situation when different sterilization methods, handling issues, and sealing mechanisms are employed is tenuous at best. One container substitution that is always valid is the use of a container that allows the most effective and less intrusive reading of the results. For example, clear containers of identical dimensions should always be substituted for opaque containers provided closure feeding and/or sealing are not affected.

Type of product

The process simulation should encompass the procedures used in the entire filling process. Thus, for lyophilized product, the aseptic loading of the freeze dryer should be a part of the simulation. A suspension product that utilizes a recycle loop around the filling machine would be validated using an identical set-up even though the media being filled does not require such a set-up. Similarly, the validation of a powder filling process should include a placebo material passed through the powder handling system and then filled into the container. When placebo materials are used development tests to ensure that the ratio of placebo to media does not result in a failure of the placebo/media mixture to support microbial growth are necessary.

Any special filling or handling activities that are specific to the product being simulated should be a part of the media fill. It is acceptable to add additional steps, such as liquid filling, to a powder fill process to allow for direct incubation of the filled units. Such additional steps may increase the potential for contamination of the filled units in the process simulation relative to the production filling process, but their inclusion is often unavoidable and represents an additional worst case challenge to the process. In some instances, the use of filling of control units, i.e., vials filled with liquid media but not the placebo powder may be beneficial as a means of assessing these add-on activities, which are not a routine part of the aseptic filling process.

In complex processes, the process simulation may be divided into steps. Provided that the steps overlap, they can cover the entire process and allow for isolation of contamination to a specific portion of the overall aseptic process. This practice is employed commonly for freeze drying, where an number of vials can be filled and sealed without transfer to the freeze dryer as a means of distinguishing between contamination derived from the aseptic filling and contamination derived from the lyophilizer loading and freeze drying process. Detailed advice on the more common product types can be found in PDA's most recent document of process simulation testing.

Filling speed

The extremes of filling speed on the line should be considered in the validation planning. The use of the slowest normal filling speed may increase the potential for contamination ingress via deposition from the surrounding environment. The use of the fastest normal speed may increase the potential for human intervention by increasing the number of routine and non- routine line interventions. The likely impact of fill speed will depend upon personnel population, proximity of personnel to the sterile field, and number of interventions. A rationale should be developed for the process simulation strategy chose. For example, in the initial validation of a filling line, one fill might be performed at the slowest speed, and two at the highest speed. In routine evaluation of the line, the speeds would be alternated.

Container size

The size of the containers being filled is viewed in a manner similar to fill speed. The largest container (often filled at the slowest speed because of its large fill volume) often has the largest opening, so the potential for microbial entry from the environment should be the greatest for that size. At the other extreme, the smallest container (often filled at the highest speed by virtue of its lower fill volume), represents the greatest handling difficulty. Smaller containers are generally more fragile, and less stable, and thus would be more prone to breakage and jamming in the equipment. Any container that presents additional handling steps or is more prone to breakage or instability should be included in the validation program, as it may represent a greater challenge to the aseptic process than either the largest or smallest container processed on the line. As such it may represent an additional worst case to be addressed.

Closure system

One of the more common differences between products is the closure system. Closure systems are selected for compatibility with the formulation, and in some cases differences in formulation may be create differences in handling difficulty. A stopper that is more prone to clumping or jamming in the tracks of the stopper bowl will necessitate additional interventions not present with other stoppers of similar size and thus would be considered worst case situations. There are a number of specialized closure systems designed to facilitate the delivery of an aseptically filled product. As these systems have sealed interstitial spaces where product contact can occur during administration of the drug product, the simulation procedure for these product configurations should include this space and media should be allowed to contact these surfaces during the incubation.

Fill volume

The volume of media filled into the containers need not be the routine fill volume for the container. It should be of sufficient volume to contact the container-closure seal surfaces and sufficiently large to allow for easy inspection of the filled units postincubation. Despite the lower fill volume, the speed of filling should match that used for the routine filling of the product being simulated. Smaller containers should not be over-filled as sufficient air must be available in the container headspace to support the growth of aerobic organisms and problems have been encountered where the liquid media essentially fills the entire container.

Filling Process Related Considerations

Filling lines

Considering the number of permutations of container, closure system, and other product attributes that must be encompassed in a process simulation program, it should be evident that only in the simplest of situations would a single set of media fills be adequate to provide coverage of all aseptic processes performed. Where multiple lines are present in the facility, each should be considered independently. Process simulation results of one line are not predictive of results on another because the contamination rate is primarily dependent upon human performance. Even identical equipment in two clean rooms designed to the same standard will not give uniform results unless the aseptic technique of the operators is at the same level of performance.

Duration of fill

The duration of the media fill is one of the more contentious issues. In general, media fills should be sufficiently long to include all of the required interventions. Using that requirement alone, a typical media fill might be at least 3–4 h long. Ideally a media fill should utilize more units than are in the product being simulated. This approach is normally followed for all batches up to 5000 units. As the number of units in batch increases current practice is to fill at least 5000 units, and increase the number as the batch size increases. For very large batches or long the campaigns common in blow/fill/seal or isolator systems, media fills interspersed with blank units (either empty or water filled) are used to maintain operating conditions during the simulation. Where this is done, media is filled before and after all planned routine and non-routine interventions, and conversion to media is performed after any unplanned non-routine interventions.

Media filled units interspersed with blank units has been a technique used to validate processes that may run for several days. In these cases media is generally filled at the beginning to evaluate set up and then again at the end to evaluate the ability of the process to maintain asepsis for the full length of the longest approved campaign. Filling a large number of units as may be possible on a high speed filling machine is not a substitute for a realistic simulation of the process. A high speed filler could fill 5000 or more units in less than 15 min of filling time, yet that would hardly be considered an acceptable practice.

Interventions

In virtually all aseptic processing activities, operator interventions are required to complete the process. Understanding the types of interventions required and how they are incorporated into the validation program is essential to protocol development.

Aseptic assembly

The first interventions performed are those that prepare the equipment for the aseptic process. This entails the removal of sterilized materials and equipment items from the autoclave and transfer to the location where the aseptic processing activities will be performed. This is ordinarily followed by the assembly/preparation of the equipment for the process.

Aseptic assembly in which sterilized parts are removed from protective materials, installed and adjusted in preparation for the aseptic process are perhaps the most potentially invasive of all of the activities which must be performed. The operator must be meticulous in their execution of these tasks to prevent the inadvertent contamination of product contact surfaces. Strict adherence to the principles of aseptic technique described earlier is essential. These interventions are a necessary part of every aseptic activity, and it is common to identify the first containers filled as they may be more indicative of potential problems with the aseptic assembly. For this reason, the validation program should include process simulations that include containers filled immediately after the set-up of the equipment.

Routine interventions

The execution of the aseptic process ordinarily requires a number of repetitive activities such as: product and component replenishment, weight checking, operator breaks, and environmental monitoring. Each of these is a required part of the process, and cannot be eliminated. They should be included in the process simulation and performed by the operators in a consistent fashion using defined methods and practices.

Non-routine interventions

During the course of the aseptic filling process there may be instances where a non-routine or corrective intervention is required. These usually occur in relation to difficulties with components or equipment aspects. Containers can break, jam in the conveyor, or fall over on a turntable. Stoppers can jam in the stopper track, clump in the bowl, or fail to seat properly. Problems with the equipment can include: weight adjustments, minor leakage, sensor failure, or rail adjustment. Each of these will require a corrective operation by the line operator to return the line to proper operation. Unlike routine interventions, these are not a required part of every process, but in order to assess their potential impact on the aseptic process the more prevalent of these should be included in every media fill. To the extent that these non-routine interventions can be considered repetitive, i.e., weight adjustments, stopper jams, etc. their proper execution should be described in a procedure and adhered to by the operators. Non-routine interventions may occur randomly or not at all during an aseptic filling process. To ensure that they are a part of the process simulation, they should be performed as if they were a required part of the simulation. Thus, even if the fill weights during the simulation are correct, the line should be stopped and an adjustment made to demonstrate the acceptability of the methods employed. Given the breadth of possible non-routine interventions, which may be possible during a batch, it may not be possible to simulate all of them. The simulation protocol should address those the firm has identified as more commonly required. Firms should make a concerted effort to minimize the number and extent of these non-routine interventions. It may be possible to reduce the need to perform them by improving component quality by tighter AQLs on incoming components, tighter controls on preparatory activities, repairs or upgrades to equipment, and similar activities. Such measures can contribute substantially to the reliability of the process and patient safety.

New interventions

If during the conduct of a batch or a process simulation, the need for an intervention not previously evaluated in a process simulation may occur. The firm should allow for this eventuality and assess the intervention during its execution via supervisory observation. Further evaluation of the new intervention in a follow-up media fill should also be considered.

Documenting interventions

It can be beneficial to define in some detail the permitted interventions for a given aseptic process in an SOP. This practice eliminates any subjectivity regarding what is permitted, and also allows for the establishment of a defined method for performing the intervention. The SOP can be employed in training of the operators and used as guidance in both routine aseptic processing and process simulation. Documentation of routine processing and process simulation should include details on the interventions (routine and non-routine) performed. The list of interventions required during routine filling can help to define the media fill program by establishing which are more common and should be given precedence in the process simulation. The required interventions can also be used as the initial justification for improvements to the procedures, components, and equipment used in the aseptic process. In the absence of such documentation during the process simulation, it is difficult to defend the acceptability of the intervention during routine processing. The use of video tapes as a means of both documenting interventions during media fills, and as a training tool for operators in the proper execution of an intervention is becoming more prevalent.

Environmental Considerations

Environmental monitoring

An aseptic processing activity is ordinarily supported by monitoring of the environmental air and surfaces in proximity to the process. The purpose of this monitoring is to confirm the acceptability of the environment during the process execution. There are a number of environmental sampling methodologies that are appropriate for this purpose each having particular advantages and disadvantages. There are also a number of regulatory and pharmacopoeial references that delineate microbial levels considered acceptable for aseptic processing environments. Each of these documents has defined the microbial conditions under which aseptic processing operations should be conducted in a slightly different manner. This situation could prove problematic for those endeavoring to comply with all of the requirements simultaneously except that in the years since the FDA's guideline on aseptic processing was published, aseptic processing capabilities have improved substantially. The microbial limits which may have once proved so daunting are now routinely observed in the majority of aseptic processing applications. Twenty years ago in this industry it was in vogue to speak of the importance of identifying trends in environmental monitoring results. It is recognized today, that trends no longer exist and that the presence of a detectable microorganism in a critical location is a rare event. With such stellar performance near routine, some change in the paradigms relative to the performance of environmental monitoring relative to aseptic processing are necessary:

1. The sensitivity of environmental sampling systems may be insufficient to detect microorganisms in critical environments with any degree of accuracy.
2. Increased sampling in a effort to detect the already low levels of microorganisms is unlikely to be successful and can actually put the product at risk by increasing personnel incursions into the sterile field.
3. Equipment and components have improved in quality to the extent, that environmental monitoring may be the most invasive intervention during an aseptic process (an undesirable situation).
4. The detection of contamination of any type in an environmental sample from a critical environment, sterility testing or a filled container during a process simulation has become a rare event.

With these views in mind, environmental monitoring must be viewed in a new light. The following insights may prove useful to the practitioner:

1. To paraphrase the Hippocratic Oath, the first rule of environmental monitoring should be "to do no harm." Sampling in a effort to detect microorganisms should not increase the potential for contamination of sterile materials.
2. No amount of sampling could ever establish the acceptability of filled containers of sterile product.
3. The sampling and enumeration of microorganisms is perhaps more prone to inadvertent contamination than the aseptic process itself.
4. The identification of a recoverable organism in the environment is a random event and may have no relationship to the integrity of the "sterile field," or the sterility of the goods being produced. In fact, given the presence of human operators (including the individual performing the sampling) how could one not expect to find occasional contamination?
5. There are no "*smoking guns*," establishing linkage between sterility test failure isolates, media fill contaminants and environmental isolates is extremely difficult.

Despite these somewhat negative perspectives, environments must still be monitored, and the levels of microorganisms controlled at levels that reconfirms the continued acceptability of the environmental conditions. Air sampling, using either active or passive sampling methods should be performed during the execution of the process. Surface sampling is best performed after the completion of the aseptic process to prevent the inadvertent contamination of product contact surfaces during the process. The vast majority of the samples taken should be devoid of contamination; however, the incidental detection of a recoverable organism from even product contact surfaces post-process should not be cause for undue alarm. The sampling of the environment is also an aseptic process, and subject to its own flaws.

Personnel monitoring

The evaluation of microbial contamination on operating personnel is a necessary part of the overall program. Sampling should be considered from a perspective similar to that described above for environmental air and surfaces. In this context samples should be taken from hands and other gown surfaces only at the conclusion of the aseptic process. It is suggested that sampling of the operators be performed on every exit from the aseptic area. Unlike environmental air and surface samples, it is unrealistic to expect that all of these samples will be free of detectable organisms, nevertheless the individuals should be able to consistently meet the levels established for them. Individuals who demonstrate a repeated pattern of non-conformance with the expected microbial levels should be subjected to corrective measures. The actions taken could include retraining, aseptic processing reevaluation and gowning recertification. Personnel undergoing these corrective measures would be assigned duties outside the aseptic processing area until they have reestablished acceptable performance.

Personnel Considerations

Preparatory training

Some firms have adopted specialized aseptic processing exercises to evaluate and prepare personnel being introduced to aseptic processing activities for the first time. These tests can take the form of hand filling, media transfers, and other procedures designed to challenge the aseptic technique of the individual in the absence of the mechanical equipment. Only after successful completion of the hands on manipulations would an individual be considered for further training as an aseptic operator. Whether this type of evaluation is performed or not, it is generally accepted that new personnel should actively participate in a media fill before they would be allowed to perform those same activities during a production batch. Additional lecture and demonstration type training of personnel is also necessary in aspects of microbiology, aseptic technique, gowning, equipment operation, and of course CGMP.

Gowning certification

Personnel assigned work in aseptic processing areas are ordinarily subjected to initial and periodic certification of their ability to gown in the prescribed manner. Gowning certification includes sampling of a variety of gown surfaces in addition to those normally evaluated during routine monitoring. For new personnel, this might be successfully performed three times before they are permitted access to the aseptic corp. Annual or semiannual sampling reconfirms that personnel are still able to gown properly. Gowning certification is generally extended to include other individuals, i.e., supervisors, maintenance workers, housekeeping personnel who must access the aseptic area, but who do not perform any activities related directly to the sterility of the products being manufactured.

Personnel participation

Virtually all aseptic processing operations require the active participation of human operators who are required to perform important tasks during the process in a manner that avoids the contamination of sterile materials, components, and surfaces. Their success in performing these tasks is assessed in the process simulation as they perform the routine and non-routine interventions, which comprise their participation in the aseptic process. In order to establish that each of the operators is capable of successfully performing their duties their periodic participation in a process simulation is required.

Set-up and line operators should be a part of not less than one process simulation per year. Individuals such as line mechanics and environmental samplers should be managed in a similar manner. Participation requires more than mere presence in proximity to the aseptic process, it must include active execution of the interventions to which they are normally assigned. Supervisory staff and others, such as maintenance personnel who do not perform process related aseptic interventions should not be considered in the validation program.

One of the personnel concerns addressed by the FDA in its guideline on aseptic processing concerned the maximum occupancy in the aseptic processing room. A simple means of accomplishing this is to designate a maximum occupancy for each room. Process simulations are then conducted at that level of staffing, and procedures are followed during routine operation in which a person must exit the room before another can enter whenever the maximum number of personnel are present in the room.

Where a firm operates on multiple shifts, the second and third shift should be included in the program as well to demonstrate the acceptability of their performance as well. Managing a large operation with large numbers of personnel, multiple filling lines and insuring that only personnel who have participated in a related media fill are allowed to perform aseptic processing can be a complex task.

Media Considerations

Media selection

The choice of a growth medium for use in the process simulation requires consideration of the organisms expected to be found in the environment, with emphasis on human derived contaminants from the operating personnel. With this in mind, the conventional choice is a general purpose medium capable of growing a wide range of common aerobic microorganisms. The usual choice is Soybean-Casein Digest Medium, also known as Tryptic Soy Broth, the same medium used in sterility testing. In some instances, other media might be appropriate. If filling is performed in an isolator under a total nitrogen environment, then an anaerobic medium such as Fluid Thioglycollate Medium might be more appropriate for the purposes of the simulation.

Use of anaerobic media

The sterility testing of parenteral products includes testing with both aerobic and anaerobic media. When media fills became common in industry during the mid-1970s the use of anaerobic media was considered a standard part of every aseptic processing validation program. Operational experience over recent years has indicated that the difficulty in establishing a truly anaerobic environment on a ordinary manned filling line are such that their execution is no longer common. Recognition that the predominant source of microorganisms in a clean room are personnel, the conduct of anaerobic media fills for other than special circumstances is unwarranted. Furthermore, anaerobic media fills are not required by any current regulatory body, as they also recognize that the focus of the effort should be on human borne contamination which can survive in air.

Media incubation conditions

An area of particular divergence in industry practice in the execution of media fills is that of incubation conditions. Cogent arguments can be made for incubation at a variety of temperatures. Some firms use only a single temperature in the range of 20–35°C. Other firms have chosen to incubate for 7 days at 20–25°C, and then move the filled containers to 30–35°C. An almost equal number have chosen to incubate for 7 days at 30–35°C, and then move the filled containers to 20–25°C. The lack of consensus suggests that the selection of incubation conditions is likely a minor concern. The suitability of the conditions employed, whatever they might be is established by the conduct of growth promotion studies. The one constant in this area is the duration of the incubation period which is almost universally set at 14 days.

Media growth promotion

The central issue in any discussion of appropriate media to use, the need to perform anaerobic media fills, selection of incubation conditions and the one that supports all of the decisions made in these areas, is the growth promotion studies. These establish that the medium used in the process simulation can successfully support the growth of microorganisms. Conventional practice is to test the media against a panel of organisms such as *Bacillus subtilis*, *Candida albicans*, *Pseudomonas aeruginosa*, *Staphylococcus epidermidis*, and *Aspergillus niger*.

The use of one or perhaps two of the most common environmental isolates in the growth promotion studies is highly recommended as these may be the most likely to be encountered in a contaminated unit. Failures of the challenge organisms to grow voids the media fill and requires a repeat of the media fill. In media challenges where a powder is added to the media, studies demonstrating acceptable growth promotion are required. Process simulations using media performed in antibiotic product facilities will sometimes require the addition of inactivating enzymes to the media in order to obtain acceptable growth promotion results as even trace amounts of antibiotics can inhibit the growth of some organisms.

ACCEPTANCE CRITERIA

Over the last 20–30 years, nothing has proven more controversial in the validation of aseptic processing than the selection of a acceptance criterion to use. The first regulatory requirements for media fills was published by WHO in the 1960s and had a criterion of 0.3%. Thus, a media fill of more than 1000 filled units would be considered acceptable if no more than three of those units were found contaminated after incubation. This limit lasted until the early 1980s when PDA prepared its first guidance on the validation of aseptic processing. The PDA document drew upon what was at that time the first survey on aseptic processing practice which had been conducted by PMA, and suggested a criterion of 0.1% of the units filled. This suggestion was at the time considered quite radical at the time as it seemingly raised the bar substantially. Interpretations of limit definition were made by Ronald Tetzlaff, at that time an employee of the Food and Drug Administration. These drew upon suggestions made in PDA's second document on aseptic processing validation where a Poisson distribution was used to project the contamination over a large batch. FDA's first official statement on acceptance criteria for process simulations was provided in their 1987 aseptic processing guideline.

The FDA guideline stated, "Test results should show, with a high degree of confidence, that the probability of a product becoming contaminated during aseptic processing is very low. In general, test results showing a probability of contamination of not more than one in 1000 are acceptable." With the publication of this document, PDA's 1980 limit had been echoed by a regulatory agency, and this limit remains FDA's current official position. PDA continued its work on aseptic processing through the conduct of industry surveys in 1986 and again in 1992. These efforts established that industry performance was continually improving and that 0.1% was almost universally accepted by industry on a global basis.

The Parenteral Society (TPS) developed its first guidance on the validation of aseptic processing, and this placed greater emphasis on statistical treatment of the acceptance criteria than prior documents. This document profoundly influenced a ISO document that was then in preparation and a second controversy was born. The emphasis placed on statistics in both these documents made many uncomfortable. While mathematically correct the extension of the acceptance criterion tables to include larger numbers of filled units created an awareness of the statistical approach that had not existed previously. Inherent in the statistics, as the number of units filled in a media fill increased, the allowed number of contaminated units increased as well. While one contaminated unit in 1000 containers seemed acceptable, it is statistically equivalent to 10 contaminated units in 16,970 units. This seemed to many as an unacceptably large number of positives units in any size batch. Official EU guidance was provided for the first time in 1996 with the publication of their annex 1 on sterile medicinal products. The annex suggested that, "The contamination rate should be less than 0.1% with 95% confidence level." This was provided without elaboration, thus while the limit was clearly statistical the implications of the TPS and ISO efforts were not addressed. The clearest response to the TPS and ISO statistical data treatment was developed by the PDA.

The PDA guidance states the following: "Despite the number of units filled during a process simulation test or the number of positives allowed, the ultimate goal for the number of positives in any process simulation test should be zero. A sterile product is, after all, one that contains no viable organisms." The PDA that originally introduced the Poisson approach for evaluation of media fills, has revised its perspective, and now believes that statistical treatment of the data is invalid. The Poisson method is appropriate for the evaluation of a low incidence of a random event, which is no longer believed to be consistent with how sterile materials become contaminated during aseptic processing. When first introduced it was assumed that contamination in an aseptic process could be derived from a variety of sources, and that any statistical approach that addressed that possibility as a random event was considered appropriate.

With the execution of many more media fills, substantial improvements in facilities and equipment, and an increased awareness of the human contribution to microbial contamination views have changed substantially. It is now a widely held belief that contamination in aseptic processing is the result of human derived contamination resulting from improper technique in the execution of a required intervention. Thus, there is nothing random about the contamination, its source is known and its elimination certainly more possible than ever. This PDA view represents the latest thinking relative to acceptance criteria.

Additional publications which have provided acceptance criteria for aseptic processing validation have been prepared by both CEN and PIC. These have attempted to reconcile the differences between the ISO document and the PDA guidance. The essence of these documents is the following. "Ideally the contamination rate should be zero. However, currently the accepted contamination rate should be less than 0.1% with a 95% confidence level." This appears to be an effort to have it both ways, and it is unclear whether the two perspectives can really be reconciled so easily.

The most recent industry survey on aseptic processing was published by PDA in 1997. It attempted to address the statistical nature of the limits as actually practiced, however the response to questions in that area are inconclusive. It did include evidence that several firms had adopted acceptance criteria tighter than 0.1%, suggesting that another round of acceptance criterion definition might be in the offing. The USP expanded upon PDA's 1996 position, and established ever tighter requirements, "The goal is zero contamination. In an individual run not more than one positive unit in 5000 filled units. In a series of three media fills, two of the three media fills should have no contamination present."

Perhaps the simplest means of establishing an acceptance criteria (and perhaps to define one's entire program) is to follow the pack, and develop a firm's entire aseptic processing validation program based upon the latest survey information. What is certainly clear is that aseptic processing performance has improved substantially over the last 20 odd years and that firms should monitor their practices against their peers and regulatory expectation on a continuing basis. What was acceptable in the past is not acceptable today, and there can be little doubt that further tightening of the criteria can be expected in the future.

Technologic Advances

The production of sterile products has benefited from at least two novel production methods: blow-fill-seal and isolation technology. Each of these can offer a substantial reduction in the amount of operator interaction with sterile materials. In blow-fill-seal (and the closely related form-fill-seal), the product container is created only seconds before it is filled and sealed. This has distinct advantages over more conventional filling where containers are exposed to the manned aseptic filling environment. A number of process simulation studies have established that the blow-fill-seal method is capable of protecting the contents of the sealed container to a greater extent than a ordinary clean room. Isolation technology enjoys similar results using an entirely different approach in which personnel are removed from the operating environment.

Isolation technology, which is a direct evolution of glove boxes, places operating personnel outside a sealed (physically or via an air pressure differential) enclosure in which the aseptic process is conducted. The enclosure can be treated with a sterilizing gas which can render the interior surfaces free of microorganisms. This treatment when combined with the elimination of direct personnel presence in the aseptic environment, makes the isolator perhaps the ideal tool for sterile drug production.

Sterility Assurance for Aseptic Processing

To this point in this effort, the validation of aseptic processing has been described as closely related to media filling or process simulation. In reality the relationship between simulation and routine production is not a direct one. A completely successful media fill program does not establish the sterility of anything other than itself. The next lot, or for that matter the previous one, may be sterile or not. The absence of contaminated units in a media fill merely demonstrate that the facility, personnel, and procedures are capable of preventing contamination in that media fill. Demonstrating that capability for routine filling is quite a different thing, and at the present time cannot be accomplished with other than a destructive sterility test of every filled unit.

Ultimately the practitioner can only infer that because media fills are successful, that similar success is also possible during routine production. There is a common misunderstanding that the 0.1% or maximum of one in 1000 units is a sterility assurance level. That is most defi-nitely not the case, it is nothing more than a maximum allowable contamination rate during the process simulation. There is no accepted means for establishing the sterility assurance level of aseptically filled products, it might be termed the "holy grail" of sterile production. We perform media fills to demonstrate a capability, and with significant limitations we infer from that effort that we can produce sterile drug products using aseptic processing.

At the present time, this is perhaps as close as we can get to the "validation of aseptic processing." Despite this most basic of constraints, media fills represent the only means of even approximating what occurs when aseptic processing is performed. Demonstrating the capability of producing sterile products will have to be sufficient for industry needs.

Demonstrating success with aseptic processing requires process simulation studies closely matching the routine production activities. As the range of sterile products manufactured by aseptic processing is quite extensive, this mandates that the practitioner be prepared to adapt the general guidance provided in this effort to their particular situation. The more closely the simulation matches the production activities, the clearer indication that success with the simulation means success in routine operation. A well founded process simulation program affords the firm confidence in their routine operation that cannot be obtained by any other means.

It is important to consider however, that at the current level of technology, particularly manned aseptic processing, uncertainty is an inherent feature. The fact that process simulation tests are merely a snapshot in time has been recognized since media fills became a standard feature of aseptic process validation in the late 1970s. Guaranteeing safety to the end user is not as simple as successful media fill tests, "good" environmental monitoring results, and successfully completed sterility tests. Even when these data appear satisfactory, uncertainty exists. Although human nature detests uncertainty, particularly in fields where numerical values are widely stated, scientific rationality requires us to recognize that we cannot test or monitor uncertainty away. Only by thorough training, supervision and reduction of human borne contamination hazards can the likelihood of contamination be controlled. Fortunately, it appears certain from the absence of data to the contrary that aseptically produced health care products are very safe when produced in accordance with current industry standards. Certainly as the industry process capabilities continue to evolve our products will become safer still, and perhaps someday the uncertainty associated with aseptic processing will be so low that we can consider these products truly sterile.

10

COMPLIANCE AND VALIDATION

GAMP (Good Automated Manufacturing Practice) has been in use from the first version in Western Europe for over 10 years. Initially supported by ISPE (International Society of Pharmaceutical Engineering) Europe, over the past few years it has been adopted by ISPE in America, with the start-up of GAMP Americas. Even more recently it has been supported by the U.S. FDA as a recognized guideline for ensuring computer systems can be validated and fit for purpose. This chapter looks at some of the fundamentals of GAMP that are now well established and can now be used by Central and Eastern European (CEE) pharmaceutical companies to allow them to ensure compliance of IT systems, which may in turn help them to gain a competitive advantage. It also discusses the evolution of IT systems over the past 10 years, and details how systems now have more compliant functionally, and can be more easily implemented and subsequently validated. As established compliance and validation practitioners who were involved with the creation of the initial GAMP guide, the writers of this chapter have been able to rely on many years practical knowledge and experience of the global market place in order to assist companies in the CEE marketplace by proactively enabling both cultural and business changes required in order to meet Western regulatory compliance. This chapter are based on a large-scale project in Poland between 2002 and 2004. Building on the principles laid out in GAMP and previous implementation skills, this ensured that a quality-driven system development lifecycle was enforced from the beginning. By starting with an approved validation master plan (VMP) all quality and validation tasks were clearly identified and used as the driving force behind the project and the deliverables. This example of good planning based on the GAMP guidance is the basis for future successful projects and implementations throughout Eastern Europe and beyond.

MARKETPLACE

Pharmaceutical companies that manufacture in the CEE zone can only supply their products on a more global market if their systems are compliant and validated in accordance with U.S. and current EU (European Union) regulations. Also, current global organizations are looking for expanding markets, with the possibility of reducing research and development, and manufacturing costs, and may consider transferring operations, or subcontracting drug manufacture to the CEE zone. The entry of the 10 new member states, detailed below, into the EU in May 2004, opened an expanded market population of approximately 100 million and a collective EU economy close to 9.3 trillion euros (approaching the same level as the U.S.A.). There has been an increased emphasis on the subject of compliance within the pharmaceutical and biotech healthcare industry throughout all companies in the CEE, and access to these localized manufacturing, storage, and distribution facilities will only be possible if the quality and compliance standards in the CEE zone match up to current U.S. and EU regulations.

Healthcare Spending in Western Europe

Maintaining a balance between costs and income is the biggest challenge faced by all companies in any marketplace. In line with various Western European government efforts to curb rising healthcare debts and costs, the proportion of gross domestic product (GDP) allocated to healthcare spending has remained either static or has fallen in recent years. This trend is likely to continue in most Western European countries in the near to medium term.

Healthcare and IT Spending in Eastern Europe

In the CEE region the trend is somewhat more optimistic, with compound annual growth rate (CAGR) of 13.5% expected in the larger countries. The following 10 countries joined the EU by signing The Treaty of Accession 2003: Czech Republic, Estonia, Cyprus, Latvia, Lithuania, Hungary, Malta, Poland, Slovenia, and Slovakia. Other countries that have applied to become members but not yet signed up are: Bulgaria, Romania, and Turkey. CEE pharmaceutical organizations are therefore being targeted for acquisitions, mergers or involvment in partnerships with current global companies, such as GlaxoSmithKline, Pfizer, and Novartis. These global companies bring over 10 to 15 years experience in IT compliance. Existing knowledge, experience and policies and procedures, based on the GAMP principles, are available to the CEE organizations from central offices and headquarters, in the U.S.A. or Western Europe.

Those that are not acquired, and retain their independence, will need to get up to speed rapidly on their own to ensure that they are competitive in both local and wider markets. It has been estimated that 41 billion euros will be invested by the EU in the 10 new members states between 2004 and 2006; of this it is estimated that 5–7%, i.e. 2–3 billion euros will be on IT spend. It is thought that a good deal of this IT spend will be on a secure information infrastructure, to meet general EU regulatory requirements by 2005. It is also a fact that 80% of this money will be spent on new systems, whereas over the past few years, 80% of IT budgets in Western Europe have been spent on legacy systems and their interface with new systems, year 2000 upgrades (rather than new functional upgrades) and retrospective validation and assessment in respect of recent regulation such as 21 CFR Part 11.

It is clear therefore that a new wave of IT implementations will take place in the CEE in the next 3 to 5 years. It is imperative, therefore, that these organizations embrace GAMP to establish policies and procedures as quickly as possible. They have a good opportunity to implement a brand new IT strategy based on a new and qualified IT infrastructure, with modern, functionally rich, software. These organizations will not have to spend millions of pounds on retrospective validation, and will not have to go through the 10 year learning curve. They will not have to spend time training and educating the software suppliers to provide validatable software, and encouraging them to include pharmaceutical functionality such as electronic records and electronic signatures (ERES) which comply to 21 CFR Part 11. The following sections detail areas where we believe focus should be given to ensure an organization can increase the level of compliance and validation of IT systems, and thus conform to the Western European, U.S., and other regulations in a speedy manner.

Key Areas of GAMP for Emerging European Countries

IT and Automated Systems

The continuous development and availability of high technology systems and equipment means that organizations within CEE will be less reliant on people to manufacture and produce goods and more dependent upon IT and automated systems. A global business system will increase efficiency by providing fully integrated and efficient processes, while not compromising quality standards. Companies that have the vision to implement such systems will become more efficient and therefore more successful, giving themselves a more competitive edge.

It is not practical or realistic to expect Eastern European companies or countries to immediately ascertain the levels of experienced Western entities, but in order to supply products in the European or global marketplace a pragmatic and realistic approach to validation and compliance must be taken. This is particularly true for IT Infrastructure, as an unstable and nonvalidated platform effectively invalidates any system that operates upon it. In many instances the business system often referred to as an enterprise resource management (ERP) system is interfaced to other business critical systems such as a laboratory information management system (LIMS), manufacturing execution system (MES), electronic document management system (EDMS), enterprise asset management system (EAMS), and also to numerous plant, equipment, and laboratory systems, such as filling and packing lines, sterilizers, coaters, granulators, etc. Ten years ago most of these systems were bespoke or custom developed systems, and were specific to each client. They were classed as GAMP *category 5* systems. Not only was the supplier documentation poor, but a 100% on-site validation exercise had to take place. This was very expensive on top of the software and hardware costs. The software products contained only partial required functionality, and the functional requirements were added onto the system via bespoke code, or bespoke reports, again all requiring validation.

Table 10.1 Software categories

Category	*Software type*	*Validation approach*
1	Operating system	Record version (including service pack). The operating system will be challenged indirectly by the functional testing of the application.
2	Firmware	For nonconfigurable firmware record revision. Calibrate instruments as necessary. Verify operation against user requirements. For configurable firmware record version and configuration. Calibrate instruments as necessary and verify operation against user requirements. Manage custom (bespoke) firmware as category 5 software.
3	Standard software packages	Record version (and configuration of environment) and verify operation against user requirements. Consider auditing the supplier for critical and complex applications.
4	Configurable software packages	Record version and configuration, and verify operation against user requirements. Normally audit the supplier for critical and complex applications. Manage any custom (bespoke) programing as category 5.
5	Custom software packages	Audit supplier and validate complete system.

Over the past 10 years, focussed user groups and special interest groups have worked together with the suppliers to ensure that critical functionality, along with good software quality practices are built into the software. A key example of this is the 21 CFR Part 11 functionality. However, some companies are now stuck with older versions, as they are working and validated. They cannot be upgraded as IT budgets have been high in recent years with the year 2000 problems and retrospective validation costs. Therefore this new compliance functionality is not available to the users.

CEE countries can take advantage of all this effort by the suppliers over the past 10 years by implementing software and systems today that are more often *category 3* or *4* Systems. This gives organizations an opportunity to have a speedy and cost-effective implementation. From our experience and involvement over this period we can now help these organizations to implement a "vanilla" system, where the system is configured to meet requirements and not tailored or customized. In this way the CEE countries will then not be caught in the trap of many existing companies where they have older software but cannot upgrade to new versions to include new functions and features which may provide financial benefits. With new member states in the enlarged EU coming under the scrutiny of external regulators, they will effectively have to control their business growth and new systems and ensure that quality and compliance is never compromised. This will take time due to various financial, cultural, and language differences. Such changes within the new EU mean tremendous practical changes for staff, who have been used to more labor-intensive operations with minimal automation. New regulatory initiatives from organizations such as the U.S. Food and Drug Administration (FDA) are set to minimize manual systems and encourage the use of technology in order to improve the quality and traceability of business and system processes.

Communication, Training, and Education

Regulatory awareness and training in validation processes and techniques using tools such as GAMP is essential. Knowledge of the pharmaceutical business and good practices are vital. Continued education and training of human resources is therefore of paramount importance. This can be said for all companies, either east or west. It is impossible to recruit a fully qualified team with local language skills, so consultants are often the prime deliverer of one-to-one and on-going training as projects progress. Effective communication channels, good project infrastructure, and team building adds to the success of any project. It is important that project team members can work together and include developers, users, and validation staff. All team members should be aware of risks and issues that can potentially impact upon the project by carrying out daily and weekly progress updates and reviews. Representation on technical subcommittees, and attendance at seminars and exhibitions, including those of organizations such as ISPE should be encouraged. This provides networking opportunities for staff to develop compliance and validation skills by sharing experiences.

IT Infrastructure

While each country has its own particular culture and problems, the key underlying element for each is the infrastructure, which is sometimes taken for granted in more established western countries. This can also be true with respect to IT infrastructure, without which no system would function. Established, documented, and tested platforms with backup processes and uninterruptible power supplies (UPS) are considered a must, as many of the new countries and markets have problems with power-cuts and have traditionally not considered validation or compliance issues which can arise around these areas. CEE countries are often in the position to build new facilities on greenfield sites, and a key part to this is the planning and specification of the cabling and network hardware such as routers and hubs. These must be documented and tested as part of the build program, removing the need for costly and expensive rework as part of a retrospective qualification process. If we look at the analogy of building a house, a good builder would not build a house on weak foundations. The IT infrastructure is the foundation of all IT systems. If an ERP business system is implemented and validated on an IT infrastructure that is not documented, tested, and ultimately qualified, then the ERP system itself is not validated!

Validation Planning

Validation planning and the creation of a validation plan (VP) or VMP is a method of building quality into your implementation at an early stage. This will ultimately prevent costly rework and ensure that the system is validated in a controlled and sequenced manner. For the recent project undertaken in Poland, policies, practices, and principles from GAMP were adopted. Effective validation planning is the key to successful compliant and validated systems. By linking this plan to the overall implementation plan, completion of tasks with predefined timescales were carried out within time and on budget. The VP therefore becomes the key *driver* for the project. The VP described the validation approach and activities for the project by dividing the system implementation into phases. Key to all successful validated and compliant systems are the people involved. Roles and responsibilities assigned within the VMP are therefore vital, and the project undertaken in Poland was no different in this respect. By carefully defining key project deliverables within the VMP and assigning responsibility, both the supplier and the user agreed on key activities and the sequence upon which they were to be conducted. While this process is well- established within existing markets in Western Europe, the application of this proved to be somewhat more difficult and required much more focus and attention.

Sufficient allocation of validation resource to projects is a key factor and there is a distinctive need for cooperation between users and suppliers at all stages of implementation using a documented and approved system development life cycle. Misunderstanding of project tasks proved to be a major risk to the efficiency of the project timescales. When agreeing the validation project team and the definition of roles and responsibilities it is essential that key staff have the required skill sets and are competent to undertake the key validation activities. For example, during the testing phase of the system, testing that the system worked within its normal operating limits was easily explained and understood. However, testing that the system operated as expected under certain conditions, i.e., negative or challenge testing, boundary and limit testing, was more difficult to explain and justify. Detailed documentation creation, review, update, approval, and issuing throughout the project life cycle to provide documentary evidence as required by regulatory authorities was even more of a challenge, but was accepted by all eventually.

Supplier Audit

This is a fundamental part of any new IT system implementation. The organization should follow the GAMP guidelines rigorously, *before* agreeing to buy the software product. Historically organizations had already invested heavily, implemented systems and were committed to software suppliers, and therefore audits of the current software and of new releases were not carried out. Over the past 10 years IT software and equipment suppliers have been encouraged to provide documented and validatable systems. There are many software products available on the market and the organization should be able to purchase a system today that meets most of the GAMP guidelines. The organization should be encouraged to use the PDA Audit Repository Centre (ARC) to check if an audit report exists for the software under review. If the package has not been audited and included in ARC, then the organization should encourage ARC to perform the audit on the organizations' behalf, as this saves time and money.

Obviously the cheapest solution may provide the organization with the most risk, whereas a more expensive system enables a less risky, more speedy, and ultimately more economical option, i.e., the system *can* be validated. This is due to the complete software development lifecycle and associated quality management system and documentation available. Departments within companies that monitor and manage elements of quality assurance should always be included in the supplier selection process from the beginning wherever possible.

Risk Management

By using risk-based analysis and management, categorization of criticality throughout the lifetime of the project was implemented. By adopting this process, project managers are able to validate the critical areas of the business system. The result is a lower probability of noncompliance and resulting regulatory action. Current trends in approach from the regulators, and embodied in GAMP, is that risk assessment and management is another key driver. A traceability matrix was developed in order to map the requirements specified within the user requirements specification (URS) and functional design specification (FDS) down to the system design specification (SDS) and ultimately to software modules or units, on which the qualification testing was conducted. This ensured that all the user's requirements, including any requirements to comply with specific regulations were met and properly tested. Equally, where gaps existed, future enhancements to the core product were fed back to the supplier. The traceability matrix can then be used as a vehicle to assist in identifying potential risks. Each risk identified can then be reviewed and extra tests or standard operating procedures or other actions can be used to mitigate or minimize the risk. Specific consideration was also given here to the U.S. FDA ruling covering ERES, often referred to as 21 CFR Part 11.

Software Engineering Techniques

There are still several software engineering techniques of a system implementation that while used in other industries, such as the defense industry, have not really been used extensively in pharmaceutical organizations. Three such examples of this are requirements management, software configuration management, and automated testing. The adoption of these software engineering techniques would provide better traceability from logical requirements definition, through functional design and then onto mapping of test cases. Software configuration management is essential in understanding monitoring and controlling the many versions of systems and software that are part of an organization. Automated testing enables companies to create a suite of test scripts on initial implementation, so that when upgrades to operating systems, package releases, and patches or minor changes are made, the tests can be rerun automatically to ensure consistent performance and hence validation.

CEE organizations would be well advised to adopt some of these techniques as part of their IT strategy so that *all* systems can be developed, controlled and tested in a consistent manner at the very start of their IT life cycle. The information in this chapter provides a summary of the past 1015 years in the development of compliance and validation in the pharmaceutical industry and in particular in relation to the development of GAMP. By adopting good practice and validation principles specified within GAMP, the project implementation was successful and within specified timescales. More importantly the CEE pharmaceutical organization has an IT compliance and validation platform and foundation for its staff and organization to build on. The endorsement of GAMP by regulatory authorities such as the U.S. FDA provides the company with a high degree of assurance that by adopting this it will be able to withstand rigorous inspections as well as having a much more robust system which will enable the organization to progress in the next 5 to 10 years.

Some key points discussed were:

1. Validation planning as the driver of the project.
2. Use GAMP risk management guideline to pinpoint areas of concern, where focussed validation effort can be conducted. This reduces costs and timescales, by ensuring that time and money is not spent on areas that are not seen as GMP critical.
3. IT infrastructure should be planned, specified, and tested during the initial building phase of new facilities.
4. Category 3 and 4 systems are now available and can be purchased and implemented in a speedy and compliant manner by ensuring the scope is limited to configuration and not customization.
5. Communication, training, and education is important for the CEE countries to get their organizations to a base platform level of knowledge.
6. Both suppliers and users should build quality into systems from the beginning, while conducting quality and design reviews throughout the lifecycle.
7. Where possible use the ARC and encourage sharing of audits.
8. Review the use of current software engineering techniques as part of the lifecycle to provide better traceability, control of software, and better test repeatability and coverage.

11

VALIDATION PLANNING AND REPORTING

The purpose of this chapter is to provide an overview of the key initiation and ending phases for the validation of GxP-critical computerized systems, namely the use of formal validation plans and the associated close out documentation related to validation reporting. It will also cover how to go about managing and creating such documents. At the same time it attempts to clarify the roles and responsibilities in both validation planning and reporting, and draws attention to the benefits that good planning and reporting activities bring to the implementation of a successful project. Finally, the chapter provides checklists to aid the user in developing validation plans and reports that are suitable for any specific application to which they may be applied.

We discuss the principles (both regulatory and business related) behind the need to create validation plans and reports and go on to identify where they fit within the typical project life cycle. These principles should be applied whenever there is a requirement to validate either a specific computerized system or a group of related computerized systems in an area or site. In particular these requirements should be formally applied when the system under consideration has been identified as being GxP-critical. It is worth noting that the methodology may also be applied to other business-critical systems if deemed necessary following an assessment of business risk. This chapter is divided into two subsections. The first covers validation planning, and the second covers the closely related activity of validation reporting.

Both of these documents are internal user-generated documents, the content of which must provide an accurate summary of the proposed validation strategy or activities (*validation plan*) and the actual history and events surrounding the whole validation effort (*validation report*). They must be of a suitable standard to allow them to be presented to outside regulatory agencies such as the U.S. Food and Drug Administration (FDA) and the Medicines and Healthcare Products Regulatory Agency (MHRA) in the U.K.

VALIDATION PLANNING

Overview of Planning in the Validation Life Cycle

There are as many differing depictions of the project life cycle that can be applied to the validation of computerized systems as there are books written on the subject. The key observation note that the creation and approval of the validation plan is one of the earliest, if not one of the very first, activities undertaken in a project. In reality, and due to the tight time-scales often imposed upon modern day implementations, the development of the validation plan generally occurs as a parallel activity with that of requirements definition.

Before looking at the activities, inputs, roles, and other elements surrounding the creation and management of this document, it is necessary to define exactly what is meant by the expressions "*validation plans*" and "*validation master plans*." Are these documents one and the same or do they represent different things to different people?

The difference is really determined by their scope. Generally the term "*validation master plan*" (VMP) will refer to the more generic validation activities associated with a corporation, single facility or a large site-wide (or multisite) system or group of systems. The term "*validation plan*" (VP), on the other hand, is generally used to refer to the document defining the specific validation activities associated with an individual given system or a piece of equipment within an area or department. Due to the fact that the VMP is more generic in nature and does not provide a high level of detail regarding specifics, this guideline will concentrate on the VP. The guide will indicate, where necessary, any additions or omissions that would be relevant when creating a VMP.

Purpose of the Validation Plan

The VP is the key document in the overall validation process. Its importance is not only relevant for internal project control but is also of specific interest to external regulatory bodies, for example, the U.S. FDA and the U.K. MHRA. It is by examination of this document that these authorities can see how organizations intend to control the implementation of a new computerized system from the initial requirements definition, via the build process, installation, acceptance testing and through to ongoing operation and maintenance. Furthermore, the authorities can understand the controls employed to ensure that the system not only meets its user requirements (and will continue to do so in the future), but that the company can formally demonstrate how the implementation has complied with the requirements laid down in the relevant cGMPs. A VP will therefore define certain critical aspects of the project. These include, but are not limited to:

1. Project background and system definition.
2. Organizational structure of the project team — both internal and external (if applicable).
3. Life cycle definition.
4. Overview and justification of validation approach and testing strategy.
5. Standard operating procedures to be followed.
6. Project team roles and responsibilities.
7. Key milestones and deliverable items required at each stage.
8. Clearly-defined set of acceptance criteria by which to measure the success of the implementation.

Once developed, the VP can be utilized as part of the selection process for both the system components and suppliers (including third party implementation services if applicable). It is generally accepted that during the selection process the prospective suppliers will be forwarded a copy of the user requirements specification (URS) (usually as part of a request for proposal (RFP)). However, the suppliers should also receive a copy of the VP for the proposed system as this will define what additional services and roles they may be required to supply within the project. For example, the plan will most likely identify the requirement for a functional specification which has been developed either for a specific bespoke system or is readily available for "*configurable off-the-shelf*" software. The readiness of the supplier to be involved in the creation of such a document or its availability will have a critical bearing on the decision making process during selection, and possibly a bearing on the success of the final implementation.

Relationships with Other Life Cycle Phases and Documents

In trying to understand the relationship of VPs with other life cycle phases and documents, it is useful to consider a more complex view of the life cycle. An extension of the "V-model," found in

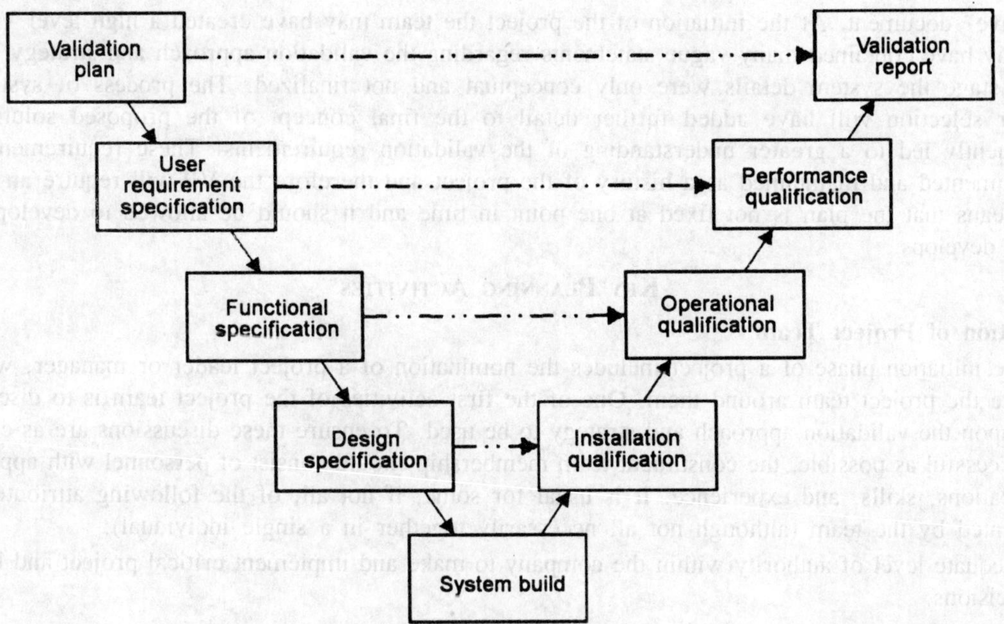

Fig. 11.1. Extended "V-model."

the GAMP 4 provides one such view. The illustration shows that there is a *direct relationship* between the VP and the validation report. In practice this means that the requirements and activities for validation proposed within the validation plan need to be adequately documented by the resultant project output generated and discussed or summarized in the validation report. Further information on the purpose and content of the validation report will be found elsewhere. At this point it is sufficient to state that all the deliverables, activities, or milestones identified as required within the VP must have some form of evidence documented in the report that either confirms successful completion or justifies an acceptable status when not fully meeting the original requirements.

When one considers the overall purpose of a VP it can be said that it is a formal statement of those activities, that when combined, have the ultimate intent to ensure:

1. The computer system delivered is that which was originally required by the users.
2. The delivered system performs as required under the operating conditions specified.
3. The delivered system will continue to perform as required in the future.

Deeper interpretation of these statements shows there is a stronger relationship between the VP and the URS than at first meets the eye. Consider that the URS is the formal documentation of what the proposed system should do and the business processes it may replace. Therefore, not only is it a statement of intent, but it is also a means to measure the success of an implementation. The URS, like the VP, should be developed prior to system selection or build. Some would even argue that a comprehensive system VP could not be created and approved without the determination of system requirements. Hence the relationship between these two documents is closer and more parallel in nature than that suggested by the V-model.

Further reflection on the purpose of the VPs shows that it must have either a direct or indirect relationship with *all* other phases in the life cycle. The plan is designed to cover the requirements and activities for design, build, testing, acceptance and long term operation and control of the computer system. A further consequence of this project term relationship is that the VP must also be maintained as a "live" document. At the initiation of the project the team may have created a high level VP. This plan may have contained many vague statements regarding the validation approach and strategy because at this stage the system details were only conceptual and not finalized. The process of system and supplier selection will have added further detail to the final concept of the proposed solution and consequently led to a greater understanding of the validation requirements. These requirements must be documented and maintained as a history of the project and therefore the VP will require an update. This means that the plan is not fixed at one point in time and it should be allowed to develop as the project develops.

Key Planning Activities

Formation of Project Team

The initiation phase of a project includes the nomination of a project leader or manager, who will organize the project team around them. One of the first activities of the project team is to discuss and agree upon the validation approach and strategy to be used. To ensure these discussions are as complete and successful as possible, the constituent team membership should consist of personnel with appropriate qualifications, skills, and experience. It is usual for some, if not all, of the following attributes to be represented by the team (although not all necessarily together in a single individual):

1. Adequate level of authority within the company to make and implement critical project and business decisions.
2. Suitable knowledge of the business areas affected by the project scope.
3. Extensive knowledge of international regulatory requirements covering cGMP and computer systems validation.
4. Computer literacy and reasonable knowledge of current IT trends.

The composition of the team may change depending upon the size of the project, the length of time it has run, or the current stage. However, each team must contain at least one member of the quality assurance department (and the validation department if separate), one member of the IT department, and one user. The project team membership will vary depending upon the size of the organization involved (due to availability of resources) and the scope of the project. However, it is generally possible to summarize the team membership in the following terms:

1. Project manager.
2. Process owner.
3. Facilitator.
4. Users.
5. Quality assurance.
6. Information technology.

Analyze the GMP Implications

At the start of any computer systems implementation project, the most commonly asked question is: "How much validation is necessary?" This is not such an unreasonable question given that since the early 1990s the regulatory bodies have focused an immense amount of attention upon computer systems validation. The result of this attention has been a number of well- documented citations against some of the industry's major global companies. These citations have covered a large variety of noncompliance issues ranging from inadequate retrospective validation documentation, poor project management and control, insufficient evidence of validation activity, poor specification and testing of error messages and the lack of controls surrounding system security. The result of this attention has been that the industry has reacted, or possibly overreacted, to ensure that the gaps are closed. It has done this mainly by producing mountains of paperwork documenting and specifying the smallest detail of a system, all backed up with an immense and complex series of test protocols. The situation toward the end of the 1990s was that more often than not the practice of validation resulted in a major spend item on the project budget and was seen to add considerably to the project timescales and for very little perceived benefit. All of this can be avoided by spending a little time planning the validation carefully and adequately for the particular project to which it is being applied. To aid this process ask the question: "What are GxP implications of this project?"

Whether the regulatory inspector is from the U.S. or the EU, the prime motivator in questions regarding validation is to ensure that the computer system will not adversely affect the product quality and, ultimately, patient safety. Hence, they will focus very clearly on the statutory regulations and guidelines as their source of reference. This leads to the conclusion that one of the initial activities of the project team must be to fully disseminate the *direct* GMP relationships that many of the system components (software *and* hardware) may have. More recently, the regulators have expressed their wish to see a more "risk-based" approach to meeting GxP compliance, and this provides the team with a key tool to aid the development of a suitable validation approach. There are many different ways in which risk can be assessed, and a good introduction can be found by reference to the ISO14971 — "Medical devices—Application of risk management to medical devices."

Once this information has been distilled, the team can better visualize the extent of the problem in front of them. This puts them in a position to develop a testing strategy of the appropriate level of detail and depth according to the GMP implications revealed by the analysis.

One problem area is that most systems implementers see computer systems as business tools and do not fully appreciate the direct GxP relationship that many of the system modules have. This is the reason for ensuring a wide knowledge base in the project team. This should therefore include people with experience in regulatory compliance who can help negotiate the complex web of rules and regulations that may be applied to the project. As an example of such an analysis is one of the more complex and convoluted of business systems, namely a MRPII system. Most modern-day MRPII systems are modular. Each module generally deals with a different aspect of the business, with some element of crossover between the modules. Some of these modules include inventory control, quality control lot control and traceability and storage and distribution. The validation of any system functionality surrounding the transaction and collection of the above data is of critical interest to the regulatory bodies. They will require adequate documentary evidence of the tasks performed in obtaining that validation.

Develop Validation Approach and Strategy

The analysis of the GxP aspects of a system helps define the approach to validation, but before finalizing the strategy it is also worth considering those elements of the system that could be classified as *business-critical* functions. After all, an organization's objective is to achieve, upon implementation of the new system, one that functions successfully to meet as fully as possible *all* the business needs originally defined. For example, it is necessary to take into account the requirements of the company financial auditors, customs and excise, and other government agencies (e.g., the U.K. Home Office in relation to controlled drugs). All must be considered and included in plans for validation.

A useful tool for carrying out this task is to perform a *risk assessment* of the processes within the scope of the project. Risk assessment is a process that allows the project team to focus on the likelihood and the potential impact of all forms of possible failure and disruption so that appropriate measures can be taken to reduce or even eliminate them. When applied to computer systems validation the risk assessment process must address the ways in which differing types of activity could be disrupted, stopped, or have their performance degraded to unacceptable levels. Some examples are:

1. Readiness and operation of business processes required as obligations under GMP regulations or under statute (e.g., health and safety).
2. Readiness and operation of normal business processes that directly affect product quality and therefore patient safety.
3. Readiness and operation of business processes that support business reputation or cost of operations.

There are many different ways in which risk assessment can be carried out and it is outside the scope of this chapter to describe them. However, all forms of risk assessment follow a similar route, which indicates the main steps to be applied in the risk assessment process. The key to performing successful risk assessment for a validation project is to follow a formal procedure and ensure that all conclusions are fully documented. It should be noted that risk assessment should occur more than once throughout the life cycle of the project. The primary activities are as follows.

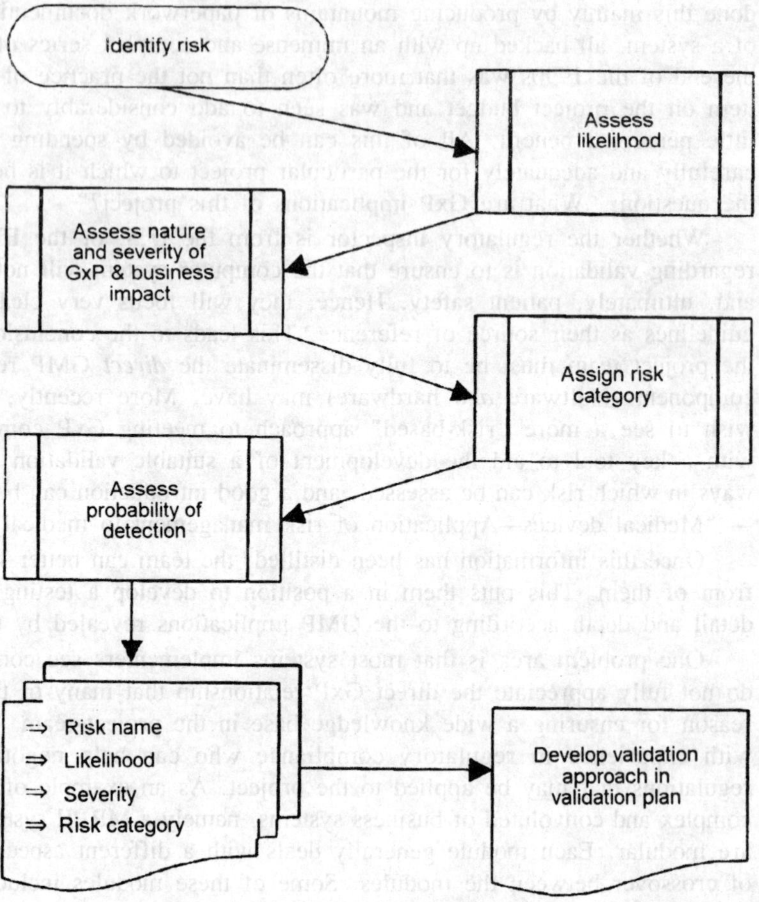

Fig. 11.2. Overview of a risk assessment process.

Identify risk

In assessing the types of risk to which the project may be subject, it is important to ensure that the assessment is well informed and based on verifiable evidence. Where possible and appropriate, the views of acknowledged experts should be called upon to ensure that the assessment of the nature and likelihood of a particular risk is as realistic as possible.

At this stage it is only necessary to record summary details for each risk. These details should include a name, which should convey something of the nature of the risk, and a one- or two-sentence description of the nature of the risk.

Assess likelihood

The most straightforward way to define the likelihood of a risk occurring is to use some simple criteria.

Low: probability of the risk occurring perceived as less than 10%.

Medium: probability of the risk occurring perceived as between 10% and 50%.

High: probability of the risk occurring perceived as between 50% and 80%.

Very high: probability of the risk occurring perceived as over 80%.

Assess nature and severity of business impact

The risk assessment process should result in the identification of the immediate effects of the risk happening and also the impact on the business of those effects. For example, the immediate effect of a hard disk problem may be the corruption of some inventory and distribution data stored on that disk. However, the longterm effect will impact upon the ability of the business to have a high level of assurance that GMP- and business-critical data relating to product distribution is accurate. This is a significant noncompliance with the regulatory requirements that could lead to the withdrawal of the company's manufacturing license and hence will adversely affect the company's ability to continue trading. As a minimum, risk assessment should consider the impact on:

1. Product quality and safety.
2. Regulatory compliance.
3. Health and safety (employees and public).
4. Financial performance.
5. Company reputation with customers, suppliers, staff, and investors.

A simple grading system can be used, ensuring that the assessment is well informed and based upon verifiable evidence.

Low: a minor negative impact, having no long term detrimental effects.

Medium: a moderate negative impact, with short- to medium-term detrimental effects.

High: a significant negative impact, having significant medium- to long-term effects.

Very high: an immediate and very significant negative impact, having significant long-term effects and potentially catastrophic short-term effects.

Assess probability of detection

The probability of risk detection can be graded using a simple scheme as follows:

Low: probability of risk detection perceived as less than 10%.

Medium: probability of risk detection perceived as between 10% and 50%.

High: probability of risk detection perceived as between 50% and 80%.

Very high: probability of risk detection perceived as over 80%.

Another factor to be considered when defining the validation strategy is the construction of the software in the system itself. One approach is to categorize the system components (software and hardware) to segregate those that are common and have a low risk of failure from those that are less common and have a higher risk of failure.

Does the implemented solution consist of software based on standard or bespoke code?

One such approach is defined in the GAMP 4 Guide, which classifies software commonly found in manufacturing systems into five types. These categories may then be used, along with the GMP and business criticality factors previously discussed, as a basis for determining an appropriate validation approach. At the lower end of the scale the validation effort will be restricted to simple recording of the name and version number in the hardware acceptance tests or equipment IQ. However, at the higher end of the scale the requirement is more likely to be for following a full life cycle for all parts of the system.

The five categories defined within the GAMP 4 Guide are as follows.

Operating systems

Where the application software is operating on an established, commercially available operating system, the operating system may be validated as part of the validation process for the application software. Currently the U.S. and EU regulatory bodies do not require operating systems to be specifically validated other than as part of particular applications that run on them. The recommended validation approach is to use only well-known operating systems and record the name and version number as part of the installation qualification. Before implementation and use of a new version of an operating system, a thorough review must be undertaken to consider the impact of any new, amended, or removed features upon the application running on it. Such a review could lead to formal retesting of the application, particularly where a major upgrade of the operating system has occurred.

Firmware

This group of systems includes equipment like weigh scales, bar code scanners, label printers. Because of their standard nature hard coded programs or "*firmware*" drives them. These programs, while non user-programmable, are configurable and the approach during validation of such items is to formally record the configuration in the equipment installation qualification. As with Category 1, the unplanned and informal introduction of new versions of firmware during maintenance must be prevented by the application of rigorous change control. Again it is important to assess the impact of new versions on the validity of the IQ documentation and the necessary corrective action planned, initiated, and confirmed.

Standard software packages

Typical examples include Lotus 1-2-3, Microsoft Excel and other spreadsheet packages, Microsoft Access and other database packages (SAS). They are sometimes also referred to as canned or COTS (commercial off-the-shelf) configurable packages. There is no requirement to validate the software package, however new versions should be treated with caution. Validation effort should concentrate on the application, which includes:

1. System requirements and functionality.
2. The high level language or macros used to build the application.
3. Critical algorithms and parameters.
4. Data integrity, security, accuracy, and reliability.
5. Operational procedures.

As for other categories, change control should be applied stringently, since changing these applications is often very easy, and with limited security. User training should emphasize the importance of change control and the validated integrity of these systems.

Configurable software packages

Such systems include MRP packages, LIMS, manufacturing execution systems (MES), distributed control systems (DCS), and supervisory control and data acquisition packages (SCADA). A typical feature of these systems is that they permit users to develop their own applications by configuring or amending predefined software modules and also developing new application software modules. Each application (of the standard product) is therefore specific to the user process, and maintenance becomes a key issue, particularly when new versions of the standard product are produced.

The full life cycle approach should be used to specify, design, test, and maintain the application. Particular attention should be paid to any additional or amended code and to the configuration of the standard modules. A software review of the modified code (including any algorithms in the configuration) should be undertaken.

In addition, an audit of the supplier is required to determine the level of quality and structural testing built into the standard product. The audit needs to consider the development of the standard product that may have followed a prototyping methodology without user involvement. In such cases it is recommended that suppliers use a formally documented quality management structure and documentation during the development of the standard product. If the system and platform are not well known and mature, it may be more prudent to consider them in Category 5 rather than in Category 4.

Custom (bespoke) software

The full life cycle should be followed for all parts of such systems. An audit of the supplier is required to examine their existing quality systems. The VP should only be finally prepared after this audit to document precisely what activities are necessary, based on the results of the audit and on the complexity of the proposed bespoke system.

Use of the above categorization regime provides invaluable aid toward defining a suitable and appropriate validation approach in the VP. Nevertheless, care should be exercised as complex systems will most often have many layers of software, each with its own degree of categorization, and therefore one system could exhibit several or even all of the above categories. One such example is that of the MRPII system that could be constructed as follows:

1. Application layer regarded as a configurable software package.
2. Running on a commercially available operating system.
3. Utilizing bespoke interfaces to other corporate systems.
4. User interfaces via standard desktop PCs, label printers, weigh scales, and barcode readers.
5. Based upon a corporate network built from standard software and hardware.

Write the Validation Plan

The first section of this chapter indicated that there are two types of plans we could consider creating — the VMP and the VP. This section will concentrate upon the creation of the VP, but first it is wise to briefly consider some features of the VMP. The VMP is an *internal* user company document, written at a high level, the purpose of which is to document the areas, systems, and projects to be managed. Because it is a high-level document it should only indicate:

1. The level to which these systems require validation. – *Primarily based on the GxP impact.*
2. Whether they are "old" or "new" systems. – *Consideration of handling legacy systems, for example.*
3. Who has responsibility for owning the system. – *Specifying the person or department that will retain responsibility for the implementation and management of the implemented system.*
4. Who is managing the validation and change control. – *Enable clearer definition of roles and responsibilities.*
5. The timescales anticipated for completion of the stated tasks. – *Providing for improved management of resources.*
6. Who is responsible for approval of the validation. – Designate specific responsibility for project completion and sign off.

The style of this document is often no more than an expanded Gantt Chart or project plan, with the additional feature of formal maintenance in a quality assurance system and approved by senior management. However, other styles are more formal, with structured paragraphs, diagrams and tables, and follow the strict rules applied for the control of compliance critical documentation. Whatever the style, the prime concern is the availability of a plan. This plan should provide an overview of the company's approach to validation, show that they know the extent of the challenge (an inventory of the systems under consideration for validation, and even those not considered for validation) and have a planned way for resolving it.

The individual systems identified in the VMP inventory will have their own VPs. As with the VMP, the VP is an *internal* user company document and should be provided by the customer organization to the supplier or implementor of the system. This type of plan will indicate, in detail:

1. What validation must be done.
2. How this validation will be achieved.
3. When it is anticipated the validation (and phases within) will be completed.
4. Who is responsible.

These validation requirements must be communicated to the supplier or implementor at the start of the project because it will help determine the mix of activities required, assignment of resources and project timescales. To achieve this, the user organization will supply the approved VP to the supplier or implementor, together with the URS. These combined documents will provide the supplier or implementor with all the basic information required to understand both the technical requirements (URS) and the regulatory constraints (VP) to be imposed on the project.

Who should actually write the VP? Conventional wisdom indicates this is best driven by and assigned to the QA department, or, if applicable, the compliance and validation department. Members of these departments will have the specific knowledge enabling them to interpret the regulatory requirements, together with the analysis of GMP impact to produce a suitable plan. However, these groups cannot perform this task in isolation and it will be necessary for them to consult with other key team members such as the users and the information systems and technology department. This process will eventually produce the first issue of the VP, and it will be this version of the document that will be used in early discussions with the supplier or implementor. Commonly this revision undergoes further refinement following these discussions, as the technical design becomes clearer and the implications for the original validation approach become obvious. For more complex systems (i.e., MRPII) it is not unusual at this stage to define parallel life cycles of activity for different aspects of the system (standard application software, bespoke software, hardware, peripherals). Each cycle will have its activity emphasized at different parts of the V-model depending upon the GxP criticality assessment identified during the earlier planning of the project.

What about the scope that the VP will cover and what should the content look like? These issues will be discussed more fully in Section 3, but it is sufficient to state that the document should cover the following aspects.

1. Project team and validation team organization.
2. Life cycle to be followed.
3. Standard operating procedures to be followed.
4. Roles and responsibilities of different parties.
5. Activities and phases.
6. Deliverable items.
7. Overall project acceptance criteria.

Review the Validation Plan

One of the important factors for consideration when creating and managing validation plans is to make certain that the validation approach, related activities, and deliverables called for by the plan are agreed upon by as wide an audience as possible. This ensures that those responsible for overseeing (or even performing) the stated tasks and providing the deliverables are committed to their successful completion. Clearly the best way to achieve this is to carry out a thorough review of the VP with these parties involved. In most cases this may not prove too difficult because it is usual to find that many of the reviewers may have already participated in the writing of the plan. It is also imperative that this audience has the appropriate levels of authority and responsibility within their relevant organizations to make approval decisions about the VP.

Approve the Validation Plan

When a company is subject to regulatory inspections of computer systems validation, it is usual for the inspectors to begin the review by understanding what validation activities were planned initially. In order to find the clearest demonstration of this, they will request to see a VP and they will expect it to be adequately approved and controlled. The approval of the plan should be clear and unambiguous, and should have been performed by suitably expert and experienced persons. Each individual should sign the VP as appropriate, with the approval signature indicating their name, job or function and the date the approval was given.

As for who should be involved in this approval process, the list is similar to the list for reviewing the plan given in the "Review the Validation Plan" section of this chapter. The approval process followed should be exactly the same as that for any other compliance critical document managed by the company's QA documentation control system.

Document Management and Control

It is not unusual for the approach defined in the VP to change as the project progresses and more is understood about the issues surrounding the system's implementation. Also the length of time it takes for some projects to reach completion means that invariably there will be personnel changes or even job or organization restructuring. Once approved, the VP must be formally controlled by a documentation control system to ensure such changes happen in an organized manner. While documentation systems can vary from company to company, the features to be aware of are generally encapsulated in the following basic principles.

1. Documents to be assigned a unique reference code.
2. Version control from one edition to the next to identify when a document has been superseded.
3. Laid out in an orderly format so as to ensure unambiguous and clear content.
4. Ability to conduct formal review process and update document as required.
5. Change control process to track change requests who, why, when.
6. Clear document approval, involving only those with suitable authority to approve.
7. Approvals to be dated.
8. Control of document issue and return or destruction of old versions.
9. Documents should be subjected to regular documented review and amended as necessary in order to stay current.

Within the U.K. (and the EU) the requirements for documentation control are contained within the rules and guidance governing GMP and are as applicable to validation documents as they are to any other compliance critical document. The responsibility for managing and controlling documents is generally given to the quality assurance function and this applies equally to VPs. However it is important that the project or validation team is conscious of the need for document control and the team should be given the necessary training to build and improve this awareness.

FORMAT AND CONTENT OF THE VALIDATION PLAN

This section defines the typical contents of the VP. While all the sections listed here should not be regarded as mandatory, careful consideration must be given to the scope of the project when deciding which ones to omit. If any sections are excluded from the final plan it is recommended that some form of justification be provided. The primary sections for inclusion in a VP are:

1. Introduction and project overview.
2. System description.
3. Validation approach.

4. Validation documentation.
5. Validation documentation procedures.
6. Training requirements.
7. Validation organization.
8. Validation activity schedule and timeline.
9. Maintenance of validation status.
10. Constraints and assumptions.
11. Appendices.

Introduction and Project Overview

The author of the VP should use this section to set the scene for the content of the remainder of the document and provide the correct context for the reader to understand the approach taken. It is therefore important that this section contain information relating to some, if not all of the following topics.

1. Background to, and reasons for, the project.
2. Who produced, reviewed, and approved the document, under what authority and for what purpose.
3. The scope of validation for the system.
4. The objectives of the validation.
5. The period within which the plan will next be reviewed.

An example of such text is as follows:

Currently the Novocastrian Pharmaceutical Company Limited (NPCL) uses a wide range of computer systems for the day to day running of the business. These range from manufacturing inventory and planning systems to finance systems, collectively known as the "MYOPE" system. In addition the company operates office automation packages. The "MYOPE" system is now old and is not easy to upgrade. In addition, the system contains large amounts of important data that could be of use to management to improve the business. However, the constituent parts of the system are based on different operating systems and databases, and hence it is very difficult to access this data in a simple way. It has also been recognized that there is an issue regarding the regulatory compliance of this older system to current MCA/FDA computer systems validation guidelines.

To resolve the above problems, and to gain business improvement through the use of new electronic computer systems, NPCL have decided to introduce a series of new computer systems that will all form part of an integrated strategy. This VP defines the strategy to validate these new computer systems for the production and financial management processes. These processes are defined in the URS (reference URS-NPCL-001) and include, but are not limited to:

1. Production planning.
2. Manufacturing and filling and packaging.
3. Quality department.
4. Engineering.
5. Warehousing.
6. Purchasing.
7. Production costing, nominal ledger, sales ledger, purchase ledger, fixed assets.

This document was produced under the authority of the production director at NPCL and has been reviewed and approved by the head of information systems and the head of quality assurance. It follows the standard company procedure for the preparation of a VMP and complies with the company validation policy.

This VP is to be regarded as an active document. It controls the generation of all validation related documents, and this documentation will be produced in stages during the phased implementation of the chosen software packages, therefore it may be necessary to review this VP at regular intervals or as and when major changes to the documentation occurs. Such updates will be reviewed and issued as a new version of the VP under standard company change control procedures.

System Description

The URS will have already described in some detail the process that the computer system will automate, support or replace. This needs to be reinforced by a high-level description of what the proposed system will be like. In earlier versions of the VP this may only be a sketchy overview of some conceptual designs, but as the project progresses through the tendering process, a more tangible proposal will emerge. It is useful to include such a description in the VP in order to allow the reader to comprehend the structure of the approach defined in the remainder of the document.

The usual form of a system description is a text description of the system as in the example below. The computer systems to be installed will cover the following functional areas:

1. Manufacturing and inventory.
2. Purchasing.
3. Sales.
4. Finance.

Over the last 2 years NPCL has been creating documents outlining the way in which the current manufacturing and financial functions operate on a day-to-day basis, both computer and noncomputer related. This was then followed by documenting, in a comprehensive user requirement document, the functionality ideally desired in a new series of computer systems.

As part of the initial stages of application software selection, many varying packages were reviewed. It was decided that no single package met all the requirements, and an integrated approach was needed to provide the overall functionality required. Reliability and ease of integration is gained by use of the Hewlett Packard (HP) computer systems as the hardware standard, and the HP Unix operating system is the basis on which all the packages will operate. The Oracle database is the base relational database package on which the application software will run. Microsoft Windows NT is the preferred client operating system, the overall company IT strategy based on client/server architecture.

The final application packages selected are:

Oracle GEMMS	– Manufacturing requirements planning.
Oracle Financials	– Financial management.
Base 10 FS	– Dispensary system.
Documentum	– Enterprise document management system.

However, this can be simplified by using a flowchart, showing the main systems and the links and interfaces between them, the hardware, the users, and peripherals. The key to creating these descriptions is to keep them as simple as possible. They should be easy to understand by a reader with little or very limited knowledge of computer systems, but they should also be sufficiently detailed for the more expert eye to be able to comprehend the objective of the project.

Validation Approach

The purpose of this section is to document the life cycle model that has been decided upon following the analysis of the system GxP criticality. In addition, it should note any special validation requirements accounting for any compliance issues that may have been identified following further investigations into software suitability and the adequacy of the development processes. The opening paragraphs of this section ought to cover the overall definition of the approach taken. For example, the text must indicate whether the validation is performed prospectively, concurrently, or retrospectively.

The discussion in subsequent paragraphs must be designed to consider whether the software applications purchased will be implemented as modified or unmodified packages. Emphasis should be placed upon the use of any bespoke software, and the development process behind it, together with how compliance will be assured. Indication should be given as to the exact nature of these developments, what they are being used for and what impact they have from a GxP or business critical viewpoint.

One area often overlooked in writing VPs is that of data transfer. Usually when a modern system updates or replaces an older or obsolete system, there is a great deal of critical business and GxP data that may need to be transferred. The same is true if a new computerized system is brought in to replace a manual one. In such cases the VP must describe the approach proposed to verify successful data transition, and indicate whether this process will be manual or electronic.

Quite often the approach taken in many plans is to concentrate solely on the GxP critical areas of the system. Such an approach should be clearly stated together with reasons provided as to why it is deemed acceptable. It is often valuable to define the life cycle and support this with diagrams or examples to illustrate the particular model chosen (for example the GAMP V- model). This should be further developed by discussion of the use of any categorization of hardware system, peripherals and software, showing the categories assigned by the team to each item in the project. It is also valuable at this stage to outline any planned project phasing and system environment management to support system development, testing, and go-live. As a final point, this section must identify any special requirements to be undertaken due to issues raised during vendor assessments. For example, the software development process of a standard COTS software package may be found to have some compliance issues with it during the vendor assessment process. The project team may still decide to purchase the software for many other valid reasons. Consequently the validation team may decide to perform some additional testing to close out any potential shortfalls that may be perceived to exist within the package.

Validation Documentation

The purpose of this section is to list documents that the team feels will be required to provide sufficient evidence of compliance and control over the entire validation process. Clearly this means that the eventual listing presented in the VP is entirely dependent upon the particular life cycle model chosen for the specific project under discussion. Therefore, for the purposes of this chapter consideration is given to the documents that could be generated if following a generic life cycle. It should be noted that no discussion regarding these documents is considered at this point as they will be encompassed elsewhere.

1. Planning phase: –URS.
   - Invitation to tender, response to proposal.
   - Company searches, vendor questionnaires, audit reports.
   - VPs.
   - Quality and project plan.
2. Specification and design phase:
   - Functional specification.
   - Hardware design specifications.
   - Mechanical and electrical diagrams.
   - Software design specifications.
   - Software module design specifications.
   - Network design specifications.

- Minutes of design review meetings.
- Change notices.

3. Building phase:
   - Hardware manufacture and assembly records.
   - Peripherals and equipment manufacture and assembly records.
   - Software code reviews.
   - Network manufacture and assembly records.
   - Change notices.
4. Testing phase:
   - Hardware testing protocols and records.
   - Software module testing protocols and records.
   - Software integration testing protocols and records.
   - Peripherals and equipment testing protocols and records.
   - Change notices.
5. Installation phase:
   - Hardware installation qualification protocols and records.
   - Software installation qualification protocols and records.
   - Peripherals and equipment installation qualification protocols and records.
   - Network installation qualification protocols and records.
   - Hardware acceptance testing protocols and records (OQ).
   - Network acceptance testing protocols and records (OQ).
   - Change notices.
   - Acceptance reports and certification.
6. Acceptance phase:
   - Factory acceptance testing (FAT) protocols and records (OQ/PQ).
   - System acceptance testing protocols and records (OQ/PQ).
   - Go-live testing protocols and records (OQ/PQ).
   - Change notices.
   - Acceptance reports and certification.
7. Reporting phase:
   - Final validation reports and sign off.
8. Ongoing operation:
   - Standard operating procedure
   — user manuals and data center operations.
   - Change control procedures.
   - Configuration management procedures.

Validation Documentation Procedures

Why does the VP need to have a section covering the procedures applicable to the validation documentation? There are several reasons for this. The most obvious reason can be seen from the listing in the above section. It shows that the range of validation documentation can be very wide. Some of these documents are very technical and complex in nature. Second, these documents will not all be produced by the same person or group of people. Some of them are likely to be generated internally by the project team (e.g., URS, acceptance protocols) while others may be produced externally depending upon the complexity of the project (e.g., functional specification, design specifications, assembly records). The third reason for defining rules and guidelines around validation documentation is to ensure consistency in both document format, content, and management procedures. All documentation must have some form of unique coding and version or date control. They must undergo a formal documented review and approval process, resulting in the unambiguous signature of approval by suitably qualified and authorized personnel, either internal or external to the company. The definition of controls around document content reduces the risk of information being erroneously omitted.

The most successful way to deal with such issues is to ensure that at the outset of a validation project it is clearly stated *why* these documents exist, *what* they are expected to contain, *how* they are to be controlled, and to *whom* this responsibility will fall. For smaller projects it is usual to handle these via the normal internal company standard operating procedures, but what about a more complex project where many documents may be generated externally by a third party implementor or have already been created by the software or hardware vendor? In such circumstances the validation team should reach agreement, both internally and externally, on the basic documentation formats and control requirements and state them in the VP. Note that they should bear in mind that they must comply with company policy and GxP requirements.

Training Requirements

A critical area often overlooked when planning validation projects is that connected with training, and it is an area that tends to need attention at different times during the project. Some training needs are more obvious than others. It may be necessary to embark upon some form of training for the groups that are to produce the various different documents during the project. After all, special rules may have been generated and personnel need to be made aware of them. Another aspect of training is more obvious — the training of the users in the operation of the new system. But what does "training" mean? Quite often it can take many different forms and the VP can be used to consider this and to identify key requirements. Some members of the company may only require a high level of information about the project, as they are not direct users. This is classed as "*communication*" and it takes the form of briefings or some other form of project overview — for example the use of video presentations. Other personnel will be directly affected and must be brought up to speed in a more controlled fashion. To achieve this they could undergo a number of project awareness sessions to prepare them for the next phase. These sessions form the basis of "*education.*" Finally, they can undergo the more formal and directly applicable "*training*" process for their day-to-day interaction with the system.

The VP must be used to provide details of all the above requirements and indicate the standard operating procedures that will control and formally record the process in adequate training records.

Validation Organization

This is a key section of the VP and must give an overview of the internal (and when applicable, external organization) requirements for its the successful execution. The first important item for inclusion is a full definition of the critical roles and responsibilities for the project. These will comprise critical roles such as:

1. Phase or task ownership.
2. Documentation ownership.
3. Technical support.
4. Quality assurance.

The section should go on to identify these key persons, including an indication of job titles to aid determination of the individual qualification and authority for the role.

Validation Activity Schedule and Timeline

The purpose of this section of the VP is to allow a high-level description of the tasks and activities associated with the project, and to link them with the overall expected schedule for the successful validation of the proposed system. It should indicate the key phases of the project together with proposed planned end dates for the validation milestones in the project. It is usual to present this information in the form of a Gantt chart or some other widely recognized project- planning chart or tool. The author of the VP should be aware that when writing this section timescales provided ought to be regarded for the purposes of indication only. The main purpose of this section is to show the time-related relationships between the phases and activities in the overall plan. It is usual for a detailed analysis of resource allocation activities and timing to be provided in another document, the quality and project plan.

Maintenance of Validation Status

The aim in this section of the VP is to indicate required procedures once the system has been validated and is "live." The purpose of these procedures is to ensure the maintenance of the validation status gained through compliance with the activities listed in the VP. Such procedures will include some, if not all, of the following.

1. Change control.
2. Access and security.
3. Configuration management.
4. Business continuity planning.
5. Backup and recovery process.
6. System start-up and shutdown.
7. Help desk operation.
8. Routine system audit.
9. Upgrade strategy and plans.
10. Revalidation policy.
11. Ongoing training.

Appendices

This section should contain the following information.

1. Definition of technical terms and abbreviations used in the document or reference to a glossary.
2. References to other relevant documentation (internal company policies and procedures, regulatory guides, international standards, etc.).

CHECKLIST FOR COMPLETION OF A VALIDATION PLAN

This section provides a checklist of typical questions that the document author may ask in order to obtain the information required to populate the relevant sections of the VP.

Question	*Y/N Details (if applicable)*
1. Has a project team been formed with the relevant: - Authority? - Business process knowledge? - Regulatory knowledge and experience? - Computer literacy?	List team membership and job titles.
2. Has the team performed an analysis of the GxP implications of the project?	Quote any references to formal documentation or meeting minutes.

Question	Notes
3. Has the team defined a validation approach or strategy based upon: – GxP/business criticality? – Risk assessment? – Software and hardware categorization?	Quote any references to formal documentation or meeting minutes.
4. Does the document meet the company requirements for layout and format, including: – Approvals page – Titles page – Unique project specific code – Text format and numbering – Clear identification of author or owner	 Record code number. Record name and job title
5. Does the creation, review, approval, and control of the VP comply with the formal company document management procedures?	Record relevant company SOPs and any change control references.
6. Is there a contents page or list?	
7. Does the plan contain a detailed project overview that details the following: – Background and justification for the project? – Who produced the plan, under what authority and for what purpose? – Scope of the system validation? – Objectives of the validation? – Review periods?	
8. Does the system description include: – A process or system flow diagram? – A detailed description of components? – List of manufacturer or suppliers? – Data and information flows? – System and user interfaces? – Constraints?	
9. Does the plan contain a definition of the validation approach, including: – Strategy for package modification? – Handling of bespoke software? – Issues surrounding data transfer? – Potential for phased implementation? – Follow up from vendor assessments?	Record any reference documents used to arrive at decisions.
10. Is there a list of each possible document type that could be required to satisfy validation? – URS? – Vendor assessment reports? – Quality and project plan? – Functional specifications? – Design specifications? – Design meeting minutes? – Change control system or notices? – Hardware and equipment assembly records?	Record any documentation standards that may apply.

- Software code reviews?
- Hardware testing protocols and records?
- Software testing protocols and records?
- Hardware IQ protocols and records?
- Software IQ protocols and records?
- Hardware OQ protocols and records?
- Factory acceptance protocols and records?
- System acceptance protocols and records?
- Go-live protocols and records?
- Acceptance reports and certification?
- User manuals and SOPs?
- Ongoing operational procedures?
- Configuration management and control?
- Final validation report and sign-off?

11. Does the plan clearly state the requirements for validation documentation management? — Quote relevant SOP reference.
12. Is there a section covering the potential requirements for training, including communication and education?
13. Does the plan contain a detailed description of the team organization with respect to validation?
14. Are details provided of the overall expected timescales and activities associated with validation of the system?
15. Is there a section within the plan that provides an indication of the ongoing requirements for validation maintenance?
16. Are the relevant appendices incorporated within the plan?
17. Have the following reviewers commented upon the plan content (list only those relevant for the project):
    - Project manager?
    - Users?
    - Quality assurance?
    - Validation?
    - Research and development?
    - Information technology?
    - Engineering?
    - Supplier or implementor?
    - Others?
18. Have the following approvers provided signed acceptance of the plan content (list only those relevant for the project):
    - Project manager?
    - Users?
    - Quality assurance?
    - Validation?
    - Research and development?
    - Information technology?
    - Engineering?
    - Supplier or implementor?
    - Others?

VALIDATION REPORTING

Overview of Validation Life Cycle

It is necessary to re-examine the simplified depiction of the generic validation life cycle for computerized systems. Initial examination of this figure seems to indicate that the validation report is one of the final activities of the life cycle and as such has the apparent function of summarizing all the activities that have gone on before. It also shows that it has a particularly close link to the project VP. Closer examination and discussion of the report and its role in the validation life cycle show that this relationship is not always as simple as depicted.

Purpose of the Validation Report

While the simplified view indicates the need for a validation report at the end of the project, in reality this final report is more than likely to be one in a series of reports produced throughout the life of the project. This will particularly be the case when involved in lengthy complex implementations across several departments, with multiple applications linked together (for example, an MRPII system). In such cases it is usual for other types of reports to be produced at regular intervals throughout the project, primarily dealing with recording the progress made, issues raised, and acceptance of different phases of the project. Generally these "phase" reports are used as the formal documentation indicating completion of one phase and approval to commence the next. Hence they form a vital part of the control process surrounding the project's management. In analyzing the subject of writing the validation report, it is necessary to consider at what stage the report is written and any relationship between the various reports produced. It is important to note that there is always a need to have a final validation report, whatever the project, which summarizes the entire project and measures its ultimate success and acceptance by the user.

An often-quoted phrase regarding validation is that: "If it isn't written down then it's a rumor". This provides a major clue as to the necessity for the creation of a validation report. When attempting to determine if pharmaceutical companies are complying with the GxPs, regulators such as the U.S. FDA and the U.K. MHRA want to see written evidence of task completion and controlled written evidence in particular. It is not acceptable to state verbally that some activity has occurred without the backup of some form of written evidence. The validation report has come to be seen to be of specific interest to these external regulatory bodies, so much so that inspectors from these bodies are more than likely to request such documents during regular inspection or surveillance visits. It is through examination of this document that regulatory authorities can see how organizations conducted and controlled the implementation of a new computerized system from the initial requirements definition, via the build process, installation, acceptance testing, and through to ongoing operation and maintenance. Furthermore, the regulatory authorities can understand, via a suitably constructed report, the degree of demonstrable compliance with the requirements laid down in the relevant GxPs.

Due to the highly crucial role that it can play in providing regulatory assurance, a validation report must record certain critical items, including, but not limited to:

1. Introduction and brief project background.
2. Overview and definition of phase or testing.
3. Organizational or procedural arrangements for phase execution.
4. Prerequisites considered.
5. Environment.
6. Planned deviations from VP (including justifications).
7. Summary of phase output.

8. Detailed description of phase output.
9. Problem reporting and resolution or actions.
10. Clear statement of status at end of phase.

Relationships with Other Life Cycle Phases and Documents

The term "*validation report*" can be applied to a series of reports rather than to a single entity. But what might these other reports be? By viewing an extension of the "V-model", found in the GAMP 4, it is possible to see that there is a direct relationship between the VP and the validation report. However, it is also possible to gain an insight into the other reports that could be created during the project life cycle.

However, what is not clear from this illustration is that each of these phases will, of necessity, generate some form of output or deliverables. Take the example of the process of creating, reviewing, and approving the functional and design specifications, a vital step in the life cycle. Any errors or omissions at this stage of the project can lead to costly amendments or delays at a later stage. It is usual to document this review process formally to ensure that the initial requirements are adequately catered for by the proposed design, and any problems, variations, decisions, and exceptions raised during this time are recorded, acted upon, or carried forward. This exercise is collectively known as design qualification (DQ). The most advantageous method of summarizing these various activities is via a design qualification report. The DQ report is therefore the key deliverable from this project phase, which also shows that similar interactions exist between the other phases of the life cycle and also with the "final" report. It is possible to see that these phase reports form a subset of supporting information for the "final" validation report. As such they represent a depiction of the critical pathway from the beginning to the end of the project.

Key Reporting Activities

Review Phase Requirements

The process of transferring from one phase of the life cycle to the next is a significant milestone in the project. During the project lifetime there will be several of these phase transfers, all of which lead to the final transfer of the system into the "live" state. Such points in the life cycle provide a focal point when the project team is required to provide confirmation that one phase has been completed to a satisfactory standard, while simultaneously granting approval for the next phase to commence. These points in time are also an opportunity for the project team to review progress against the overall project plan and to manage resources accordingly. The key output from this process should be the creation and approval of a "*phase report*." The phase requirements review process should take the form of verifying that all the planned activities are complete and the planned deliverables for the phase are present and correct. This is not a detailed review at this stage, more a preparation for the subsequent collation and analysis of test results and issues. If this process reveals any unusual occurrences, deviations, or variations from the planned activities and project deliverables, they can be noted and further discussed within the main body of the phase report.

Collate and Analyze the Results Obtained

The project team should nominate an individual or, in the case of large projects, a subteam to perform this task. Generally these people should have the appropriate experience and qualifications to understand the GxP and business impact of the results and be able to present their conclusions to the remainder of the project team in a clear and concise manner.

A useful approach is for this group to tabulate the outcomes and results to make review easier, highlighting any deviations from the planned activities or outcomes at the same time. They should then prepare to summarize the outcome and conclusions to the rest of the team, using the deviations noted to stimulate discussions on possible resolution.

Collate and Analyze the Issues Raised

All deviations must be addressed to the satisfaction of the project team and within the project's scope and objectives. Each one must be assessed for any potential GxP impact. The nature and severity of the deviation could well determine the approach to its resolution. If the deviation is the result of an incomplete activity or deliverable then the reasons for noncompletion must be determined and the project team must decide if it needs to be completed before the phase can be accepted. If some critical documentation is not available, an action plan must be formulated either to obtain it or to justify its noninclusion. However, if the deviation is the result of a test failure it may be necessary to make a controlled change to the system and repeat the relevant tests. The project team must decide which, if any, of these issues must be completed in order to accept the phase, and conversely, if any may be carried forward to the next phase. All such decisions must be formally documented and approved. The phase report provides the ideal mechanism for achieving this.

Write the Validation Report

The task of writing the validation report (or phase report) is the responsibility of the project team. It is more efficient and usual for the team to nominate an individual to perform this task rather than attempt to create a report by committee. If the project has already created a number of report formats or templates, the task of creating the report will be relatively simple, with the author required only to enter the relevant information or data into predefined sections. It is advisable to begin the process of drafting the report at almost the same time as the phase begins, creating it in parallel with the activities of the phase. This will not only save time at the end of the phase when the report is undergoing the review and approval process, but it can also act as a focal point for the collation of the information required by the review team as discussed in the "Review Phase Requirements" section.

Review the Validation Report

The draft report should be presented to the project team for a review process. The entire team may not need to perform this process; an appointed subteam may well suffice. However this subteam must be made up of members who have the relevant technical expertise and qualifications, including detailed knowledge of any issues raised and the implications that they may have on the project as a whole (in particular GxP and business impact).

It may be necessary for the report to undergo two or three cycles of the review process in order to reach agreement with the whole team (including QA). This fact should not be overlooked and it is important that time is allowed in the project planning process for this. All to often a project plan will assign one day for approval of the report, with no time allowance built in for an adequate review and modification process. If the report is used to signal the end of one phase and the start of another it is entirely possible that the next phase will be delayed while the report is undergoing this process.

Approve the Validation Report

Regulatory inspectors often seek to assess the approach to and levels of compliance with the approved validation requirements by asking to review the validation activities that were initially planned. Hence they will request to see a VP, which should be adequately approved and controlled. The next logical question following this review will be to request evidence that the planned activities were satisfactorily completed. In addition they will attempt to determine that throughout the duration of the project adequate controls were in place. By providing the phase reports the company is able to demonstrate that it can meet these requirements, but these reports need to carry the suitable level of authority that can only be granted full approval. The approval of the reports should be clear and unambiguous, and should be performed by suitably competent and experienced persons. Each individual should sign each report as appropriate, with the approval signature indicating name, job or function and the approval date.

Table 11.1. Participants in the report review process

Users	Ensure the reports meet the requirements of the planned activities.
Project manager	Ensure the conclusions detailed in the report adequately reflect the status of the phase or project. Ensure issues or deviations have been resolved, justified, or corrective actions agreed and carried forward if necessary.
Validation	Ensure the conclusions detailed in the report adequately reflect the status of the phase or project and comply with current accepted industry or company standards for validation of computer systems.
Information technology	Technical expertise regarding hardware, software, and systems acceptability and compatibility. Ensure compliance with company IT strategy. Management of day-to-day IT systems operations and controls.
Engineering	Acceptance of hardware siting, cabling and peripherals, and compliance with capacity and maintenance requirements.
Supplier or implementer	Ensure the conclusions detailed in the report adequately reflect the status of the phase/project.
Quality assurance	Ensure the report complies with predefined format and structure requirements. Review all deviations and issues and ensure GxP or business impact has been assessed. Ensure issues and deviations have been resolved, justified, or corrective actions agreed and carried forward if necessary. Ensure compliance with any relevant regulatory requirements.

As for who should be involved in this approval process, the list is similar to that given in the preceding section for phase reports review. The approval process followed should be exactly the same as that for any other compliance critical document managed by the company's QA documentation control system.

Document Management and Control

Validation reports are usually classed as critical documents in the same way as one would regard a standard operating procedure or a master batch record. However, in the context of their importance in the validation life cycle as illustrated in this chapter, the author considers that such documents should be treated similarly to other "*compliance critical*" documents and should, once approved, be formally controlled by a documentation control system. This will ensure they are adequately issued and stored so as to be available for subsequent inhouse review (maybe as part of a system modification or upgrade project) or by regulatory agencies, without fear of any adulteration having taken place.

While documentation systems can vary from company to company, reports should include the following basic principles.

1. Documents should be assigned a unique reference code, linked to the original VP.
2. Version control must be in operation from one edition to the next to identify when a document has been superseded.
3. Documents should be laid out in an orderly format so as to ensure unambiguous and clear content.
4. The ability to conduct formal review processes and update documents as required must exist.
5. There must be a clear change control process to track change requests — who, why, when?

6. There must be clear document approval involving only those with appropriate qualifications and with suitable authority to approve.
7. Approvals must be dated.
8. Control of document issue and distribution should be in operation, including return or destruction of old versions.

The responsibility for managing and controlling documents is generally given to the quality assurance function and this applies equally to validation reports. However, it is important that the project team are conscious of the need for document control and they should be given the necessary training to build and improve this awareness.

Format and Content of a Validation Report

This section defines the typical contents of a validation report. While none of the sections listed here should be regarded as mandatory, careful consideration must be given to the scope, criticality, and phase of the project when deciding which to omit. If any sections are excluded it is recommended that some form of justification is provided. The primary sections for placing within a validation report, irrespective of project phase, are:

1. Introduction.
2. Summary of phase results.
3. Phase execution.
4. Problem reporting and resolution.
5. Validation phase status.
6. Glossary.
7. Appendices.

Introduction

The introduction to any formal document is vital to setting the scene for the reader and should place the main content and conclusions into their correct context. Therefore the author of a validation report should spend a reasonably significant amount of time in constructing this section and structuring it to meet these needs adequately. Examples of the typical themes to be covered by the introduction include:

1. Purpose of the report.
2. Who created it.
3. Under what authority (with cross references to key documents).
4. Definition of the phase requirements.
5. Summary of the approach adopted.
6. Scope of phase.

Although many of the items listed seem to require a high level of detail, it is possible to encompass them in a few well-chosen sentences.

Summary of Phase Results

It is normal, and aids the readability of the report, if a short section is included early on to provide a brief summary of the test results. This could take the form of a short text description of the overall outcome of the testing and activities performed, giving an indication of the levels of success or failure. More simply, the results could be tabulated to indicate the total numbers passed, the numbers failed, those tests not performed, and any with inconclusive outcomes. Finally, the summary should briefly indicate any unusual occurrences, deviations and variations from the expected outcome, and raise key issues for further discussion within the main body of the report.

Phase Execution

This section of the report will probably be the longest and most detailed. It provides a comprehensive breakdown of the outcome of all the activities required for completion of the phase, including test results, test certificates, documentation, etc. A suggested list of themes to be covered within this section is as follows:

1. Prerequisites.
2. Project environment.
3. Exclusions.
4. Details of phase execution.
5. Comprehensive results breakdown.

Each of the above is briefly discussed in the subsequent paragraphs. However this list is not exhaustive and consideration should be given to any other relevant information which can be used to provide a historical record of the events that occurred to support the implementation and validation of the system.

Prerequisites

The objective of this subsection is to present a detailed itemization of the tasks, conditions, and actions deemed to be satisfactorily completed before beginning any phase specific activities such as testing. There is no idealized list of the items that can be created as they will very much depend upon the individual requirements of each and every project. In practice not all of these items may have reached such a suitable conclusion and it may be necessary to indicate where some of these cannot be satisfied and to justify the reasons for continuing the implementation uninterrupted. In constructing the report and using a table to list prerequisite status, it is useful to indicate these actions and responsibilities at the same time. This table is constructed on the basis of the pre-requisites that may be considered necessary when moving from the FAT to the system acceptance testing (SAT) phase. The example project is a fictional ERP implementation for the Novocastrian Pharmaceutical Company Limited (NPCL), which is supported by a third-party systems implementor (SI).

Project environment

Within the context of this chapter the phrase "*project environment*" is used to refer to the different combinations of hardware and software at various stages of the project. Hence the combination may develop from that housed on a development server and simple client to the more complex client/server combination of the live system. The project environment used for the various phases should be described in sufficient detail so as to give an overview of the software configuration, master databases, hardware, and peripherals involved. The origin of this environment should be indicated, for example, where was it initially created, and when was it copied over. The text should go on to describe how and when it was finally migrated to the live server and the clients, and if any special configuration requirements were implemented. Indication must also be provided of the change control procedures applied to the software configuration and master databases.

Exclusions

Quite often it is necessary to modify the original approach taken to reach a satisfactory conclusion to the different phases of a project as a result of changing circumstances throughout the lifetime of that project. For example, because of the need to satisfy certain SAT prerequisites before executing some SAT tests, and the need to continue specific business processes in some areas, it could be found that a number of planned tests could not be executed in the manner expected, or at all. It is vital that when this happens the validation report must not only highlight these exclusions, but also justify them in terms of the overall risk to the successful completion of the project and the satisfactory validation of the system. Some example situations are:

1. Tests involving equipment that could not be tested outside its normal environment (e.g., floor-mounted balances in a dispensing area).
2. Activities associated with an area undergoing a parallel refurbishment program, that was not completed on time.
3. Activities including full operational testing of legacy system interfaces where a test legacy system could not be implemented.

Details of phase execution

It is good practice to include in the report a short description of the underlying details of the phase execution. At the outset it is customary to refer to the controlling specification for the phase (the acceptance test specification, for example). The text should then proceed to confirm that all completed tests were executed and witnessed by suitably qualified and authorized personnel, indicating any support resources that were available and specifying the names, job titles, and qualifications of those involved. As far as reasonably possible the testing and witnessing personnel should be selected on the basis of their knowledge of that area of the business under test, and past experience of the proposed solution. The description should then continue with a discussion regarding the location of the testing. This is particularly important, as it is necessary to explain the level of control exercised during the development of a system, demonstrating the reduction of any risk to existing live systems during the implementation and before acceptance. Another detail that should be considered for inclusion in this part of the report, particularly in relation to tracing the project history, is confirmation of the dates over which the phase occurred, together with explanations of reasons for delays and actions taken to resolve them. Finally it is recommended that the text include confirmation that all tests and activities are subjected to a regular project team review process, indicating the evidence to support this statement.

Comprehensive results breakdown

This section forms the main body of the report and it is important to ensure that it is both comprehensive and concise. The recommended way to achieve this is to record the summarized results in a tabular form. In designing the table format it is necessary to consider what information is conveyed to the reader. The validation report is a summary of the activities that took place during the phase. Hard copy original test records or documents containing detailed information of the activity, reference to any other documents (e.g., URS, FDS) and the outcome of those activities will back it up. Therefore the summary table only needs to indicate the test reference, what it applies to, the title of the test or activity, the outcome and a reference to the incident log for follow-up if required.

Problem Reporting and Resolution

As can be observed from the discussion in the previous section of this chapter, it will be most unusual for the activities or tests performed during a phase to complete without any problems or deviation from the expected outcome. In such circumstances it is vital that the validation report accurately reflects these issues and discusses them in sufficient detail to clarify the required actions and timescales for resolution and justification for the chosen courses of action. A full assessment of system readiness before proceeding from one phase to the next requires a review of not only the test results, but also the solutions to the issues and problems raised during the total testing period. The documentation of these issues is very much a matter of individual taste, but again the use of a tabular format provides a disciplined approach that will ensure all the required issues are highlighted for each adverse event or deviation. The use of such a simple format for recording these problems means that the author and readers of the report can quickly observe the main issues and trace the resolution during future stages of the project.

Validation Status

The opening to this section of the chapter indicated that an important feature of any formal document is the need to set the document into its correct context. It is also equally important that the status at the conclusion of the activities covered by the validation report is clearly defined. The structure of the report proposed in this chapter naturally guides the reader to this statement of the validation phase status. Such statements need not be excessively complex, but should attempt to covey the following basic messages.

1. Who has reviewed the report and under what authority?
2. What does their signature on the report represent?
3. Is the status acceptable or unacceptable?
4. Can the project proceed to the next phase?

In cases where the report is the final validation report, the last bullet point would be more akin to a statement that the system is validated in accordance with the planned activities originally defined in the VP.

Glossary

The inclusion of a glossary is a useful aid for the reader who is unfamiliar with specific terminology employed within the project or the technology adopted for the final implemented system. The glossary should limit itself to brief but meaningful definitions of technical terms and abbreviations used within the report and any other reference documentation.

Appendices

This section should contain the following information.

1. For validation reports that cover a wide number of events it may be useful to provide listings of cross-reference documentation.
2. References to other relevant documentation (internal company policies and procedures, regulatory guides, international standards, etc.).

Checklist for Completion of a Validation Report

This section provides a checklist of typical questions that the document author may ask in order to obtain the information required to populate the relevant sections of the validation report.

Question	*Y/N*	*Details (if applicable)*
1. Does the report meet the company requirements for layout and format, including:		
– Approvals page?		
– Titles page?		
– Unique project specific code?		Record code number
– Text format and numbering?		
– Clear identification of author or owner?		Record name and job title
2. Does the creation, review, approval, and control of the validation report comply with the formal company document management procedures?		Record relevant company SOPs and any change control references
3. Is there a contents page or list?		
4. Does the report contain an introduction which details the following:		

- Purpose of the report?
- Who produced the report and under what authority?
- Definition of the phase requirements?
- Summary of the approach adopted?
- Scope of the phase and report?

6. Does the report provide an easily readable summary of the results?
7. Does the report contain the following details of the execution of the phase:
   - Prerequisites?
   - Project environment?
   - Exclusions?
   - Details of the phase execution?
   - Comprehensive results breakdown?

   Record any reference documents used to arrive at decisions
8. Does the report highlight any deviations or variations from the expected results and actions for resolution or closure?
9. Does the report indicate that any deviations or variations from the expected results have been assessed for:
   - GxP and business criticality?
   - Risk analysis?
10. Are the relevant appendices incorporated within the report?
11. Is there a clear statement of the validation status of the project or system following approval of the report?
12. Have the following reviewers commented upon the report content (list only those relevant for the project):
    - Project manager?
    - Users?
    - Quality assurance?
    - Validation?
    - Information technology?
    - Engineering?
    - Supplier or implementer?
    - Others?
13. Have the following approvers provided signed acceptance of the report content (list only those relevant for the project):
    - Project manager?
    - Users?
    - Quality assurance?
    - Validation?
    - Information technology?
    - Engineering?
    - Supplier or implementer?
    - Others?

12

Computer System Validation

Computer systems validation, as established in 21 *Code of Federal Regulation* (CFR) Part 11.10(a) and defined in the recent draft United States (US) Food and Drug Administration (FDA) guideline, is one of the most important requirements applicable to computer systems performing FDA-regulated operations. It involves establishing the conformance to the intended use, user, regulatory, safety, and function allocated to the computer system. Similar to any FDA-regulated products, quality is built into a computer system during its conceptualization, development, and operational life. The quality of computer systems cannot be tested after being developed. In addition to software and hardware testing, other verification activities include code walkthroughs, dynamic analysis, and trace analysis. The documentation generated during the validation can be subject to examination by FDA field investigators. The results of a high-quality validation program can ensure with a high degree of assurance the trustworthiness of electronic records and computer systems-related functionality.

The introduction in 1997 of 21 CFR Part 11, Electronic Records, Electronic Signatures Rule (hereafter referred to as Part 11) provided the formal codification applicable to computer systems performing FDA- regulated operations. One fundamental principle in Part 11 is that it requires organizations to store regulated electronic data in their electronic form once a record is saved to durable media, rather than keep paper-based printouts of the data on file, as had been the long-term practice in organizations performing regulated operations. If information is not recorded to durable media, the stored data will be lost and they cannot be retrieved for future use. If "*retrievability*" is an attribute, then procedural and technological controls contained in Part 11 are essential to ensuring integrity. The implementation of procedural and technological controls to achieve compliance with Part 11 shall be monitored during the SLC. The approach to be used in covering computer systems validation is by presenting key elements applicable to any development/maintenance methodology. It is not intended to cover everything that computer system validation should encompass, including Part 11. A wide range of information about computer systems validation is listed in the bibliography.

Key Validation Elements

The key elements required to successfully execute computer system validation projects are as follows:

1. Selection of a development/maintenance methodology that best suits the nature of the system under development.
2. Identification of operational functions associated with the users, operational checks, regulatory, company standards, and safety requirements.
3. Selection of hardware based on capacity and functionality.

4. Inspection and testing of the operational functions.
5. Identification and testing of "worst case" operational/production conditions.
6. Reproducibility of the testing results based on statistics.
7. Documentation of the validation process.
8. Written design specification that describes what the software is intended to do and how it is intended to do it.
9. A written validation plan based on the design specification, including both structural and functional analysis.
10. Test results and evaluation of how these results demonstrate that the predetermined design specification has been met.
11. Availability of procedural controls to maintain the validation state of the computer system and its operating environment.
12. Any modification to a component of the system and its operating environment must be evaluated to determine the impact to the system. If required, qualification/validation is to be re- executed totally or partially.

Selection of a Development/Maintenance Methodology

The SLC is the "period of time that begins when a product is conceived and ends when the product is no longer available for use." Certain overall discrete work products are expected when evidencing the development and maintenance work of computer systems compliance to regulatory requirements. Refer to "Documentation of the Validation Process." The selected SLC specifies the overall periods and associated events. Different system acquisition strategies and software development models can be adapted to the SLC. The SLC model focuses on software engineering key practices and does not specify or discourage the use of any particular software development method. The acquirer determines which of the activities outlined by the standard will be conducted, and the developer is responsible for selecting the methods that support the achievement of contract requirements. A modifiable framework must be tailored to the unique characteristics of each project. The SLC includes the following periods:

- Conceptualization.
- Development.
- Early operational life.
- Maturity.
- Aging.

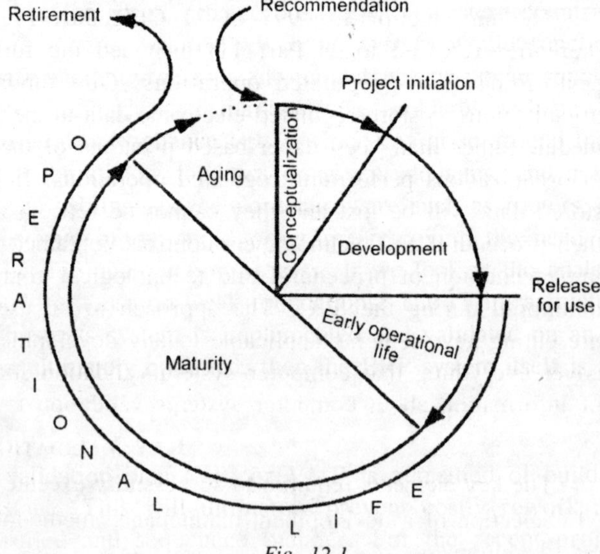

Fig. 12.1

Project Recommendation, Project Initiation, Release for Use, and Retirement are events. These events are considered phase gates or major decision points, which include formal approvals before the development can proceed to the next period. The development methodology associated with the SLC is a structured process that decomposes the engineering tasks and associated work products in support of the computer system validation effort. It breaks down the systems development process into subperiods, containing specific inspection and testing tasks that are appropriate for the intended use of the computer system. During each subperiod, detailed discrete work products are developed. This approach leads to well-documented systems that are easier to test and maintain, and for which an organization can have confidence that the system's functions will be fulfilled with a minimum of unforeseen problems. The most common development methodologies are the Waterfall Model, Incremental Development, Evolutionary Model, Object Oriented, and Spiral Model.

A critical component of the validation process is providing assurance that the development/ maintenance methodology is being followed. The SLC and associated development/maintenance methodology applicable to computer systems performing regulated operations shall be specified in procedural control(s). A project team should have the authority to select a developmental/maintenance methodology that best suits the nature of the system under development/ maintenance and that is different from the one included in the related procedural control. If this is the case, the selected development or maintenance methodology must be explained in the validation plan. It is the objective of FDA-regulated companies to select the appropriate SLC and associated development/maintenance methodology. Development and maintenance teams shall receive adequate training in the use of the chosen methodology.

Identification of Operational Functions

Using a structured process, the goal of the Development Period is to specify, design, build, test, and install the application to be automated or updated. One of the deliverables of the Development Period is the written and approved operational functions (e.g., user's, functional, design) that describe what the application is intended to do. A key activity to identify operational functions is by gathering systems requirements. The term "requirement" defines a bounded characterization of the scope of the system. It contains the information essential to support the operation/operators. These requirements include functional capacity, execution capability, safety, operational, installation, system maintenance, and regulatory compliance.

The refined scope is captured in the requirements specification, which describes what the system is supposed to do from the process/user's/compliance perspective. The requirements specification is used as part of the framework to select the computer technology supplier and/or contract developer. The system functionality must be well defined at the outset in order to provide the prospective supplier/ integrator with enough information to provide a detailed and meaningful quotation. The requirements specification is used to develop the performance qualification (PQ) protocol.

The requirements specification addresses the following:

1. The process to familiarize the developer with the user, process and data acquisition requirements, and special considerations of the project.
2. The scope of the system and strategic objectives.
3. The problem to be solved.
4. Process review and sequencing, as well as where each operation is to be completed.
5. The direction to solve the problem (e.g., device driven or may just be the mode of presentation of data, data security, data backup, data and status reporting and trending).
6. Redundancy and error-detection protocol.
7. Environmental control.
8. Interfaces (e.g., to field devices, data acquisition, reports and HMI), input/output (I/O) list, communication protocol, and data link requirements.
9. Type of control/process to be performed.
10. Operational checks and sequencing.
11. Data management.

12. Definition of the input and output formats.
13. How the data are to be collected, used, and stored.
14. How input data influence the operation of the system.
15. Retention requirements.
16. Data security requirements.
17. Audit trails and metadata.
18. Timing requirements.
19. Regulatory requirements.
20. Preliminary evaluation of technology.
21. Feasibility study and preliminary risk assessment.
22. Safety and security considerations.
23. Non-functional requirements (e.g., development standards, program-naming convention standards).

Each requirement in the requirements specification must be "testable." A "testable" requirement includes an objective criterion and it is non-ambiguous. A "testable" requirement provides the advantage that it can be recorded in quantified terms and allows for a subsequent review and independent evaluation of the test results.

Selection of Hardware Based on Capacity and Functionality

Based on the identification of operational functions and design, computer hardware technologies can be selected. Depending on available technology and cost, automated functions can be assign to the computer hardware or software. Computer hardware can be further decomposed into a number of subelements. Processor, memory, I/O and networks are some examples. Process, field instruments, control requirements, available technology and cost are some of the factors driving the selection of the hardware. This selection is specified in the requirement specification and the implementation described in the design specification. The design specification needs to be sufficiently detailed in order to familiarize the implementation team (e.g., engineering) and the hardware vendor with the requirements and special considerations of the process, field instrument, and control requirements.

- The requirements include, but are not limited to, the following:
- Purpose of the system.
- Regulatory requirements.
- Information and material inputs. Preliminary block diagrams.
- Data processing requirements (e.g., supervisory control and data acquisition).
- Number and type of I/O cards.
- Instrumentation and cabling.
- Control and information outputs.
- Operating modes.
- Alarms and alerts.
- Safety features.
- Error checking.
- Reporting.
- Redundancy requirements.
- Environmental requirements.
- Network requirements.
- Supporting utilities requirements.

- Hardware/human machine interfaces.
- General plan and acceptance criteria.

The critical field instrumentation must support accuracy and reliability requirements over the entire process range conditions.

Inspection and Testing of the Operational Functions

Software engineering practices may include documented unit testing, code reviews, explicit high-level and low-level design documents, explicit requirements and functional specifications, structure charts and data flow diagrams, function-point analysis, defect and resolution tracking, configuration management, and a documented software development process. These are the same quality principles that the FDA expects to be used during the development and maintenance of computer systems. These quality principles shall be contained in procedural controls. Inspections and testing are part of these principles. Testing and inspections are activities performed as part of the development methodology. Numerous inspection steps are undertaken throughout the system development and operational life to determine whether a computer system is validated. These include static analyses such as document and code inspections, walk-through, and technical reviews. These activities and their outcomes help to reduce the amount of system-level functional testing needed in the operational environment in order to confirm that the software meets the requirements and intended uses.

Reproducibility of the Testing Results Based on Statistics

Testing is not just executing a program using a test data file or randomly selected test cases just prior to implementation. It is an on going process using techniques based on Statistical Process Control (SPC) principles and product quality concepts implemented as components of a Statistical Quality Control (SQC) program. If software systems are viewed as a manufacturing facility that produces the desired output products, then statistical sampling procedures and statistical inference can be used to predict the reliability of test results. Instead of paying too much attention to the development of the application, another factor that requires attention is the data (raw material) to be converted into information (product). Information flow is a design technique that may be helpful in achieving this task.

Concerning testing, the input and output domains must be strictly defined. This suggests a response to the following: (1) What sampling technique will ensure an adequate subset of possible input values that will provide as complete a test of the software as possible? and (2) What information sampling procedures will allow the developers to determine product reliability? It is suggested that White and Black box test cases design strategies be used to sample the data (input domain), including Equivalent Partitioning, Boundary Analysis and Error Guessing, Cause–Effect Graphing, and Structural Tableau. The basics of Software Testing must be understood before the more abstract principles of statistical inference are tackled.

Documentation of the Validation Process

Design specification

System requirements are allocated to the software design. During the technical design it is described how each specification described in the system specification deliverable is to be implemented. This includes also developed subsystems components and interfaces, data structure, design constraints, algorithms and system decomposition. This activity is very critical to medical device companies. Design inputs are contained in the requirements of the computer system, and design output(s) can be included as part of the specification of the design. This design is the input for developing integration test and operational checks. Design according to the development methodology and specific procedural controls

1. Computer hardware and software architecture. Data structures.
2. Flow of information.

3. Interfaces.
4. Put together the design.
5. Perform design reviews. Verify whether the risks previously identified were mitigated as part of the solution presented in the design.
6. Finalized the test planning.
7. Design Part 11 technical controls.
8. Approve the design specification deliverable.
9. Conduct in-process audit activities associated with the technical design.
10. Re-visit the risk analysis.

Begin the planning of development of procedural controls for those Part 11 requirements not covered by technology.

Validation plan

Validation plans are documents that tailor a firm's overall philosophies, intentions, and approaches to be used for establishing performance adequacy to a specific project. They state who is responsible for performing development and validation activities. They identify which systems are subject to validation, define the nature and extent of inspection and testing expected to be done on each system, and outline the protocols to be followed to accomplish the validation. In summary, validation plans describe the following:

1. Organizational structure of the computerization project.
2. Responsible departments and/or individuals. Resource availability.
3. Risk management.
4. Time restrictions.
5. SLC and development methodology to be followed.
6. Deliverable items.
7. Overall acceptance criteria.
8. Development schedule and timeline.
9. System release sign-off process.
10. Sample format for key documentation.

Test results and evaluation

Although installation qualification (IQ)/operational qualification (OQ)/PQ terminology has served its purpose well and is one of the many legitimate ways to organize computer system testing tasks in FDA- regulated industries, this terminology may not be well understood among many software professionals. However, organizations performing regulated operations must be aware of these differences in terminology as they ask for and provide information regarding computer systems.

Once the qualification protocols have been completed, test results and data need to be formally evaluated. Written evaluation needs to be presented clearly in a manner that can be readily understood. The report should also address any non-conformance or deviation to the validation plan encountered during the qualification and resolution. The outline of the report parallels the structure of the associated protocol. The qualification testing should be linked with relevant specification's acceptance criteria, such as PQ vs. system requirements specification deliverable, OQ vs. system specification deliverable, and IQ vs. technical design specification deliverable. If applicable, it is included as part of the summary of the results of inspections and technical review of all technologies that are elements of the systems. In very large validation efforts, a report references (by title and document reference number) other documents that satisfy the protocol requirements. In smaller validation efforts, actual evidence is incorporated as appendices to the report. The documentation and results of the qualification efforts are assembled and reviewed by appropriate and qualified personnel. Following the review, the personnel responsible for the criticality of the system, including QA, approve the qualification effort. The approval of all qualification reports is a confirmation that the computer system as a whole has been proven to fit its purpose and that all essential elements of documentation are available. On computer systems controlling manufacturing equipment (process control systems), the approval of all qualification reports indicates the release of the computerized systems to the Process/Product Performance Qualification. On other computer systems, the approval of all reports indicates the release of the system to the user. Test results on Part 11 shall be addressed in the associated qualification report.

The Project Report summarizes the outcome of each activity performed to develop or maintain computer systems and the verification of critical checkpoints throughout the entire development process. The end- result is to verify that good quality development procedures were adhered to as established in the project plan. All verification and testing results completed during the project shall be addressed in the Project Report as well. The approval of the project report is the event to be considered prior to the release of the system for operation.

Validation maintenance

After the system has been released for operation, computer system maintenance activities take over. The maintenance activities must be governed by the same procedures followed during the Development Period. The validated status of computer systems performing regulated operations is subject to threat of changes in its operating environment, either known or unknown. Adherence to security, operational management, business continuity, change management, periodic review, and decommissioning provides a high degree of assurance that the system is being maintained in a validated state. It is the objective of organizations to have procedures in place to minimize the risk of computer systems performing regulated operations out of validated state. Maintenance in computer systems becomes an essential issue, particularly when a new version of the supplier-provided standard software is updated. A change control procedure must be implemented whereby changes in the software and computer hardware may be evaluated, approved, and installed.

If necessary, additional analysis may be needed to evaluate the changes (e.g., impact analysis) to the computer systems. The procedure should allow for both planned and emergency changes to the system. This procedure must include provision for updating of pertinent documentation on the system, including procedures. Records of changes to the system must be kept for the same period as any other regular production document.

Evaluation of Modification to Computer Systems

As required by regulations, all maintenance work must be performed after the evaluation and approval of the work and must be consistent with the selected SLC methodology. Maintenance to a software system includes, among other things, the following:

1. Perfective maintenance or correcting the system because of new requirements and/or functions.
2. Adaptive maintenance or correcting the system because of a new environment, which could include new hardware, new sensors or controlled devices, new operating systems, new regulations.
3. Corrective maintenance or correcting the system because of detection of errors in the design, logic, or programming of the system. It is essential to recognize that the longer a defect is present in the software before it is detected the more expensive it is to fix it.
4. Preventive maintenance or correcting the system to improve future maintainability or reliability in order to provide a better basis for future enhancements.

Change management procedural control is in place when the validated system is released for use. The change management procedural control provides for the following activities:

1. Identifying and specifying the change.
2. Assessing risk, criticality, and impact of change.
3. Specifying testing requirements and acceptance criteria.
4. Implementing change after authorization.
5. Performing regression testing.
6. Reviewing of change(s) with an independent reviewer.
7. Updating system and user documentation to reflect implemented change(s).
8. Establishing of provisions for the management of "*emergency change*," including expeditious documentation modifications.

System Development Files

One key element to support the SLC is the availability and maintenance of system development files. The developer shall document the development of each system unit, system component, and configuration items in software development files.

The developer should establish a separate system development file for each unit or a logically related group of units. The developer should document and implement procedures for establishing and maintaining system development files. The developer should maintain the system development files until the retirement of the system. The system development files should be available to the agency review upon request. System development files may be generated, maintained, and controlled by automated means. To reduce duplication, system development files should not contain information provided in other documents or system development files. The set of system development files shall include (directly or by reference) the following information:

1. Design considerations and constraints.
2. Design documentation and data.
3. Schedule and status information.
4. Test requirements and responsibilities.
5. Verification and test procedures, and results.

The validation of computer systems in the U.S. FDA-regulated environment is an ongoing process that is integrated with the entire System Life Cycle (SLC). Quality to a software system is introduced by following the system life cycle and following the key validation elements.

13

TONICITY

Parenteral formulations, both large and small volume, have been discussed in depth in Volume 11 of the Encyclopedia of Pharmaceutical Technology. However, no discussion of parenteral formulations is complete without an adequate description of tonicity. Tonicity is an important factor in the formulation of products intended for application to sensitive mucous membranes of organs such as eye, ear, and nose. In this article, an attempt is made to first introduce tonicity with respect to its physiological significance, followed by a discussion of the physicochemical basis for tonicity and colligative properties. Then, a brief review of methods of measuring and/or calculating tonicity is given, followed by the established methods of adjusting tonicity and the examples illustrating each of the methods.

Dosage forms are drug-delivery systems designed to deliver drug to the systemic circulation or to a localized region of the human body. These dosage forms should ideally be free of any undesired adverse effects from the drug and from the formulation components. Reasonable risks associated with the drug substance are sometimes tolerated with an objective of realizing significant therapeutic advantages, as in the case of cancer chemotherapeutic agents. However, any untoward side effect, even as minor as irritation, resulting from an excipient or the finished dosage form cannot be accepted and should not be tolerated. This concern is particularly important to parenteral formulations that breach the normal defensive barriers of the human body to deliver the drug. Therefore, any formulation that comes in contact with sensitive mucous membranes of organs such as the eye should not result in tissue irritation and pain attributable to the formulation itself. One of the physicochemical means by which a formulation may result in pain and tissue irritation is caused by the non-physiological concentration of dissolved solutes coming in contact with sensitive tissues. Tonicity is a formulation property that has a direct influence on the ability of the formulation to result in tissue irritation, as described by the following example.

If a small quantity of blood defibrinated to prevent clotting is mixed with a solution containing 0.9% w/v of NaCl, the red blood cells remain intact and retain their normal size and shape. The NaCl solution is considered to be isotonic and has essentially the same salt concentration as does the red blood cell. In contrast, if the blood is mixed with 1.8%w/v NaCl solution, erythrocytes shrink and become wrinkled or crenated as if the cell content has been sucked out. The salt solution that causes this is considered hypertonic with respect to the red blood cell contents. It is because the red blood cell contains a lower salt concentration than the surrounding 1.8%w/v salt solution and as if the water from the erythrocytes passes through the cell membrane to dilute the surrounding salt solution to equalize the two salt concentrations across the membrane. The opposite phenomenon occurs if blood is mixed with 0.45% w/v NaCl solution. Water from the surrounding salt solution enters the erythrocytes, causing them to swell and finally burst, with the liberation of hemoglobin. The 0.45% w/v salt solution is considered hypotonic, and the phenomenon is known as hemolysis. The physiological significance of hemolysis was reconfirmed recently by the report of 10 episodes of hemolysis among patients who received hypotonic 25% human albumin because of dilution with sterile water instead of isotonic sodium chloride. Two of these 10 recipients exhibited significant hemolysis and adverse pathological conditions, with one resulting in death. Also, it has been observed that hypertonic and hypotonic salt solutions tend to irritate sensitive mucous membranes of the eye, the nose, and the muscle when applied. However, an isotonic solution causes no tissue irritation when it comes in contact with the tissue. The crenation and the hemolysis of red blood cells in hypertonic and hypotonic salt solution, respectively, can be explained by the movement of water across the cell membrane. A membrane is defined as semipermeable if it allows only the movement of solvent molecules across it.

The process of diffusion of a solvent through a semipermeable membrane from a less-concentrated solution to a more-concentrated solution is known as osmosis. The pressure that must be applied to the concentrated solution side of the membrane to prevent the flow of pure solvent across the membrane from the diluted solution is known as the osmotic pressure. In crenation, water diffuses from the inside of the erythrocyte across the membrane into the exterior hypertonic salt solution. Hemolysis occurs when water diffuses from the exterior hypotonic solution into the erythrocyte, causing it to swell and burst.

An isotonic solution is an aqueous solution that generates the same "tone," or osmotic pressure, as the body fluids across biological membranes and thus prevents water flow in either direction and hence is non-irritating when injected, instilled, perfused, or brought into contact with sensitive mucous membranes. When a solution is hypertonic or hypotonic, osmotic water flow occurs and tone of the membrane is affected. Thus, formulators need to adjust the tone, or tonicity, of the solution to be isotonic with physiological fluids. To be able to adjust the tonicity of a formulation to the isotonic state, one has to understand the principles behind the generation of the osmotic pressure resulting from the dissolved solutes and how it can be altered to that of the physiological fluids.

Osmotic pressure is a colligative property unlike the additive and constitutive properties of solution. Simply stated, the colligative properties of a solution are dependent solely on the number of non-solvent (solute) particles (molecule/ions) dissolved or in a true solution form in a given solvent and are independent of the specific physicochemical characteristics of the non-solvent dissolved substance(s). For example, two non-electrolyte solutes A and B when prepared as 0.1 M solutions will exhibit the same osmotic pressure irrespective of the chemical nature of A and B. Experimentally, it has been found over the years that the colligative properties are indeed independent of the solute nature and dependent solely on the number of independent particles in dilute solutions for a wide variety of solutes, provided the number of particles is properly assessed. An implicit assumption in the statement above is that the solute is non-volatile relative to the solvent and the reasoning will be clear from the discussion that follows. The colligative properties of solution are vapor pressure lowering, boiling-point elevation, freezing-point depression, and osmotic pressure. These four properties are effects of solute on the solvent, in that it reduces the escaping tendency of the solvent, and all of them can be related to vapor pressure lowering of the solution. Osmotic pressure is of primary importance from the formulation standpoint; however, it is cumbersome to measure, and therefore other colligative properties are determined because they are all interrelated.

Raoult's and Henry's Laws as Basis for Colligative Properties

Raoult's law states that in an ideal solution, the partial vapor pressure of each volatile constituent is equal to the vapor pressure of the pure component multiplied by its mole fraction in the solution. Thus, for two constituents A and B in solution:

$$P_B = P_B^o X_B \quad ...(1)$$

$$P_A = P_A^o X_A \quad ...(2)$$

where P_A and P_B are the partial vapor pressures of constituents A and B over their solution when the fractional molar concentrations are X_A and X_B, and the vapor pressure of the pure constituents are P_A^o and P_B^o. Therefore, it can be inferred that the vapor pressure of B above the solution by dilution with A is reduced relative to its vapor pressure in pure state and vice versa for A. This diminishes the escaping tendencies of each component, leading to a reduction in the rate of escape of the molecules of A and B from the surface of the solution. This law is valid only in ideal solutions in which there are no intermolecular interactions between components A and B (adhesive interactions) or in which interactions between the two components A and B are identical to the interactions of the pure components A and pure B (cohesive interactions between A and A and between B and B). In essence, the molecule of each component sees an environment identical to its molecular environment in the pure state. This refers to an infinitely dilute solution in which a component's thermodynamic activity is equal to its concentration. However, in the real solutions, the assumption noted above may not apply, and negative deviation from Raoult's law may occur when adhesive attractions between A and B are greater than cohesive attraction within pure A or pure B molecules; i.e., the vapor pressure of the solution or the partial vapor pressure of each component is lower than that expected based on Raoult' s law applied to ideal solution. Similarly, positive deviations from Raoult's law can occur when interactions between A and B are less than the cohesive interactions of pure A or pure B, resulting in vapor pressures higher than that expected based on Raoult's law applied to ideal solution. In general, Raoult' s law states that when a component A is diluted with another component B, the partial vapor pressure of A is reduced; in essence, a dilution effect.

Raoult's law does not apply over the entire concentration range in a non-ideal, real solution. However, when one component is in a large enough excess to be considered a solvent, Raoult's law may be expressed as:

$$P_{\text{solvent}} = P_{\text{solvent}}^o X_{\text{solvent}} \quad ...(3)$$

in such a dilute solution and is valid only for the solvent component of a non-ideal solution that is sufficiently dilute for the other component, i.e., the solute in a dilute non-ideal solution. In such a dilute solution, the solute molecule is completely surrounded by solvent molecules such that the solute molecule can interact only with the solvent molecules because there are very few solute molecules. Further dilution beyond this point does not alter a solute molecule's environment and, even if the solute molecule interacts with the solvent molecule, the solute's partial vapor pressure or the thermodynamic activity becomes proportional to its fractional molar composition as:

$$P_{\text{solute}} = K_{\text{solute}} X_{\text{solute}} \quad ...(4)$$

Eq. (4) is known as Henry's law, and K_{solute} is the Henry's law constant, which is less than P_{solute}^o. Therefore, Henry's law applies to the solute in dilute solutions, and Raoult's law applies to solvent in dilute non-ideal solutions. Note the similarities between Eqs. (1) and (2) and between Eqs. (3) and (4) for the non-ideal dilute solution case. When the solution is ideal, Henry's law becomes identical to Raoult's law, and K_{solute} becomes identical to P_{solute}^o. When the partial pressures of the solute and the solvent are directly proportional to their molefractions over the entire range, the solution is ideal. In a non-ideal solution, Raoult' s law will apply to the solvent over the entire concentration range, whereas Henry's law will apply to the solute in a limited concentration range in which it is in a sufficiently diluted form.

When a non-volatile solute is dissolved in a solvent, the partial vapor pressure of the solvent above the solution is equal to the vapor pressure of the solution. And because the mole fraction of the solvent is $X_{\text{solvent}} = 1 - X_{\text{solute}}$. Eq. (3) can be rewritten as:

$$P_{\text{solution}} - P_{\text{solvent}} = P^{o}_{\text{solvent}}(1 - X_{\text{solute}}) \qquad ...(5)$$

for the dilute solution of a non-volatile solute of mole fraction X_{solute}. Therefore, the important conclusion from Raoult's and Henry's laws is that the thermodynamic activity of a solvent as measured by its vapor pressure is proportional solely on the mole fractional composition of the solute, irrespective of the physical and chemical nature of the dissolved species. The vapor pressure of the solvent above the solution thus depends solely on the number of particles (molecules/ions) of the dissolved solute and not on the weight concentration of the solute in solution. Therefore, the vapor pressure of a solvent above a dilute solution that obeys Henry's law is a colligative property of the solution. Henry's law has been found to be applicable to non-electrolyte-type solute mole fractional concentrations of 0.1; however, the range is much smaller for electrolyte type solutes owing to the long-range nature of interionic interactions as noted above. Its impact is evaluated later below.

Colligative Properties

Raoult's law forms the basis for the colligative properties, and Henry's law sets the limits of the applicability of Raoult's law to colligative properties of a solution as increasing amounts of solute are added to solution. As noted above, colligative properties are a consequence of the number of dissolved particles in solution and are all related to the escaping tendency of the solvent from solution.

The four colligative properties that are of importance are: (1) the vapor pressure lowering; (2) the elevation of boiling point; (3) the freezing-point depression; and (4) the osmotic pressure. An attempt is made below to describe qualitatively and quantitatively each colligative property of solutions, with an emphasis on their interrelationship and their application later in measurement and adjustment of the tonicity of solutions, with particular reference to parenteral formulations. Although theoretical derivations based on thermodynamics can be used to show how each of the colligative properties of solution arises and relate to each other, textbooks on physical chemistry for theoretical derivations are recommended.

Lowering of Vapor Pressure

The addition of a non-volatile solute to a solvent leads to a reduction in the vapor pressure of the solvent because of a reduction in thermodynamic activity of the solvent. Also, because the solute is non-volatile, the vapor pressure of the solvent is the vapor pressure of the solution, as seen from Eq. (5). Qualitatively, one can imagine that fewer numbers of solvent molecules are escaping per unit surface area of the solution than from the pure solvent because fewer solvent molecules are present per unit surface area of the solution owing to displacement by solute molecules. However, these solute molecules will not affect the condensation of solvent molecules with insufficient kinetic energy present in the vapor phase. The result is a net reduction in escaping tendency of solvent molecules on the surface, causing a lowering of vapor pressure and, consequently, the rate of vaporization. The resulting vapor pressure lowering ($P^{o}_{\text{solvent}} - P_{\text{solution}}$) and the relative vapor pressure lowering as a function of mole fractional concentration of solute can be obtained by rearranging Eq. (5) to Eq. (6):

$$\frac{P^{o}_{\text{solvent}} - P_{\text{solution}}}{P^{o}_{\text{solvent}}} = \frac{\Delta P}{P^{o}_{\text{solvent}}} = X_{solute} \qquad ...(6)$$

The left term is the relative vapor pressure lowering, which is solely dependent on the mole fraction concentration of a single solute or the sum of mole fraction of each solute dissolved in the solution. Thus, the relative vapor pressure lowering is a direct measure of the total number of dissolved solute particles, irrespective of their physicochemical nature. The mole fractions can be converted into molality (m moles of solute per 1000 g of solvent) to result in the following equation for water as the solvent:

$$\frac{\Delta P}{P^{o}_{\text{solvent}}} = X_{\text{solute}} \cong \frac{m\,M_{\text{solvent}}}{1000} \cong 0.018\,m \text{ for Aq. solutions} \qquad ...(7)$$

where m is the concentration of solute expressed in molality, and $M_{solvent}$ is the molecular weight of the solvent in grams. For water, M = 18, and because the density of water is close to 1, for dilute aqueous solutions, the molality and molarity (moles/liter) can be used interchangeably, and Eq. (7) can be used to calculate the relative vapor pressure lowering from the molar concentration of the non-electrolyte solute.

Elevation of the Boiling Point

The boiling point of a liquid is the temperature at which the vapor pressure of the liquid becomes equal to the external pressure acting on the liquid, which is 760 mm Hg at one atmospheric pressure. Therefore, the boiling point of a solution of non-volatile solute will be higher than that of the pure solvent owing to the solute reducing the vapor pressure of the solvent above the solution according to Raoult' s law. The solution has to be heated to a higher temperature to achieve the same vapor pressure to result in boiling of the solvent. The elevation of the boiling point ($T_{solution} - T_b^o$) is directly proportional to the relative vapor pressure lowering based on the Clausius–Clapeyron equation, resulting in an equation relating it to molality as follows:

$$(T_{solution} - T_b^o) = \delta T_b = \Delta T_b = K\Delta P = K_b m \quad \ldots(8)$$

where in K_b is called the molal elevation constant or the ebullioscopic constant, a characteristic constant for each solvent, and is the boiling point elevation of an ideal 1-molal solution of a non-volatile solute. K_b can be obtained by measuring the $\delta T_b/m$ of several molal concentrations of solute in solutions and extrapolating the $\delta T_b/m$ versus molality curve to zero solute concentration. The value of K_b for water is 0.515°kg/mole. By measuring the boiling point elevation of a solvent in a solution and knowing the K_b for that solvent, one can calculate the molal concentration of a solute in the solution. From Eq. (8), it is evident that the elevation of boiling point is a colligative property like vapor pressure lowering because it is strictly dependent on the molal concentration of the solute: the number of particles in solute and, thus, independent of the physicochemical nature of the solute.

Freezing-Point Depression

The freezing point of a liquid or the melting point of a solid phase of a pure compound is the temperature at which the solid and liquid phases are in equilibrium at a pressure of 1 atm. The freezing point of a pure compound is described by a unique point in the phase diagram of the compound, and, at that point, the solid and liquid phases are in equilibrium, and the vapor pressure of the liquid phase coincides with the vapor pressure of the pure solid phase. Because in a solution, the vapor pressure of the solvent is lowered relative to the pure solvent, no freezing (or crystallization) takes place at the equilibrium temperature of the liquid and solid phases of the pure solvent; i.e., the freezing point. The phase with the lower vapor pressure is the more stable phase thermodynamically. Therefore, cooling of the solution below the freezing point of the pure solvent results in a greater reduction in vapor pressure of the pure solid phase than the solution phase, and when the vapor pressure of the two phases eventually coincides, freezing (crystallization) of the pure liquid solvent occurs. The dissolved solute reduces the escaping tendency of the solvent molecules to crystallize, and thus the temperature must be reduced to reestablish equilibrium between the solid and liquid phases and hence the depression of freezing point. It must be noted that the dissolved solute only affects the freezing of the liquid phase and does not alter the tendency of the molecules to leave the solid phase, although both processes are occurring in equilibrium at the freezing point. Also, the solvent should form a pure solid; if the solute cocrystallizes with the solvent, the phenomenon is complex and cannot be described as a colligative property. The more concentrated the solution, the greater the freezing-point depression, and using thermodynamic principles, Raoult's law, and Clausius–Clapeyron equation, the freezing-point depression can be related to solute concentration expressed in molality as follows:

$$(T_{solution} - T_f^o) = \delta T_f = \Delta T_f = K\Delta P = K_f m \quad \ldots(9)$$

where in K_f is called the molal depression constant or the cryoscopic constant, a characteristic constant for each solvent dependent on the physicochemical nature of the solvent, and is the freezing-point depression of an ideal 1-molal solution of a non-volatile solute. K_f can be obtained experimentally by measuring the $\delta T_f/m$ of several molal concentrations of solute in solutions and extrapolating the $\delta T_f/m$ versus molality curve to zero solute concentration. The value of K_f for water is 1.86° kg/mole. By measuring the freezing-point depression of a solvent in a solution and knowing the Kf for that solvent, one can calculate the molal concentration of a solute in the solution. Freezing-point depression is a colligative property as seen from Eq. (9), because it is proportional to molal concentration of solute: the number of particles in solution, and not on the physicochemical characteristics of the solute.

Osmotic Pressure

As described in the Introduction, the process of diffusion of a solvent through a semipermeable membrane from a less-concentrated solution into a more-concentrated solution is osmosis. This results in the development of a hydrostatic pressure head on the more-concentrated solution side of the membrane. Alternatively, pressure may be applied to the more-concentrated solution side of the semipermeable membrane to prevent the diffusion of solvent. This applied pressure on the concentrated solution is identical to the hydrostatic pressure head that may develop owing to osmosis. It is known as the osmotic pressure and is directly proportional to the solute concentration in an ideal solution. A semipermeable membrane is one that allows the movement of only solvent molecules, and if the membrane is not semipermeable, osmosis may not be observed because the solute will diffuse quickly through the membrane to equalize the concentration on two sides of the membrane.

Osmosis tends to equalize the escaping tendencies of the solvent on both sides of the semipermeable membrane. Escaping tendency can be measured in terms of partial vapor pressure of solvent above the solution. Alternatively, one can see that at the beginning, the solution and pure solvents have different thermodynamic activities for the solvent because they have different vapor pressures. For the solution and pure solvent on two sides of the semipermeable membrane to be in equilibrium, they should have identical escaping tendency or identical vapor pressure and, thus identical thermodynamic activity. The equilibrium is therefore established by the generation of the osmotic pressure that compensates for the difference in solvent concentration on the two sides of the membrane, which is responsible for the different vapor pressures, escaping tendencies, and thermodynamic activity. Therefore, osmosis is a process to reach equilibrium state whereby solvent spontaneously flows from the high-free-energy (low-vapor-pressure) side of the membrane to the low-free-energy (high-vapor-pressure) side of the membrane, until the solvent's free energies on both sides of the membrane are equal and identical. Obviously, the solute will not be able to attain equilibrium because it cannot diffuse through the semipermeable membrane. Because osmotic pressure is attributable to the difference in vapor pressure of the solvent above solution, it is also a colligative property as explained below.

Using thermodynamics and considering free energy of the solvent as a function of vapor pressure, the osmotic pressure (π) that develops when a solution is separated from pure solvent by semipermeable membrane can be related to vapor pressures as shown below:

$$\Pi = \frac{RT}{V^M_{solvent}} \ln \frac{P^o_{solvent}}{P_{solution}} \quad \ldots(10)$$

where in R is the gas constant, T is temperature, $V^M_{solvent}$ is the partial molar volume, (the volume occupied by 1 mole of solvent), and π is the developed osmotic pressure when a solution with vapor pressure $P_{solution}$ is separated from a solvent with vapor pressure $P^o_{solvent}$ by a semipermeable membrane. Applying Raoult's law and substituting mole fractions for the vapor pressures from Eq. (5) into Eq. (10) results in the following:

$$\Pi = \frac{-RT}{V^M_{solvent}} \ln(1 - X_{solute}) \cong \frac{RT}{V^M_{solvent}} X_{solute} \text{ since } \ln(1 - X_{solute}) \cong -X_{solute} \quad ...(11)$$

In a dilute solution, X_{solute} is approximately equal to the molar ratio $n_{solute}/n_{solvent}$, and Eq. (11) becomes:

$$\Pi = \frac{n_{solute}}{n_{solvent} V^M_{solvent}} RT = \frac{n_{solute}}{V_{solution}} RT = mRT \quad ...(12)$$

in which the number of moles of solvent multiplied by the partial molal volume is equal to the volume of the solvent in solution. In a dilute solution, the volume of solvent can be approximated to the volume of solution, which results in the above equation relating osmotic pressure to molar or molal concentration of a solute in solution. Eq. (12) is known as Morse's expression and demonstrates how osmotic pressure is a colligative property directly proportional only on the number of particles dissolved in the solvent irrespective of the nature of the solute. van't Hoff had recognized early on that there is a direct proportionality among osmotic pressure and concentration of solute and temperature, and suggested a relationship that was similar to the equation for an ideal gas as follows:

$$\Pi V_{solution} = n_{solute} RT \quad ...(13)$$

Eq. (13) is analogous to the ideal gas equation, and van't Hoff concluded that osmotic pressure of a dilute solution was a pressure that the solute would exert if it behaved like a gas occupying that volume. Eq. (13) can also be expressed as:

$$\Pi = \frac{n_{solute}}{V_{solution}} RT = cRT \quad ...(14)$$

which shows that osmotic pressure is directly proportional to the concentration of solute expressed in molarity. This equation is similar to Morse's expression, Eq. (12); however, it has been shown theoretically and experimentally that more accurate results can be obtained when solute concentration is expressed in molality rather than in molarity. Although the resemblance of Eq. (13) to the ideal gas equation is striking, osmotic pressure is a result of differences in the escaping tendencies of the solvent on two sides of the membrane rather than of the behavior of a solute such as a gas. From Eqs. (12)–(14), one finds that 1-molar solution of any solute will generate an incredibly high osmotic pressure of approximately 24 atm at room temperature, which has been verified experimentally. Although this estimate is based on the assumption that the solution is dilute and behaving ideally, at high concentrations of solute, the theory overestimates the experimental findings. The discussion above deals primarily with the thermodynamic basis for the generation of osmotic pressure; however, it does not address the issue of how fast the equilibrium is attained or how fast the osmotic pressure will be generated. The rate of generation of osmotic pressure is a kinetic process and depends to a great extent on the characteristics of the semipermeable membrane. Red blood cell membrane or the mucous membrane in the eye are very thin and moist, and water can diffuse very rapidly through the membrane to generate the enormous osmotic pressure. However, the osmotic pressure may develop very slowly across synthetic and semisynthetic polymeric membranes, across which the diffusion is very slow.

Colligative Properties of Electrolytes as Compared with Non-electrolyte Solutes

The colligative properties, by definition, should be independent of the nature of the solute. Therefore, 0.1-molal solutions of sucrose and NaCl should exhibit similar colligative properties. It was observed by van't Hoff that colligative properties of dilute solutions of non-electrolytes such as sucrose were expressed satisfactorily by the equations above. However, solutions of strong electrolytes such as salts gave osmotic pressure twice or three times as large as would be expected based on Eq. (14), depending on the electrolyte investigated. To account for this anomaly, van't Hoff proposed the following modification of Eq. (14) as shown below:

$$\Pi = i\,c\,\mathrm{RT} \qquad \ldots(15)$$

in which i can be considered to be a factor to account for the deviation of concentrated solutions of electrolytes and also non-electrolytes from Raoult's law as applied to ideal solutions. After Arrhenius developed the theory of ionization or dissociation of salts into ions, van't Hoff and others recognized that the value of i approached or equaled the number of ions into which the electrolyte or the molecule dissociated as the solution was made more dilute. For example, a dilute 0.1 M solution of NaCl would be twice as active osmotically as a 0.1 M solution of sucrose, and i for NaCl was two. Similarly, 0.1 *M* solutions of $CaCl_2$ and $MgCl_2$ would generate three times the osmotic pressure of 0.1 M sucrose solution, and i for both is equal to three. Therefore, it was realized that i reflected the number of ions the electrolytes dissociated into and, thus, electrolytes at equimolar concentrations were more effective in generating osmotic pressure based on the number of ions they produced on dissociation. However, it was also observed that at moderate concentrations of electrolytes, osmotic pressures were less than that expected based on complete dissociation. In fact, this led the scientific community to suggest partial dissociation for even strong electrolytes and to use colligative properties as a measure of degree of dissociation. However, we know now that strong electrolytes do dissociate completely even in concentrated solutions from other measurements such as conductivity techniques. The lower-than-expected values of osmotic pressure in moderate concentrations of electrolytes is attributable to the influence of long-range ionic interactions that come into play as the solution gets increasingly concentrated. The basic assumption in Raoult law was that there was no interaction between solute particles and, even if there was any, it should equal that between the solute and the solvent. However, the strong attractive forces between ions of opposite charges do predominate in increasingly concentrated solutions of electrolytes, and their thermodynamic activity is reduced relative to that in an infinitely dilute solution. Also, the effect of ionic strength of a solution has been shown to influence the activity of electrolytes, and thus, it is the interionic forces rather than the partial dissociation that seems to influence the colligative properties of electrolytes being lower than expected based on complete dissociation.

All the colligative properties of all solutes with the modification by the van't Hoff factor i can be expressed as:

$$\Delta P = iP^{o}_{\text{solvent}}\,m;\ \Pi = iRT\,m;$$
$$\Delta T_f = i\,K_f\,m;\ \Delta T_b = iK_b m \qquad \ldots(16)$$

where in i for non-electrolyte should be 1 and for strong electrolytes equal the number of ions formed on dissociation. For example, i should be 2 for NaCl, 3 for $CaCl_2$, and 4 for $FeCl_3$. However, in reality, i is less than that calculated, based on the number of ions produced in concentrated solutions, but will approach the theoretical number in infinitely dilute ideal solutions. When the i value is calculated, for a number of solutions with increasing concentration of the solute and then extrapolated to zero concentration of the solute, one can obtain the theoretical i value. The van't Hoff factor has also been considered the ratio of any colligative property of a real solution to that of an ideal solution of a non-electrolyte.

Physiological and Clinical Significance of Tonicity

Osmotic pressure becomes important from a physiological standpoint because a majority of biological membranes are semipermeable, and body fluids such as blood and tears exhibit significant osmotic pressure owing to a number of solutes dissolved in them. As noted above in the Introduction, if a small quantity of blood is mixed with a solution containing 0.9%w/v NaCl, the red blood cells remain intact and retain their normal size and shape. The NaCl solution is considered to be isotonic because it maintained the tone of the membrane of the red blood cell. In contrast, if the blood is mixed with the hypertonic 1.8% w/v NaCl solution, cells shrink and become wrinkled or crenated owing to its content being sucked out. It is because the red blood cell content exerts a lower osmotic pressure than does the surrounding hypertonic 1.8% w/v salt solution, and the water inside the cells diffuses through the cell membrane to dilute the surrounding salt solution to equalize the osmotic pressure across the membrane. The exact opposite phenomenon occurs if blood is mixed with hypotonic 0.45% w/v NaCl solution. Water from the surrounding salt solution enters the cells, causing them to swell and finally burst with the liberation of hemoglobin, and the phenomenon is known as hemolysis. The crenation and hemolysis of red blood cells in hypertonic and hypotonic salt solution, respectively, are explained by the movement of water across the cell membrane owing to the osmotic pressure differential. However, it is well-known that the different physiological membranes are different with respect to their permeability characteristics. The red blood cell membrane has been found to be permeable to small polar and semipolar solutes such as alcohol, boric acid, and urea, etc. Thus, the erythrocyte membrane is not truly semipermeable, and although 2% boric acid solution is iso-osmotic with erythrocyte cell contents, it causes hemolysis because boric acid moves freely across the membrane and its solution being hypotonic acts like pure water in its effect on erythrocytes. However, the same 2% boric acid solution is both iso-osmotic and isotonic with eye secretions and causes no irritation when instilled in the eye because the mucous membrane of the eye is a true semipermeable membrane. To resolve the confusion created by different permeability characteristics of biological membranes, the word isotonicity was created. The word isotonic refers to solutions that are isoosmotic with the cell contents, across a specific membrane, and in addition, maintains the tone of the membrane, i.e., no solvent movement across the membrane. Thus, 2% boric acid solution is iso-osmotic with blood but it behaves like a hypotonic solution with erythrocytes while it is both iso-osmotic and isotonic with respect to the mucous membrane of the eye.

It has been also observed that hypertonic and hypotonic salt solutions tend to irritate sensitive tissue and cause pain when applied to mucous membranes of the eye, ear, and nose, etc., whereas isotonic solution causes no tissue irritation when it comes in contact with the tissue. Obviously, the tonicity of formulations that come in to direct contact with blood, muscle, eye, nose, and delicate tissues is critical. Therefore, the issue of tonicity is important in small- and large-volume injectables, ophthalmic products, and products intended for tissue irrigation. The degree of tissue irritation or hemolysis or crenation observed depends on the degree of deviation from isotonicity, the volume injected, the speed of injection, the concentration of the solutes in the injection, and the nature of the membrane. The parenteral and ophthalmic formulations are therefore adjusted to isotonicity if possible.

Hypotonic solutions can be easily adjusted to isotonicity by adding solutes such as dextrose or sodium chloride, commonly used for this purpose. However, at times, the formulation may be hypertonic and may have to be diluted with water to maintain isotonicity. This dilution of the hypertonic solution may be precluded owing to other limitations such as poor aqueous solubility of the drug. In such a case, the hypertonic solution can be administered slowly in small volumes into a large vein such as the subclavian vein in which the formulation will be diluted and distributed rapidly, minimizing chances of crenation of erythrocytes, pain, and tissue irritation on injection. It has also been observed that minor deviations such as 10% from isotonicity may result in no effect or only temporary effects at the site of injection. However, the effects of deviation from isotonicity of large-volume parenterals can be fairly severe and, thus, parenteral nutrient solutions and infusions of large volume need to be adjusted to isotonicity. Large-volume infusion of hypotonic solutions has been observed to cause effects ranging from hemolysis to water-retention problems such as convulsions and pulmonary edema. This was exemplified by the recent report of 10 episodes of hemolysis, with two patients exhibiting significant hemolysis and renal insufficiency resulting in one death. These severe episodes of hemolysis occurred because of the large volume infusion of 25% human albumin diluted with sterile water instead of with isotonic sodium chloride for therapeutic plasma exchange. In contrast, large-volume infusion of hypertonic solutions can result in severe conditions such as intracellular dehydration, osmotic diuresis, hyperglycemia, glycosuria, dehydration from loss of water, and coma. Also, hypertonic solution infusion should be terminated gradually to avoid sudden changes in osmotic pressure. In summary, any formulation that comes in to contact with sensitive tissues of the human body needs to be adjusted to isotonicity to minimize any adverse effects. To be able to adjust the formulation to isotonicity, a method to measure the tonicity and/or the osmotic pressure of the formulations has to be used.

Measurement of Tonicity of Solutions

The most direct method for measurement of tonicity obviously would be to observe changes in erythrocytes on mixing solution with blood. If hemolysis or crenation or a marked change in the appearance of erythrocytes occurs, the solution is not isotonic. If the cells retain their normal size and shape, the solution is isotonic. Grosicki and Husa used this method early on; however, one has to be mindful of the fact that solutions may be iso-osmotic with erythrocyte contents, yet may cause hemolysis because solutes such as boric acid are permeable through erythrocyte membrane and, thus, solution is not isotonic. Therefore, Grosicki and Husa recommended that the word isotonic should be used with reference to solutions having equal osmotic pressures with respect to a particular membrane. Because hemolysis due to hypotonic solution results in release of oxyhemoglobin directly proportional to the number of cells hemolyzed, a quantitative method has been developed to calculate osmotic pressure and the van't Hoff *i* factor noted above. A limitation of observing changes in erythrocytes as a measure of tonicity is the fact that the specific chemical interaction of the solute with the cell, pH of the solution, presence of solvents, lipid solubility of the solute, and denaturant activity of solute may have influences on the cell membrane and, thus, osmotic pressure differences alone are not responsible for hemolysis. Furthermore, it was shown recently that hemolysis is related to the contact time in addition to hypotonicity of the formulation. To overcome this limitation, some investigators have used measurements of erythrocyte cell volumes as a function of tonicity of solution, which influence solvent (water) uptake or loss from erythrocytes. This method is more sensitive, objective, and reliable than observation of hemolysis. Recently, a method using fluorescence anisotropy for fluidity of erythrocyte membranes demonstrated differences between hypotonic and isotonic solutions. However, the method is involving, and more data need to be obtained to correlate tonicity with fluidity of the membrane to be reliable.

An alternative approach is based on the theoretical foundation described earlier for the colligative properties. If the solution is isotonic with blood, its osmotic pressure, vapor pressure, boiling-point elevation, and freezing-point depression should also be identical to those of blood. Thus, to measure isotonicity, one has to measure the osmotic pressure of the solution and compare it with the known value for blood. However, the accurate measurement of osmotic pressure is difficult and cumbersome. If a solution is separated from blood by a true semipermeable membrane, the resulting pressure due to solvent flow (the head) is accurately measurable, but the solvent flow dilutes the solution, thus not allowing one to know the concentration of the dissolved solute. An alternative is to apply pressure to the solution side of the membrane to prevent osmotic solvent flow. In 1877, Pfeffer used this method to measure osmotic pressure of sugar solutions. With the advances in the technology, sensitive pressure transducers, and synthetic polymer membranes, this method can be improved. However, results of the search for a true semipermeable membrane are still elusive, and this method is still cumbersome and inconvenient. The measurement of osmotic pressure using this method has been applied successfully to colloidal solution of proteins to measure their molecular weight because they are of relatively large molecular weight and are impermeable across number of membranes. Numerous instruments, known as osmometers, are commercially available to measure osmotic pressure. Only the Knauer membrane osmometer and colloid osmometer are true osmometers using a semipermeable membrane. Vapor pressure osmometers such as the Wescor osmometer, using the principle of vapor pressure lowering should not be called osmometers. These types of instruments measure the vapor pressure using the isopiestic method, or the thermoelectric method, or the measurement of the dew point of unknown solution in comparison with a standard, and then calculate osmotic pressure and osmolality using the theory of colligative properties. These instruments require a few microliters, and the method is fairly precise, simple, and totally automated. The presence of a volatile solvent such as ethanol will create problem with this method because the inherent assumption is that only water is present in the vapor phase. This can be a serious limitation because many parenteral and, ophthalmic formulations contain organic solvents for the purposes of drug solubility and, sometimes of stability. Commercial osmometers of this type have been found to measure osmolalities in the range of 100–3000mmol/kg reliably.

Boiling-point elevation can also be used to measure osmotic pressure and tonicity of a solution using just a reflux condenser and a thermometer. The commercially available instrument is the Cottrell boiling-point apparatus. However, this method is affected by the ambient barometric pressure and the presence of volatile solvents in the solution.

Osmometers based on the freezing-point depression are the most commonly and widely used instruments for measurements of tonicity because of the simplicity, reliability, and ease of use. Freezing-point depression of solutions of a number of drugs at various concentrations has already been determined, and thus, an extensive database is available for adjustment of tonicity of solutions of these drugs, as addressed below. The freezing-point depression of a solution can be simply measured using a salt–ice bath, Dewars flask, and Beckmann's thermometer. Numerous commercial instruments requiring small quantities of solution such as Osmette from Precision Systems that use the principle of Beckmann's freezing-point method are now available. One of the problems with this method is the disengagement of ice and the need for determination of the actual equilibrium freezing point. The latter limitation can be overcome by use of the equilibrium method, in which solid solvent (ice) is placed in contact with solution (aq.) and the freezing point measured and compared with that of the pure solvent (water) in contact with the solid solvent (ice). Also, one has to consider the presence of other solvents in influencing the freezing-point depression. The freezing-point depression method is precise to the extent that the differences in freezing points of two systems within ±0.0002°C can be measured. Freezing-point osmometry can be used for all samples with osmolalities less than 550 mmol/kg, including those that contain volatile solutes. Once the freezing point of the solution is known, inert solute such as sodium chloride is added to match the freezing point of solution with that of blood and lacrimal fluids. After considerable debate and experimentation, it is now well-established that –0.52°C is the freezing point of blood and lacrimal fluids, following the work of Lund, Nielsen, and Pedersen-Bjergaard. This is also the freezing point of 0.9% sodium chloride solution, which is therefore considered to be isotonic with both blood and lacrimal secretions. Therefore, to determine the tonicity of a solution, one has to measure its freezing-point depression and compare it with that of blood (–0.52°C). An important consideration when using this method is that although all the solutes present in solution contribute to its freezing-point depression, those that permeate the biological membrane will not maintain the tone, for example, boric acid. In addition, association of solute molecules by processes such as complexation and micellar association, which are temperature-dependent, may have to be considered. The viscosity and presence of suspended particles can also affect the freezing point by altering the crystallization of the solvent. Nevertheless, freezing-point depression has become popular because of its simplicity, reliability, and availability of commercial instruments. The methods of osmometry, the technology, and the limitations inherent in each method have been reviewed recently and should be consulted for more details.

Based on the theory of colligative properties and the principles of osmometry, it is understood that osmometer will read osmolalities and not osmolarities because colligative properties are directly proportional to the total solute concentration expressed in molality. The relationship between osmolality and osmolarity and its significance can be found in the Remington's Pharmaceutical Sciences and in a review article by Deardorff. However, it is more convenient to use osmolarity because it is based on weight/volume rather than on weight/weight as in osmolality. The U.S. Pharmacopeia also recommends that the labeling of parenteral and ophthalmic formulation should list osmolarity while the experimentally determined quantity is osmolality. Methods to convert osmolality to osmolarity using determinations of solution density and solute content or using partial molal volume of solute and solvent have been described.

Theoretical Method to Calculate Tonicity Using L_{iso} Value

In the discussion above of colligative properties of electrolytes, the equations were modified by introduction of the van't Hoff *i* factor as shown in Eq. (16). Because the freezing-point depressions of strong and weak electrolytes are always greater than those calculated from Eq. (9), because of different degrees of ionization and interionic interaction, a new factor, $L = iK_f$, is introduced. The *L* value obtained from freezing-point depression of a solution of a particular type of electrolyte at a molar concentration (c) that is isotonic with blood is defined as L_{iso} (L_{iso} = 0.52°/c). For example, the L_{iso} value for an isotonic sodium chloride solution (0.9% w/v) is 3.4, and its freezing-point depression is 0.52°C. Because the colligative properties are independent of the chemical nature of the electrolyte and the interionic interactions in dilute solutions are similar, all electrolytes of the same type will have identical L_{iso} values. Therefore, all non-electrolytes have L_{iso} = 1.9, whereas uni-univalent electrolyte's L_{iso} = 3.4 and triunivalent electrolyte's L_{iso} = 6.0. Thus, if the ionic nature of the solute and its molecular weight are known, using the appropriate L_{iso} value, freezing-point depression can be calculated for a solution of a given concentration. The average Liso values for all types of solutes are available in the literature. This method is simple and does not require experimentation, but it is only approximate, with potential for some error. Also, one has to know the ionic nature of the solute, which can be difficult to determine for a new drug compound with a complex structure.

Methods of Adjusting Tonicity

From the theoretical background presented above, one can easily devise his or her own methods to adjust tonicity of solutions using the principles of colligative properties. However, in the practice of pharmacy, a number of simple methods to adjust tonicity of formulation in a prescription order on an extemporaneous basis were developed to help the pharmacist. The methods of adjusting tonicity could be classified into two types. In class I methods, some inert substance such as sodium chloride or dextrose is added to the solution to lower its freezing point to match that of blood (–0.52°C) i.e., made isotonic by the addition of inert excipient. In class II methods, a calculated quantity of water is added to the total solute content (drug) of the prescription to make it isotonic, which is then diluted with sufficient isotonic diluting solution to bring it to the final volume. These methods are explained below, followed by a simple example illustrating the method. However, the assumptions inherent in all the methods need to be considered carefully. The first assumption is that colligative properties are additive for mixture of solutes and that they are related linearly to their concentration expressed in molarity, molality, or in percentages. This assumption is true in dilute solutions of non-electrolytes and electrolytes. However, when dealing with concentrated solutions, this assumption may not be valid. In cases of chemical interaction, association, complexation, or micellar interaction among solutes in solution, the colligative properties of solutes may not be additive. The second assumption is that they consider all solutes present in solution to be contributing to its tonicity. However, it is known from the discussion above that all biological membranes are not truly semipermeable, and thus, some solutes will not contribute to the tonicity of the solution across that membrane, for example, boric acid across erythrocytes membrane. Nevertheless, the errors introduced are small, and slight deviations from isotonicity on either side do not result in significant adverse effects. In the literature, one may also find methods known as the L value method or the L_{iso} method, which are identical to the theoretical method described above for solutes, for which one can calculate the freezing-point depression based on molecular weight and ionic nature. By knowing the freezing-point depression, any of the class I or class II methods can then be used to adjust their solution to isotonicity.

Class I Methods

Freezing-point depression method (cryoscopic method)

The freezing-point depression of a number of drugs and excipients, either experimentally determined by the method described above or calculated theoretically using the L_{iso} method, is available in the literature. Basically, from the percentage of drug present in solution, the freezing point of the solution is calculated. This number is then subtracted from the freezing point of blood (–0.52°C) to obtain the freezing-point depression to be achieved by the addition of sodium chloride. Knowing that 0.9% sodium chloride is isotonic and freezes at –0.52°C, the amount of sodium chloride to be added is calculated as shown in the example below.

Example 1

Calculate the amount of sodium chloride needed to prepare 100 ml of 2% isotonic physostigmine salicylate solution.

Freezing-point depression of 2% physostigmine salicylate = 2 × 0.09°C = 0.18°C. Therefore, the freezing-point depression to be achieved by adding sodium chloride = 0.52°C - 0.18°C = 0.34°C. Sodium chloride (0.9%) produces a freezing-point depression of –0.52°C; therefore, the percentage of sodium chloride needed = (0.34°C/0.52°C) × 0.9% = 0.59% = 0.59 g/100 ml.

Sodium chloride equivalent (E) method

The sodium chloride equivalent (E) is the amount of sodium chloride equivalent to 1 g of the drug in exerting the same osmotic effect. The E value for a new drug can be calculated from its L_{iso} value or from the freezing-point depression as shown below.

The freezing-point depression of a 1 g/L-solution of a new drug can be expressed as:

$$\Delta T_f = L_{iso}\frac{1g}{MW} \quad ...(17)$$

By definition, E gram of sodium chloride (MW = 58.45 and L_{iso} = 3.4) in 1 L will have similar freezing-point depression as shown below:

$$\Delta T_f = 3.4\frac{Eg}{58.45} \quad ...(18)$$

Therefore, equating Eqs. (17) and (18), results in the following equation for E:

$$E = 17\frac{L_{iso}}{MW} \quad ...(19)$$

Wells developed a nomogram based on the above equation to readily calculate E values from the MW and L_{iso} value of the drug. Thus, the E value for physostigmine salicylate (MW = 413.46) calculated using L_{iso} = 3.4 for a uni-univalent electrolyte is equal to 0.14, which is close to 0.16 (E value). This small deviation is attributable to the difference between the experimentally determined L_{iso} (3.9) of physostigmine salicylate and the theoretical value of 3.4 for a uni-univalent electrolyte. By knowing the E value, the solution can be adjusted to isotonicity as shown below.

Example 2

Calculate the amount of sodium chloride needed to prepare 100 ml of 2% isotonic physostigmine salicylate solution.

Physostigmine salicylate (2 g/100 ml) is equivalent to 2 × 0.16 (*E*) = 0.32 g/100 ml of sodium chloride. Therefore, 0.58 g (0.9–0.32 g) of sodium chloride has to be added to 100 ml of this solution to make it isotonic. Note that the answers given by the two methods are not identical, but very close.

Class II Methods

The class II methods involve the calculation of a quantity of water needed to make an isotonic solution for a given amount of drug, followed by dilution with an isotonic solution to make up the volume. These methods were developed to enable pharmacists to prepare parenteral and ophthalmic formulations with simplicity and ease.

White-Vincent method

In this method, the weight of the drug (*w*) is first multiplied by its sodium chloride (*E*) to obtain the quantity of sodium chloride osmotically equivalent to weight per gram of drug. Because 0.9 g of sodium chloride dissolved in 100 ml results in an isotonic solution, the volume of isotonic solution that can be prepared from weight per gram of drug is given by the following equation:

$$V = wE\frac{100}{0.9} = 111.1wE \qquad ...(20)$$

Thus, dissolving weight per gram of drug in V ml of water will result in an isotonic solution that can be further diluted with isotonic solutions such as 0.9% sodium chloride or isotonic dextrose solution to make up the volume. The method can be illustrated by the following example.

Example 3

Prepare 100 ml of 2% physostigmine salicylate solution isotonic with blood.

Using Eq. (20) and *E* of physostigmine salicylate = 0.16, the volume of water needed to prepare isotonic solution, V = 2g × 0.16 × 111.1 ml/g = 35.55 ml. This solution can be diluted with 64.45 ml of any isotonic diluting solution to obtain 100 ml of 2% isotonic physostigmine salicylate solution. To verify the results, if we assume that we dilute the above solution with 64.45 ml of isotonic sodium chloride solution, the equivalent amount of sodium chloride added is 0.58 g, which matches with results obtained using the class I methods.

Sprowls method

In the early days of pharmacy practice, many prescriptions were written to prepare one fluid ounce of a 1% drug solution, thus, the amount of drug (*w* = 0.3 g) and the final volume were fixed (one fluid ounce or 30 ml). Sprowls, recognizing this fact, suggested a modification of the White-Vincent method to further simplify the calculations for the practicing pharmacist. In this method, the amount of drug is fixed at 0.3 g (30 ml of 1% solution), and the volume of water required to prepare the isotonic solution is calculated using Eq. (20) for all drugs that are commonly used in parenteral and ophthalmic formulations and for which sodium chloride equivalents are known. The pharmacist then makes up the volume of the preparation to 30 ml with an isotonic diluting solution to fill the prescription. For example, if one fluid ounce of 1% physostigmine salicylate solution is to be prepared, we recognize that 5.3 ml of water is required for 0.3 g of physostigmine salicylate to prepare an isotonic solution. After the preparation of this 5.3 ml solution, it can be diluted with any isotonic diluting solution to make up the volume to one fluid ounce. If one needed to prepare 100 ml of a 1% solution, the volume of water (V) should be multiplied by 3.33 to obtain the amount of water necessary to make it isotonic.

The theory of colligative properties is well-understood and successfully applied to parenteral formulations for making them isotonic and, thus, safe and acceptable. The techniques of osmometry have been refined, and now instruments that can estimate freezing-point depression, vapor pressure, or osmotic pressure from microliter quantities of samples in a few minutes are commercially available. At the same time, very few pharmacists are required to compound prescriptions requiring the knowledge of the various methods of adjustments of tonicity. Because of ever-increasing complexities in the structure of new drug entities, there is an increasing problem of their inadequate aqueous solubility, exemplified by drugs such as Cyclosporine and Taxol. A number of organic solvents and new classes of surfactants are being developed and used to aid in solubilization and, thus, in the formulation of these drugs for parenteral administration. The issue of tonicity needs to be addressed from this perspective because organic solvents and the surfactants behave differently in solution than do the traditional solutes whose characteristics in solution are well-understood. Also, dispersed systems such as nanocapsules, liposomes, and microemulsions are being developed as parenteral formulations. The colligative properties of these systems need to be investigated too. There is an increasing concern regarding tissue irritation and muscle injury at the site of injection resulting from formulations. With the advent of biotechnology, more peptide and protein drugs are in clinical trials than before, and, also, gene therapy is being considered for few diseases. The parenteral formulations of these newer drugs are more complex to maintain the integrity of their higher-order structure. Therefore, the issue of tonicity needs to be revisited with a newer approach and from a different perspective.

14

VALIDATING LEGACY SYSTEMS

Automation is now part of everyone's life. Today's economy would cease to function without computers, and to blame this on the computers themselves is not entirely fair; they were after all, designed and put into use by man. We have only ourselves to blame when and if automated systems malfunction and we cannot understand why. When we design and implement new systems, we are ideally placed to define them, test them, and approve their functionality. But most computer systems are existing installations and known as "*legacy*" systems, where we have a totally new situation. There may be no formal description of the system, the code may have been changed or replaced many times. Manuals will possibly have disappeared long ago.

Now we need to deal with the reality of such a situation, providing step-by-step guidance for those faced with assessment of legacy systems, for whatever reason that may be perhaps to gain a better understanding of how a system operates, because of changed regulatory requirements, or simply to assess its performance and usefulness. Much is written on new systems, with interest groups focussing on the "how to" element of system selection and installation. Little guidance can be found on legacy systems, guidance written in "plain English" rather than in technical terms. We try here to put that right, using a bullet point summary at the end of each section.

We refer frequently to the healthcare and pharmaceutical and allied industry sector, but we are not writing entirely for the life sciences professional. The principles discussed here, such as system assessment and evaluation, identification of remedial action and validation thereof, apply to all industries. Pharmaceutical, chemical, beverage, electronic, nuclear, cosmetic, animal health, and food personnel will all gain some benefit from the guidance, showing the steps which can lead to a fully-understood computer system, which does the job for which it was designed and intended an eminently worthwhile result. Since this chapter was first drafted, a number of significant changes have occurred within the U.S. Food and Drug Administration (FDA), from both organizational and regulatory perspectives. The most significant change, introduced as part of FDA's initiative "cGMPs for the 21st Century," was the publication of the final guidance for industry document "Part 11, Electronic Records; Electronic Signatures—Scope and Application" in August 2003. In this document the FDA now makes significant concessions with regards to Part 11 compliance requirements for legacy systems; it does not, however, renege on the demand for fulfilling the requirements of the applicable predicate rules. In the strictest sense of this guidance document, a legacy system is one that meets all the following criteria for a specific system.

1. The system was operational before the effective date.
2. The system met all applicable predicate rule requirements before the effective date.

3. The system currently meets all applicable predicate rule requirements.
4. You have documented evidence and justification that the system is fit for its intended use (including having an acceptable level of record security and integrity, if applicable).

If a system has been changed since August 20, 1997, and if the changes would prevent the system from meeting predicate rule requirements, Part 11 controls should be applied to Part 11 records and signatures pursuant to the enforcement policy expressed in this guidance.

There are indeed such systems still in use, although most applications will have had some upgrades or patches installed, not least to receive continued vendor support, or because upgrades became necessary with the migration to new or upgraded operating systems and changed hardware. There is a high risk of failure associated with such legacy systems; a dual risk, one of failing to work and one of no longer having a validated status. These "true" legacy systems are more of a curiosity than the norm.

Most users still consider any automated system already in operation as a legacy system, distinguished from new installations or upgrades to a new software version. As it is necessary to assess all existing systems for their validation status and whether the system has to comply with 21 CFR Part 11, it is only understandable to call them "legacy" systems. The scope of this chapter has thus not changed, and only minor amendments were made to ensure conformance with current guidance and regulations.

Despite FDA's initiative to reform the good manufacturing practices (GMPs) and with it 21 CFR Part 11, it is fair to assume that this guidance will be in place for the coming years, as it takes considerable effort to change the law, and to obtain buy-in from industry. Doing nothing or waiting for things to change soon is not an option if one wishes to stay in compliance. Where there are existing systems that have not yet been assessed and brought into compliance, this should be initiated and performed without delay. Following the advice and the processes outlined hereafter provides the reader with a pragmatic, proven and useful approach to achieving compliance for legacy systems.

It is hard to imagine finding a facility or a sector within the life science industry in this 21st century without some sort of automation and use of desktop computers. We are all involved in the deployment of information technology (IT) to complete our everyday activities satisfactorily. Automated and computer and IT systems improve business processes, ensure health and safety, and enable a company to function. The IT revolution has brought about an enormous change in both the way we work, and the way we document such work. This exponential evolution also means that today's computer or IT system is outdated tomorrow, whereupon it will become a "legacy system," or an inherited system. Existing automated systems fulfil their role and run for many years, before replacement by new technology. Some of these systems fall under the regulations governing the healthcare (i.e., drug substance, drug product, and medical device manufacturers), food, cosmetics and nutraceuticals industries. Legislation extends beyond manufacturing and associated laboratory activities; it encompasses all aspects of a product life cycle. Typical examples for IT applications which must comply are:

1. A simple spreadsheet for yield calculations.
2. An enterprise resource planning software package used as a worldwide manufacturing planning tool.
3. A programable logic controller on a filling line.

This gives a flavor of the immense variety of systems with which a company must work successfully. This chapter is aimed at the regulated life science industry, in order to assist management from all disciples in the assessment, qualification, and validation of their IT systems. It aims to provide a common understanding of the requirements for all parties involved, such as the IT, manufacturing, administration, quality control, and regulatory affairs. Although most companies have implemented commissioning, qualification, and validation programs for their equipment and processes, some systems (such as servers, networks, or archiving systems) have often been excluded, particularly if not associated with processing or analytical equipment. The regulatory authorities no longer tolerate this negligence. This has resulted in many inspection report citings for deficiencies in this particular area in recent years. Although industry started to look at ways in which automated systems should be commissioned, qualified and validated, it was only when the U.S. FDA published the "Blue Book" in 1983, that the regulators provided rules and guidance. This was followed in 1997 by the requirements for electronic records and electronic signatures (ER/ES) in the U.S. Code of Federal Regulations, 21 CFR Part 11. This regulation, which was first published on March 20 1997 and came into force on August 20, 1997, provides the current impetus for industry to assess IT systems and take remedial action to attain this goal.

Because automated systems were not purchased and installed with this regulation in mind until recently, many companies have little or no knowledge of the compliance level of their automated systems. Companies not producing for or exporting to the U.S. market may think that they are excluded from these rules and regulations. This is a gross misconception. Regulatory authorities worldwide are in the process of adopting the guidelines laid down in 21 CFR Part 11. The latest release of the European GMPs mandates audit trails for electronic records, which goes beyond even the latest FDA requirements. The PIC/S inspection guideline is now the *de facto* global inspection standard for automated systems, irrespective of the fact that the FDA will not be able to formally adopt the standard for legal reasons. All guidance and legislation have the same principles in common and by complying with the GMPs and 21 CFR 11 one will comply with most or all other applicable regulations. The focus of this chapter therefore is on Part 11 as the leading regulation.

Industries not directly impacted by 21 CFR Part 11 can also gain tremendously from understanding and implementing the principles of this rule. The pharmaceutical and medical devices industry should also look at other sectors, such as the food industry, for beneficial validation approaches. While the authorities describe the *what* element of computer systems validation in their guidance documents, it is up to process owners and manufacturers to prove logically and consistently the *how* element. Consequently, sensible and affordable approaches are a *must*. What are these approaches and how can they be implemented to comply with current regulatory requirements? This chapter provides answers to these questions.

ASSESSMENT PROCESS

Software is one of the most complex items man has ever created. Compared with other complex systems, developed software has the added disadvantage that one cannot see it, listen to it or feel it. Software can be defined as an assembly of a large number of elements interrelating in a multitude of ways. Therefore complex software cannot be understood in its entirety during development, testing, or use without the application of the assessment process, the primary tool for the appraisal and categorization of automated systems. While for new systems, qualification and validation can be incorporated into the software development and implementation process, to ensure that the software can be fully understood and that quality is "programmed" into it, this is not always the case with *existing software*. The regulators would like to see the same level of documentation for existing and new automated systems, but in reality their expectations are rarely met. This is one of the main reasons why legacy systems need to be looked at from an entirely different angle. Although it may sound trivial, the first thing you must remember is — *don't panic*! Any attempt at problem-solving ahead without a strategy and sound planning is, at best, a waste of time and money. There is no "ready-made" legacy systems validation protocol, so it is quintessential to have a plan, i.e., *a strategy*. This chapter is a cookbook with a variety of recipes to choose from; whichever recipe you select depends entirely on the particular circumstances for a given automated system.

Strategy Document

Strategy should always be part of formal approved and controlled documentation, which can be changed and improved with the experience gained over time. The resulting strategy document is a vital component, and the team defining strategy and scope need to include members drawn from quality assurance, management, and IT departments.

The strategy document should define:

1. The rationale for the assessment (reasons and expectations).
2. Which parts of the enterprise shall be assessed (boundaries).
3. Which regulatory rules and regulations must be referenced.
4. Which internal guidance documents apply.
5. The company's interpretation of the rules.
6. Who will conduct the assessment.
7. How the assessment will be conducted and documented.
8. The required resources in monetary, time, and manpower terms.

The document should be written in a manner presentable to inspectorates, and also to the board of directors within the company, as it will outline the financial implications of the undertaking. Generally, the strategy is defined for an entire company or site. Careful consideration and planning at this stage is highly recommended, as the processes that follow generally take months or years to complete.

A uniform and consistent approach throughout the company is therefore advantageous from a project control and financial viewpoint. As a result of this policy, it becomes apparent that additional guidance documents such as clear standard operating procedures (SOPs), training procedures, or additional resources, are required. This approach will provide vital information on the length and breadth of the task in hand.

Recognizing the need to assess legacy systems and rectify any deficiencies may seem an obvious task to certain individuals within a company. All senior management must be made aware of the problem, must ultimately take responsibility for it, and act as sponsors for the legacy computer systems validation project. Quality assurance is a key component of automated systems validation and is the responsibility of senior management; although the task of assuring quality can be satisfactorily delegated, the responsibility for the end result may not.

It is strongly advised that a strategy document is written, approved, and ready for presentation in the event that it is required during a regulatory inspection. The strategy document provides evidence of a company's commitment and willingness to undertake the necessary steps. Without this documentary evidence, steps may be taken against the company by the regulators.

Recent citations by the FDA were based on the fact that some companies had more than one approach to legacy systems validation within different parts of their enterprise. This resulted in contradictory protocols, interpretations, and results. The favored approach must be having one approach and one interpretation within a company. The rationale for this is the adherence to existing laws and regulations, that require companies to apply qualification and validation to parts or all of their computer systems.

If this only applies to parts of the company then this must be clearly stated, reasons given, and the boundaries well defined. Although the number of regulations dealing directly with computerized systems is limited, others apply to systems supported by the automation in question. This interlink is crucial and again shows the need to ensure that the IT expert and the end user work together in a partnership. The most inconspicuous entry in the list above deals with the company's interpretation of the rule. However, this is the one with the farthest-reaching consequences. This will become clearer when we have a look at the different assessment methods and the resulting consequences. The following example will illustrate just how far-reaching the consequences of the interpretation can be.

The FDA states in 21 CFR Part 11 that: electronic signatures can be applied, and if they are then they must comply with the rule ... Clearly, the FDA does not require a company to apply electronic signatures if they do not want to. A company may now decide that they interpret those cases where signatures are applied both electronically and by hand on a printout of a document, not to be electronic signatures. In the company's view this will eliminate compliance with the electronic signature rules for all cases where there still is a 'wet ink' signature. It is obvious that this will lessen the company's workload. Whether or not this interpretation is acceptable to the authorities is an entirely different matter.

Another major benefit immediately arising from a clear understanding of the requirements for automated legacy systems assessments is through the relationship between the suppliers and the users of automated systems. Suppliers need to understand their customers' specific requests, needs or wishes with respect to their approach and the contents of their automated legacy system compliance assessment. Often the customers, i.e., the users, have a much more in-depth understanding of the regulations, whereas the supplier may be selling mainly into a nonhealth care customer base, thus mainly unaware of the specific legal requirements. Texts in advertisements and product descriptions, claiming full 21 CFR 11 compliance or FDA approval for a product should be approached with care and apprehension. Only a few companies have so far proved to have the appropriate quality systems, inhouse expertise and build the right functionality for compliance into their products. As part of the assessment and remediation process, the users will regularly contact the vendors to obtain information to either fill gaps in the system assessment documents, or to discuss remedial actions, for example, migration to a compliant release version.

The decision as to who will conduct the assessment within the company should be based on staff availability, their training and understanding of the task, and particularly on the estimated time and cost expectations. Few companies have sufficient resources inhouse to conduct the assessment process with the necessary level of expertise and within the time constraints. The process is sometimes accelerated through involvement of the regulators.

Inspections may identify deficiencies or noncompliant practices, resulting in enforcement proceedings against the company, which require immediate action. In most cases external resources will be brought in to help with either part of, or the entire, process. If this is envisaged, it should be planned for in the strategy document. In most cases, the overall validation process for both legacy and new systems stretches over months, or even years. It is therefore prudent to distinguish between immediate, i.e., short-term measures, and long-term activities.

Immediate activities are aimed at achieving compliance through measures implemented with limited effort, often resulting in "*hybrid*" systems. The term hybrid system is generally used to describe a system that fails to fulfil all sections of the FDA ruling; those parts which fail are substituted by administrative or technical measures. The immediate aim is to secure the ongoing use of the system.

Long-term actions should always result in a fully compliant system, and this can ultimately mean replacing the system. There are a variety of good reasons why some tasks will take a long time, such as replacements not being available immediately, which then need to be handled as part of a long-term strategy. Retrospective validation work is acknowledged to be considerably more expensive than prospective activities. The cost estimates included in the strategy document should also be included in the company's financial planning documents. Failure to do so may jeopardize the success of the project and could result in citations from the regulators. As mentioned many times before, the regulators only believe in documented evidence, not in "lip service."

System Assessment Documents

The assessment process for legacy automation systems is comparable to the risk assessment process, something with which people from other departments may already be familiar with, such as manufacturing or production, health, safety, or the environment. As in these other areas, it is equally important to define the process, tools, deliverables, and associated documents. With regard to the computerized legacy systems assessment process, these activities are encompassed in the inventory and the assessment protocols. Without a complete, accurate, and constantly updated inventory no work should start; you will either find that you have to go back and do additional work (at inflated cost), or that an inspector will find those systems you have overlooked, and will challenge you. You do not want to be in either position. Thus the first step is the creation of the system inventory.

System inventory

IT infrastructure within a company comprises both software and hardware. For all existing legacy systems, a complete inventory is a prerequisite for any type of assessment. From experience this is an ideal opportunity to update or create the documentation for the IT infrastructure in a suitable manner for both internal and external presentation. Inventory tables should be complemented by graphical illustrations, where appropriate. The IT network configuration is a good example, where several layers of increasingly detailed maps provide a quick and efficient overview, both of the existing and the planned infrastructure.

Many companies in 1999 put much effort into creating comprehensive inventories in preparation for the Year 2000 (Y2K) problem; these inventories are today an excellent source of information for legacy systems. However, a word of caution is appropriate here. The Y2K assessment process focused on date fields and calculations based on (or for) yielding dates.

The legacy system assessment has a much wider focus and its consequences are more far-reaching. There is no easy fix for legacy systems, such as setting the clock back a number of years to fool the system. If we take an example such as Lotus Notes, the Y2K assessment would have been fine; but the legacy system assessment must pay attention to all applications created within Lotus Notes. The most striking difference between the Y2K problem and computer systems validation is simply this: there is no end date for computer systems validation.

Identifying those systems which fall under the GMP, good clinical practice (GCP), or good laboratory practice (GLP) regulations (generically known as GxPs), requires the assessment team to recognize whether a particular system can or will influence product quality. It is also prudent to simultaneously assess the impact of a system on business performance (e.g., a finance software package). Even if not GxP critical, it may still have a profound impact on business operations and the company may therefore decide to qualify it too. Knowing which of the product- quality critical systems is also business-critical will make it easy for the company to assign priorities. It is unlikely that the critical systems will be in compliance with regulations, so remedial work should start on systems assigned the highest priority. Those who do not have to comply with any of the GxP regulations may want to assess their systems with regards to the business impact only.

Information for the inventory is likely to be based on existing information, and is usually stored in either a spreadsheet or database form. Manufacturing, for example, is likely to maintain an up-to-date and complete inventory of all of its computerized systems. However, this may not be the case within administrative sections, although they are likely to handle quality-critical product data, such as customer shipment information. When deciding on the format for the inventory, it may be advantageous to make use of existing formats. Care should be taken to only use those formats that can be handled with ease, and are widely acceptable and suitable for all sites in all countries.

Even a "simple" paper document can cause endless problems. If for example, the original was designed in Europe in DIN A4 format, this can result in missing information on printouts on American standard format paper. When using electronic formats, care should be taken to allow for all alphabets and symbols in use in the company. Most modern software packages incorporate Unicode, which allows representation of any language, and by converting outputs to a generic format, such as PDF, shortcomings of other program outputs can be overcome.

Once the inventory is generated it will be subject to change as systems are added, modified and retired. As the inventory is a crucial document for continued compliance with regulations, as it provides an overview of all of the systems owned by the company, these changes should be managed under a formal *change management* procedure. It is not uncommon for companies to stop changes to the inventory immediately prior to the assessment process. If this were not done then, apart from the risk of missing certain changes, the inventory would itself become another legacy system, something that should be avoided if at all possible.

The authorities are very reluctant to accept noncompliant legacy systems and their patience is fast running out when they find new unqualified and unvalidated systems. For the authorities, it is no longer acceptable to find that companies are developing and implementing nonvalidated automated systems with quality critical components. It is bad business practice to permit the uncontrolled development and use of any computerized system, irrespective of GxP criticality.

Whether the inventory is generated first, followed by the assessment, or whether the two tasks are carried out in parallel, is a decision based on practical considerations; most companies will attempt both tasks simultaneously. This is partially because the compilation of the inventory, and the assessment of the items it contains, requires the input of users and local support functions. As always, spare time is hard to find and it is often more economical to divert resources to this exercise once, if feasible. For examples of inventories see the sections on the assessment protocols.

Companies complying with GxP regulations and suppliers of software and hardware solutions regularly refer to and apply the guidance found in the Good Automated Manufacturing Practices (GAMP) documents.

GAMP categorization

The GAMP documents have proven very popular with many companies for several reasons. In the absence of more detailed regulatory guidance, these guidelines provide the only international guidance documents. There are other guidance documents available, but they are all limited either to particular countries or regions, or cover only one specific legacy computer system topic. The GAMP Guide provides guidance for users and suppliers, slotting all types of software into categories. This simplicity makes this guide very attractive to industry.

The GAMP Guide is currently in its fourth edition. Although GAMP is not an official guidance document it has been endorsed by all the major regulatory bodies, and is considered an international reference. The guide is not designed specifically for the retrospective assessment and validation of existing systems and is therefore limited in its usefulness for legacy systems. GAMP at present classes automated systems within five categories.

1. *Operating systems*. Established, commercially available operating systems, which are used in pharmaceutical manufacture.
2. *Firmware*. Instrumentation and controllers often incorporate nonuser-programmable firmware. Examples include weigh scales, bar code scanners, three-term controllers. They are configurable.
3. *Standard software packages*. These are commercially available, off-the-shelf standard software packages. Examples include statistical analysis packages and laboratory instrumentation software

4. *Configurable software packages*. These provide configurable standard software interfaces and functions. Examples include distributed control systems (DCS), supervisory control and data acquisition packages (SCADA), manufacturing execution systems (MES) and some laboratory information management systems (LIMS) and management resource planning (MRP) packages. A typical feature of these systems is that they permit users to develop their own applications by configuring or amending predefined software modules and also developing new application software modules. Each application (of the standard product) is therefore specific to the user process.
5. *Custom (bespoke) software*. There are many instances of this type of system in the pharmaceutical industry that meet the specific needs of the user.

GAMP category application

It should be noted that complex systems often have layers of software, and one system could exhibit several or even all of the above categories. An off-the-shelf LIMS will require configuration, but links to existing applications are likely to call for customized solutions.

This classification strongly correlates with the suggested qualification, validation levels and efforts for each category. So this guide may seem to be the right thing to use. Before jumping to that conclusion, however, one should bear in mind that the above was written for new systems. Even the latest edition of GAMP does not cover legacy (in the meaning of already existing) systems in detail; written for the pharmaceutical industry, it has a slight bias toward U.S. regulations. And last, but not least, it does not offer universal and easy-to-apply solutions to all legacy system problems. It is a valuable tool which should be used, as appropriate, in the qualification and validation of computer systems.

The completion of this matrix will allow the grouping together of systems that require a particular level of validation. For legacy systems, this categorization is much too broad and simplistic to be of any significant value. The assessment protocols require a lot more refinement and the following chapters will detail how these assessment protocols can be developed and put to good use. Obviously, a breakdown of the automated systems inventory into segments such as LotusPage for your notes applications, process logic controllers associated with equipment in manufacturing, gas chromatographs in the laboratory, etc., can provide a much more manageable structure to the assessment process.

General and detailed assessment protocols

The deliverable from the assessment process, initiated by the strategy document and based on the inventory, is a document providing details for all existing computerized systems, their level of compliance with the rules and regulations (in the understanding of the company), and any remediation work necessary. It should be noted that all inspectorates expect to find descriptions for all inspectable systems (their use, purpose and validation status, as a minimum). Often for existing systems this information has become outdated or is even missing.

The decision on whether the assessment process is divided into a general assessment and a detailed assessment, or whether only a detailed assessment will be carried out, is largely dependent on the size of the task, the available resources and is ultimately a management decision. As both approaches are successfully followed by industry, it would be difficult to make a recommendation on which to choose. As a result, this chapter will present both ways in order to provide complete coverage. From a practical viewpoint the assessment protocols should be organized into categories, and grouped by department area, etc. For example, it is most likely that the automated analytical systems are assessed by qualified computer systems validation personnel, backed up by appropriate operators, scientists, and technicians from each area.

It is initially sensible to test more than one version of the assessment protocol to find the one most suitable for the company. It will become clear within a very short time which approach suits the business best, or is the most practical solution. This decision should then be recorded in the strategy document, and any deviations from this approach avoided, if that is possible. Any changes at a later stage in the process will have a knock-on effect, impacting on cost and efforts. It must be reiterated at this point that the hardware is as much a part of the assessment process as the software. The hardware platform and its architecture has a profound impact on many regulatory aspects, such as security, access protocols, etc. Hardware is typically maintained by the IT department and may not have been assessed for compliance in the past. To answer some questions, one has to look beyond the software and hardware aspects, and consider the system environment, such as facilities, company documentation procedures (including system manuals), or training programs.

General assessment protocol

The assessment itself is often named a gap or risk analysis. The terminology is ambiguous and each company should define, either in the policy document or in the quality manual, the terms and acronyms used in connection with this task. If it is desirable to gain a general overview or to collate a limited set of data for further refinement of the assessment process, then this general or high level assessment is the process of choice. As a minimum, it will identify and classify the systems into the following three categories:

1. Computerized systems requiring qualification and validation because they impact on product quality.
2. Computerized systems that do not impact on product quality but have a significant impact on business performance.
3. Computerized systems that do not have an impact on either of the above.

These categories assume that systems affecting product quality implicitly also impact on business performance. From a regulatory standpoint, no further action is required for systems that impact neither of these areas. It may, however, become apparent that there are gaps in the documentation of these systems and the company may wish to correct this.

Systems not impacting product quality do not require qualification and validation. It is, however, prudent to determine if the existing procedures (e.g., backup, archiving, access control, etc.), and the life cycle documentation are of sufficient standard to enable system maintenance to be carried out under change control. Often yes or no answers are replaced by more fine-tuned terms, such as: in full, to a greater part, partly, to a lesser part, not applicable. Another method is to assign numerical values to each term, thus providing a means for creating a "weighed" answer.

Although this is a simple query matrix, completing it requires additional clarification and explanations. In this case such details should be found in the SOP referenced on the assessment protocol. The example document indicates that separate assessment protocols were created for each site and each building. In other cases it may be more sensible to break the documents down by department. A managed protocol numbering system is advisable for tracking and reconciliation purposes. System boundaries may not always be easy to identify. One may define physical boundaries or base the boundaries on system drawings. Printing system identification numbers may be helpful for grouping systems. We must remember that this protocol is mainly concerned with automated parts of the system.

So here inventory completeness refers to the inventory document, which must detail all automated system parts. The questions on impact on product quality and business operations are usually straightforward. If either or both of these questions are answered with "yes" a detailed assessment will be required. More detailed questions may be included in the general assessment, and while providing a wealth of information, collating the answers may be too time- consuming. The assessments require a sound understanding of the issues, the company's interpretation of the rules and a certain amount of pragmatism. This may be beyond the requirements for the preceding questions.

The question of whether an electronic record is created may already be difficult to answer if the data is only stored transiently. The FDA guidance on "*Scope and Application*" provides some pragmatic views, challenging the users to define whether the use of the automated system is purely incidental or whether an electronic record is created that the users rely upon. It may not always be easy to find an answer when carrying out the assessment and one should rather err on the safe side (consider it an electronic record), especially if the use of the record has not yet been defined in a written document.

Also, whether a legacy system is qualified or validated is never a trivial question. Even if archived validation protocols did not include testing for compliance with 21 CFR Part 11 (FDA's rule on electronic records, electronic signatures) it is normal practice to consider the systems to be in a validated state. The shortcoming of not addressing the issue of e-records and e-signatures is the logical conclusion and result of the assessment process. Again, one should consult the FDA's "Scope and Application" guidance, which explicitly requires compliance with all rules and regulations in force at the time, i.e., compliance with the predicate rules, the current GMP. As judgement and probably bias is unavoidable, it is good practice to provide comments with all entries to document the reasons for the choice of entry. More detail can, of course, be included in these tables and other aspects such as impact on safety, health, and environment (SHE) are also sometimes added. This all depends on the particular needs of each company, and no one example will suit everyone.

Where does a general assessment end and a detailed one start? The previous examples are suitable for high-level assessments. Although the systems are assessed and categorized, the high level assessment does not provide an answer to the question of what exactly is noncompliant with a particular system and what must be done about it! An assessment without this information would be like a mechanic stating that there is something wrong with your car, but not what it is and how it can be fixed.

Detailed assessment protocol

In-depth information on a system is obtained by conducting a detailed assessment. This allows the assessor to find deficiencies in compliance, identify recurring gaps and problems, and enables the analysis and design of remedial actions. It is clear that the completion of these protocols requires a thorough understanding of the assessment process and the automated systems concerned, including their use within the company. The topic of training becomes very important here and more information on this is given in the next section. These detailed protocols can take different forms, e.g., spreadsheets, tables, and can be completed either manually or electronically. The following examples are suggestions and are by no means universal solutions. The selection criterion was the GAMP category 9 and for each separate category individual check sheets were created. The text of the applicable guidance document is included and extended to provide additional guidance to the assessors, and to include the company's interpretation of the requirements.The previous examples provide an insight into how detailed the assessment questionnaires should be. The development of the questionnaires on which to base the necessary qualification and validation activities for compliance purposes or to satisfy internal business needs, is the most important step in the entire assessment process. Everything that follows is a direct consequence of these protocols. Now it is time to execute these protocols and it is vital that as much effort is put into their completion as was needed to initially create them. Only specially trained (internal and external) staff should be employed in the delivery of this task. Personnel training requirements are described in more detail hereafter.

Training

With the strategy document and the general and detailed assessment questionnaires available, it is time to think about executing the assessment, collating the information, judging what actions may be necessary as a result of the assessment process and, most importantly, decide who will do it. The system user generally has the best knowledge about the computerized system's use, but may lack knowledge or understanding of the underlying IT structures. Many staff will also have a deficit in understanding the requirements for regulatory compliance. In order to overcome these problems, it would seem sensible to adopt a team approach when executing the assessment.

There should be a core team of assessors who do understand the issues and have been trained in the applicable regulatory compliance guidelines. Depending on the size of the company or the specific task, it will be necessary to train additional staff from within the various departments.

Faced with such a task for the first time often seems daunting, and the question arises as to who will be suitably qualified to execute the assessment and how the chosen approach can be benchmarked against industry's best practice.

Many companies do not have sufficient or appropriate resources in-house to initiate the process and specialist consultants will be hired to provide the necessary assistance. Although this is a sensible approach, care should be taken to ensure that the knowledge gained by the consultants is transferred to the team and becomes part of the knowledge pool of the company. Simply purchasing the questionnaires should also be discouraged as only an understanding of the underlying principles and rationales can lead to a useful result. Thus front-end support and training using actual examples from within the company is a highly efficient way of getting started and getting it right first time.

An observation often made is the fact that quality assurance (QA) personnel have limited knowledge of IT systems and operations and IT staff have little appreciation for the regulatory environment and its implications. This is a primary area on which to focus training. In some cases it may be advisable to consider the appointment of an IT QA manager. The training benefits are manifold. Staff training means that the workforce receives the qualifications required by the regulators. It also means that the understanding and awareness of the issues involved are improved. It is particularly interesting to see the considerable changes in the quality and numbers of entries in inventory lists once the contributors have received their training. What may have been a mere listing of hardware items will develop into a comprehensive systems inventory. The training should yield confident assessors, and users or system owners who have the knowledge to provide the right information.

Assessment

With everything in place, from the questionnaires to the training, the procedures and all of the support needed, the assessments should now get under way. Many entries on the inventory will not contain any electronic records or electronic signatures and will not be business critical.

Filling in the forms for these items will be an easy task, particularly if the inventory database and the forms are linked electronically to facilitate automatic data entry. It is an often voiced misconception that it is unnecessary to document and assess those systems that will not be inspected. Inspectors will want to see documented evidence of your decision process that leads you (the system owner) to believe that the system is out of inspection scope. Lack of such documentation can result in a deficiency citation. Where the situation is not so obvious, and where the necessity for a detailed assessment can be assumed, the team needs to plan the time and location for it. Sometimes the system owner or user is also the assessor; but more often than not the assessors will have to arrange for a meeting with the person familiar with the system. Time and progress estimates should be based on the latter scenario.

Depending on the complexity of the systems, the available documentation and information, experience shows that an assessor can complete between two and six detailed assessments per day. This will also include the time taken to formulate appropriate actions for those areas where deficiencies with the requirements have been identified. The limiting factor in most cases is the availability of the system user or owner, who is often occupied with meeting the daily needs of the business, which must be given first priority.

For a medium-sized establishment this assessment process will therefore take, on average, from several weeks to a few months. Multisite and multinational companies will probably need several months to complete the task. More likely, this will be an ongoing exercise, as there seem to be no relenting in the number of takeovers and mergers, which regularly create the need for additional assessments or reviews of those already completed. The time consumed by the assessment process will have significant financial implications, and these costs are often not included in the company's financial projects and budget forecasts.

Not all assessments will be as straightforward as was first thought, and the guidance documents may not give the answer, or at least not the detail, sought. In these instances it is advantageous to have a designated person (the project manager?) or a committee that will deal with any queries. In addition to providing guidance and answers to the assessors, there is also an opportunity to refine the internal guidance literature and to consolidate methods and solutions within the company. The most efficient way to consider and decide on remedial actions for any type of deficiency identified is during the assessment itself. Often the system users or owners will already have deliberated on systems or procedures improvements and they should be aware of any limitations that would favor one solution over another. The completed and signed-off assessment forms are collated and grouped, for example, by system type, department, deficiency profile, suggested remedial actions and any other sensible criteria. If there are more than just a handful of systems, such an approach is always preferable as it minimizes the workload resulting from the assessments.

Results and Options

With the exception of very specific systems or special circumstances, it is industry's experience that virtually no IT system is in complete compliance with the GxP regulations, and in particular with 21 CFR Part 11. This statement has several important implications.

1. Pharmaceutical companies are using noncompliant IT systems and they are aware of it.
2. So are the regulators, and they want industry to take action on this matter. That is what this chapter is about.

First we need to look at the options available to a company when the assessment comes up with a noncompliant system. There are five standard approaches:

1. Redefine the use of the system — is it necessary for the application or is the use of the system purely incidental?
2. Add procedural controls — this is often only a short-term solution.
3. Upgrade the system — the preferred solution if cost and timescales are reasonable.
4. Replace the system — a clean, but drastic solution.
5. Retire the system — the medium- to long-term solution for systems that will never be compliant.

All options are open to a user but the implications vary widely. These are best explained using practical examples. A laboratory is running an analytical test method and the result is calculated using an MS Excel spreadsheet which is stored on a networked PC with no particular access restrictions. All laboratory staff can use the spreadsheet when needed. The mathematical result is used in the release procedure for the product. There are clearly a number of deficiencies here that require immediate action. Retiring the system would mean using paper again and using a second person to check the calculations. This may well be a suitable option in this case.

There is no obvious need to replace or upgrade the system as the spreadsheet itself is well suited for carrying out the calculations, and another system would probably require the same effort for bringing it into compliance. Adding procedural controls may be a good option here. The spreadsheet could be password protected, it could be stored on a nonnetworked PC, and a standard operating procedure

(SOP) could detail further control aspects. Redefining the use of the system does not seem to be an option as the result would remain product quality critical.

A document management application is used for creating controlled documents, such as SOPs. The present program version does not have audit trail functionality. One option would be to consider this system as purely incidental use of a computer system ("typewriter rule"). This will require the company to rely on the paper documents for daily use. In this case no further action is required. If, however, the documents are distributed and accessed in their electronic format on a regular basis, then these will be electronic records and 21 CFR 11 applies. Retiring the system would mean reverting to paper again; not a likely solution. Implementing a paper-based audit trail is an enormous effort, particularly as a logbook alone cannot satisfy the requirements for complete contents and version control, including date and time stamps. As the system obviously satisfies most of the users' needs and the regulators' expectations, a good solution would be to approach the vendor for an updated version that provides the required functionality. Clearly, each system must be analyzed for its merits and to determine the most appropriate way forward to achieve compliance or the users' requirements. This is a project in its own right and requires serious planning and the allocation of resources. This is discussed in detail in the following sections.

Managing Legacy Systems

With few exceptions, there will be a short-term activity followed by a long-term strategy, that will bring the existing computerized systems into compliance with current legislation or users' requirements. It is now time to execute these plans and we will look at the issues around the various options that may have been selected, and the associated project needs. From the assessments, all of the information is now available: the number and particular types of systems, the associated deficiencies, necessary remedial actions, and the urgency with which these should be implemented. All of this information, when entered into a suitable planning tool, provides the company with an action plan, information on the project duration and milestones, plus associated cost and manpower estimates. This plan is exactly what the regulatory authorities are looking for. It is also the tool that management must have for the purposes of planning, budgeting, and project control. It does, however, make any weaknesses in the company's assets or procedures highly visible. To overcome or rectify these weaknesses, it is necessary to choose from one of the five options mentioned in the results and options section. Here we want to look at each option in detail to evaluate the pros and cons. Ultimately, the choice of action will determine the quality, cost, and time of the resulting solution.

Decommissioning (System Retirement)

When an IT system is obsolete, superfluous, inappropriate or unsuitable for validation, then decommissioning is the right choice. Again, this should be performed in a planned and documented manner. Depending on the type of computerized system and the volume of data, the archiving or migration of data should be considered. It is unlikely that none of the data are relevant to the business, which would be the only circumstance in which data deletion and system destruction is the straightforward option. If the use of the system is discontinued, the data will need archiving, using a suitable storage media and location. This procedure may either follow an SOP on data archiving or a specific protocol for the application concerned. In either case, data retrieval and the completeness and accuracy (trustworthiness) of the data should be tested on a representative sample. The verification process could employ check sums, file size figures, comparison of printouts, etc. The suitability of the archiving format should be assessed in advance. Following the data archiving the obsolete software application should be deleted from the system. Specialists from IT should ensure that the software application has been completely removed. If the data are still required, then migration of the data to a new software application must be evaluated.

A typical example would be the replacement of workflow information stored as text and tables, which was created using standard text and spreadsheet software applications by an enterprise management system. Such a system can store information on batch sizes, status, location, etc. This information would have been held in numerous locations, on different systems, and in potentially incompatible formats by various people. Rather than having to address a large number of systems, these would be decommissioned and replaced by just one (new) system. The benefits are obvious and the applications would still be available, although in a different environment and format. Systems that are especially prone to retirement are those that are only kept alive by the common notion that "We always do it this way." Where progress can provide improvement, progress should be made.

Redefining the System

Instead of retiring or decommissioning a system it may be possible, or desirable, to redefine its use or role. This would allow the continued use of the system without the need for potentially extensive remedial work. In the context of 21 CFR Part 11, for example, the requirement to maintain records under predicate rules or submitted to FDA, and that are maintained in electronic format *in place of paper format*, are considered to fall under the rule. A laboratory may be used for the analysis of drug substances and for research purposes. If there are several systems serving this dual purpose, it may be possible to dedicate just some of these to analysis only. The regulators would not be concerned with any of the other systems. With this "simple" move the situation is simplified and savings are achieved. Clearly it is necessary to incorporate this procedure into the relevant SOPs and to train and audit staff working under these changed circumstances.

Where both electronic and paper records are created, it is now permissible to define (preferably in an SOP), which of these the master record is. This must reflect actual business practice. The system owner should be challenged if loss of the electronic record is acceptable. The answer should of course be yes. Where paper records can be defined as the master records, compliance with 21 CFR 11 is no longer a requirement.

Replacement or Upgrade?

This is probably the solution that first springs to mind when discrepancies are found with a system. However, unless the company using the system is producing its own hardware or programming its own software, obtaining a solution will be entirely dependent on vendor offerings. In most instances the latter will be the case. Few vendors will have a suitable upgrade or replacement available when needed. This is partly because many software packages or programs are written for clients from a wide range of industries, that typically are far less regulated than the pharmaceutical industry, and also because equipment or hardware vendors prefer to sell particular models in large numbers before they make available any new or substantially altered models.

It is not uncommon to encounter vendor claims of a "*fully compliant*" solution to whatever problem is most current in industry. These are often exaggerated and sometimes unsubstantiated or even false. Why should equipment and software producers have a better understanding of the regulatory requirements than the regulated industry itself? How can they know what the user really needs without having seen a user requirements specification? In conclusion, only the close cooperation of the vendor and the purchaser will allow a proper assessment to be conducted, whether a suitable upgrade or replacement is available.

No matter, whether a company chooses to replace or to upgrade a system, one is looking at new software or hardware, which will require formal qualification and probably validation. All of the relevant documents like the user requirements specification (URS), functional specification (FS), design specification (DS), and the test protocols, must be established and executed. Code reviews and supplier audits must be conducted, change control procedures followed and other associated activities completed, as applicable, for the systems concerned. It is likely that the request for bid documents, together with the supplier selection process, will need to be redefined due to the experience gathered during the legacy computer systems assessment process. Such an action is not a "*quick fix*" and is rarely a short-term solution. In many instances replacements or upgrades are associated with substantial capital spending and will have to follow time-consuming internal procedures.

A number of factors may make it impossible for a company to obtain either an upgrade or a new system which fulfils all requirements, and not least the regulators' expectations. The reasons for this may be technical limitations, price, availability, unwillingness, and others. As always in such cases, a risk analysis should be performed, establishing the benefits compared with the risks of not upgrading or replacing the system. In any case, documenting this exercise will help to demonstrate to internal and external parties that everything humanly possible had been done to rectify the identified shortcomings of the existing system, even if only a partial solution or none at all can be found.

In some specific areas it is already apparent that client demand for certain features which are associated with demands from the regulatory bodies, has resulted in improved or compliant systems. At present, this applies mainly to sophisticated laboratory, enterprise resource planning, and materials or document management systems. As demand grows, more solutions will become available, which should benefit all parties, not least the patients.

Hybrid Systems and Procedural Controls

Although "disliked" and discouraged by the regulators, hybrid systems are the short- term solution of choice in many instances. As discussed before, technical solutions may not be available currently, or too far into the future, too costly to implement, or unsuitable for a particular situation. The only way forward is to establish procedures for controlling the system until such time that appropriate solutions are made available. As this is the method used most often for immediate remediation, we will need to look at some of the solutions encountered more closely. One of the most cited deviations is the lack of, or insufficient, access control. The reasons for this are numerous, for example:

1. The system has no, or limited, access control functionality (e.g., no password, one password only and no user ID, etc.).
2. The functionality is not used or enabled (e.g., one password is used by all laboratory staff, etc.).
3. The system is accessible from other applications (e.g., protected files can be modified and deleted using Windows Explorer, etc.).
4. The physical location of the system is publicly accessible.
5. There is no control over passwords and user IDs (e.g., expired user IDs are reused, etc.).
6. The vendor or maintenance contractor has a "master" password or the administrator access codes are printed in the manuals.
7. The passwords used for accessing the system never expire.

Where the system lacks access control it may be possible to physically secure the area, e.g., access by key or swipe card. In addition, it is necessary to establish a written procedure which details who has access and how this is recorded, managed, and controlled. Such controls must include any third party requiring system access. Where access control functionality is available it should be used, and SOPs must detail the associated procedures to be followed. If correctly implemented and applied this will result in a compliant rather than a hybrid system.

Audit trails are another area of widespread concern. The regulatory expectations are such that an audit trail for electronic records should also be generated electronically and must be securely tied to that record. Few systems have this type of functionality and the audit trail information is not secure.

As always, the authorities want to be able to detect fraud. For the company however, there is further interest in knowing when a particular event took place, and who was involved in it, because it may help to improve processes, avoid errors and faults, and therefore reduce system downtime.

Before the advent of electronic audit trails, paper based logbooks were used (and still are) to document sequences of events, and for providing the date and time, and the identity of the person who made the entry. In order to avoid fraud, two people had to be involved in this operation, the second person confirming the action or the observation made by the first. Automated systems were introduced to reduce the number of people involved in such operations. Modern processes are therefore no longer geared to cope with such procedures, which often prevents a company from reverting back to the old system. Clearly it is not acceptable to simply provide the operator with a logbook to fill in, as this would serve no purpose. It would be impossible to detect wrongdoing without an independent check. In essence, where it is required, companies should attempt to bring in electronic audit trails because most other solutions are proving more complicated and costly. Exemption are locked-down databases, which do not allow record editing or deletion, only entry and export of new data entries, and automatically apply a date and time stamp. Data for export are additionally secured with a hash key to prevent (fraudulent) change before reimport. The absence of an electronic audit trail should always be described in a risk assessment document.

In this connection the issues of date and time must be addressed. Even companies with a single location should accurately date and time stamp on drug products, documentation, etc. Wristwatches and computer clocks are mostly out of synchronization with the national time standards. Providing accurate time on the system is not a big challenge and should be delegated to the IT department. Accurate atomic clock time signals can be either gathered from the Internet or a clock may be purchased and installed. (Improved accuracy can be obtained by coupling the system to a global positioning system (GPS)). The time signal can also be made available via the company's internal network.

What about companies with multiple sites and systems that are used globally? In the first case local time should always be used. Where one system is used on multiple sites in different time zones, it is often practical to use one time only. This may be the time at the location of the central processor unit, or it may be an arbitrarily set time for the system, such as Greenwich Mean Time (GMT). The FDA states in its guidance document: "Although we withdrew the draft guidance on time stamps, our current thinking has not changed in that when using time stamps for systems that span different time zones, we do not expect you to record the signer's local time. When using time stamps, they should be implemented with a clear understanding of the time zone reference used. In such instances, system documentation should explain time zone references as well as zone acronyms or other naming conventions."

These few examples show that simple solutions can often be enough to improve the current situation and eliminate some of the computer system's deficiencies. Starting remedial action after the completion of the assessment process for all systems provides the opportunity to implement more far-reaching (site-wide or even global) solutions, with the obvious benefit of potential cost savings. It does not mean, however, that these procedural controls are always in full compliance with the regulators' expectations. It is likely that in many cases system upgrades or replacements must be considered as a long-term solution.

Practical Examples

The following examples are excerpts from actual assessments. They are meant to provide the reader with practical and pragmatic solutions to typical deficiencies and deviations from regulatory requirements. The examples were chosen as they represent typical and recurring deficiencies associated with legacy computerized systems.

Remediation planning and risk assessments

The completed detailed assessments for computerized systems with electronic records or electronic signatures contain the information where compliance with the regulatory requirements has already been achieved, and also any deficiencies identified. Industry's experience is that only some legacy systems are really fully compliant, and that for most systems some sort of remedial action is required. Where only a limited number of systems or deficiencies are identified, it may be possible to devise individual remediation plans for each automated system or application, without losing control over the task.

It is often advantageous to tabulate the findings from the detailed assessments, thus facilitating the information assessment process. Several advantages can be gained from this approach: similar or identical deficiencies or shortcomings can be grouped together, and a common solution can be potentially found. In addition, the deficiencies can be classified to form the basis for a risk assessment. The risk assessment process can also provide the information on the level of priority that should be given to a particular automated system or application. The plan for remedial action should take into account all of the information contained in the detailed assessments and gained from the risk assessments. Excellent articles on the risk assessment process for computer software have been published in *Pharmaceutical Engineering*. These state that consideration should be given to the following:

1. The risk that the system poses to product safety, efficacy, and quality.
2. The risk that the system poses to data integrity, authenticity, and confidentiality.
3. The system's complexity; a more complex system might warrant a more comprehensive validation effort.

The FDA guidance document, *Guidance for Industry, FDA Reviewers and Compliance on Off-The-Shelf Software Use in Medical Devices*, is much more specific about the particularities of the software risk assessment process: "Existing international standards indicate that the estimation of risk should be considered as the product of the severity of harm and the probability of occurrence of harm. On the software engineering side, probabilities of occurrence would normally be based on software failure rates. However, software failures are systematic in nature and therefore their probability of occurrence can not be determined using traditional statistical methods. Because the risk estimates for hazards related to software cannot easily be estimated based on software failure rates, CDRH has concluded that engineering risk management for medical device software should focus on the severity of the harm that could result from the software failure. Because risk analysis for software cannot be based on probability of occurrence, the actual function of risk analysis for software can then be reduced to a hazard analysis function."

Although this document specifically deals with medical devices, the FDA's conclusions are applicable to the software risk assessment process in general. It should be noted though, that there is no specific FDA guidance for computerized legacy systems. GAMP details the risk assessment process for a given system function or system subfunction. Both the risks to GxP and the business are identified, and their respective likelihood and severity of impact assessed. The risk assessment process described is closely tied into the lifecycle and the validation process for a computerized system or application. It is therefore best suited to new systems.

The European GMP guidance document has a section on retrospective validation for computerized legacy systems, which specifically requests a risk analysis for GxP impact. As all entries were identified to represent electronic records, they are therefore all GxP critical. Additional information on past performance and experience with the automated system or application can be provided in the history column. Additional information and guidance on how to describe or assess business risk and GxP risk can be found in Appendix M3 to the GAMP Guide. In this example seventeen discrepancies from eleven systems or applications used by six departments are recorded. Closer analysis led to the following approach for remedial action.

Deficiency. No procedure for creating copies of electronic records for inspectors.

Solution. The existing SOP "Procedure for Regulatory Agency Inspections and/or Investigations" for this site was amended to include the submission of electronic records in electronic format. This ensures that the correct information is handed to the authority and by marking the data storage media label with the "Confidential Trade Secret Information" stamp, confidentiality is assured. This procedure will also cover the data format depending on the original application and the record contents.

Deficiency. Inadequate or no backup, archival, record retention, and data retrieval procedure.

Solution. A new site-wide SOP "Procedure for Data Archival" was drafted covering data storage, archival and retrieval.

Deficiency. No procedures for physical system access.

Solution. In one case the existing departmental system SOP is amended, following internal change control procedures. On one portal system physical access cannot be restricted, and there is no electronic access control facility. Replace the entire system.

Deficiency. Sequencing steps were not validated.

Solution. The existing validation protocol for the system is changed to incorporate the sequencing step tests. The protocol execution is therefore planned to coincide with the planned revalidation of the system. This is an actual example showing that, by collating the information from the detailed assessments in a risk assessment type format, it is possible to limit the time and effort for deficiency rectification and to optimize the remediation effort. Five remedial actions covered all seventeen recorded deficiencies.

Analytical system deficiency remediation

For reasons of clarity, only the comments for noncompliance are shown.

Deficiency. The ability to discern invalid or altered records was not validated.

Solution. The existing validation protocol for the FT-IR spectrometer is changed to incorporate the additional tests. The protocol will be executed during the annual system revalidation.

Deficiency. No backup or archival procedure.

Solution. Adaptation of the corporate SOP "Procedure for Data Storage, Archival and Retrieval."

Deficiency. There is no audit trail or audit trail functionality.

Solution. The system itself does not have the required functionality and a manual audit trail was not considered an acceptable solution. Furthermore, a system replacement or an application software upgrade, which would have rendered the system compliant, was unavailable. Therefore, it is necessary to acquire additional software that will make the system compliant. Various companies offer such software solutions, particularly for analytical laboratory systems. References to these can be found, *inter alia*, on the FDA website under Electronic Record — Electronic Signatures 21 CFR Part 11 Guidance Documents Dockets Established — Topics for Guidance.

Deficiency. The application developer has left and there is no qualification record for the developer or the maintainer. User training logs are complete.

Solution. The history records for recent years show that the system and its application are very stable and operate reliably. The system vendor operates to internationally accepted software development standards and this was confirmed in writing. This information was considered sufficient, as it proved impossible to obtain the required records retrospectively. The existing SOP "Procurement and Invitation to Bid" was updated to require all qualification certificates for future purchases. The system maintainer's training logs were updated to include this particular system.

Deficiency. The number of copies and the location of the system documentation are unknown.

Solution. As this is a site-wide deficiency, a SOP "System Documentation" was established, describes the steps necessary for the review, approval, distribution, and use of system documentation for GxP critical systems. The documentation covered by this SOP comprises training manuals, applications manuals, operating systems manuals, configurable software manuals, SOPs, help files, security and access lists and drawings. In the case of the FT-IR instrument all documentation was collated and is now stored with the instrument in an access-controlled location.

Deficiency. The printed names of the signatories are not on the document.

Solution. It is possible to enter the printed name of the signatories on the document before the printout and the application of the wet signature. The existing SOP for the instrument was updated accordingly.

Validation

This chapter is not intended to provide in-depth guidance on the validation process for legacy systems, as this is dealt with in great detail in other publications. However, the subject does warrant mention as one will come across the issue during the system assessment process. The question will be: Is the system validated? We would like to assume that those companies obliged to validate systems would have done so. Nonetheless, having created this new awareness within a wide audience, it is very likely that gaps will be identified within the previous validation effort. For example, many IT departments are prepared for a system crash and provide a backup service for that purpose. Few will have a system in place that allows for the archiving and retrieval of specific records for many years (often seven years or more), something that is required for electronic records, particularly under 21 CFR Part 11. Companies should assess if some or all of their existing computerized systems need to be reviewed, and the qualification or validation documents revisited in light of the newly-established requirements and needs.

Ongoing Operations

Unfortunately time does not stand still and reviewing the automated legacy systems in a company does not stop day-to-day operations or changes to, or the purchase of, new systems. The process of introducing new items and administrative controls should always consider the impact these have on the legacy systems. This may affect, for example, SOPs for:

1. Data backup.
2. Archiving.
3. Disaster recovery.
4. Data retrieval.
5. QA audits.
6. Purchasing procedures.
7. Training.
8. Error logging.
9. Software and hardware maintenance.
10. Change control.
11. Organizational structures.
12. Software and hardware distribution, etc.

Assessing and understanding legacy computer systems not only helps to improve the operation and maintenance of the existing systems, it also has a profound impact on new systems or upgrades that are introduced into the company. The assessment effort and the associated training and awareness-

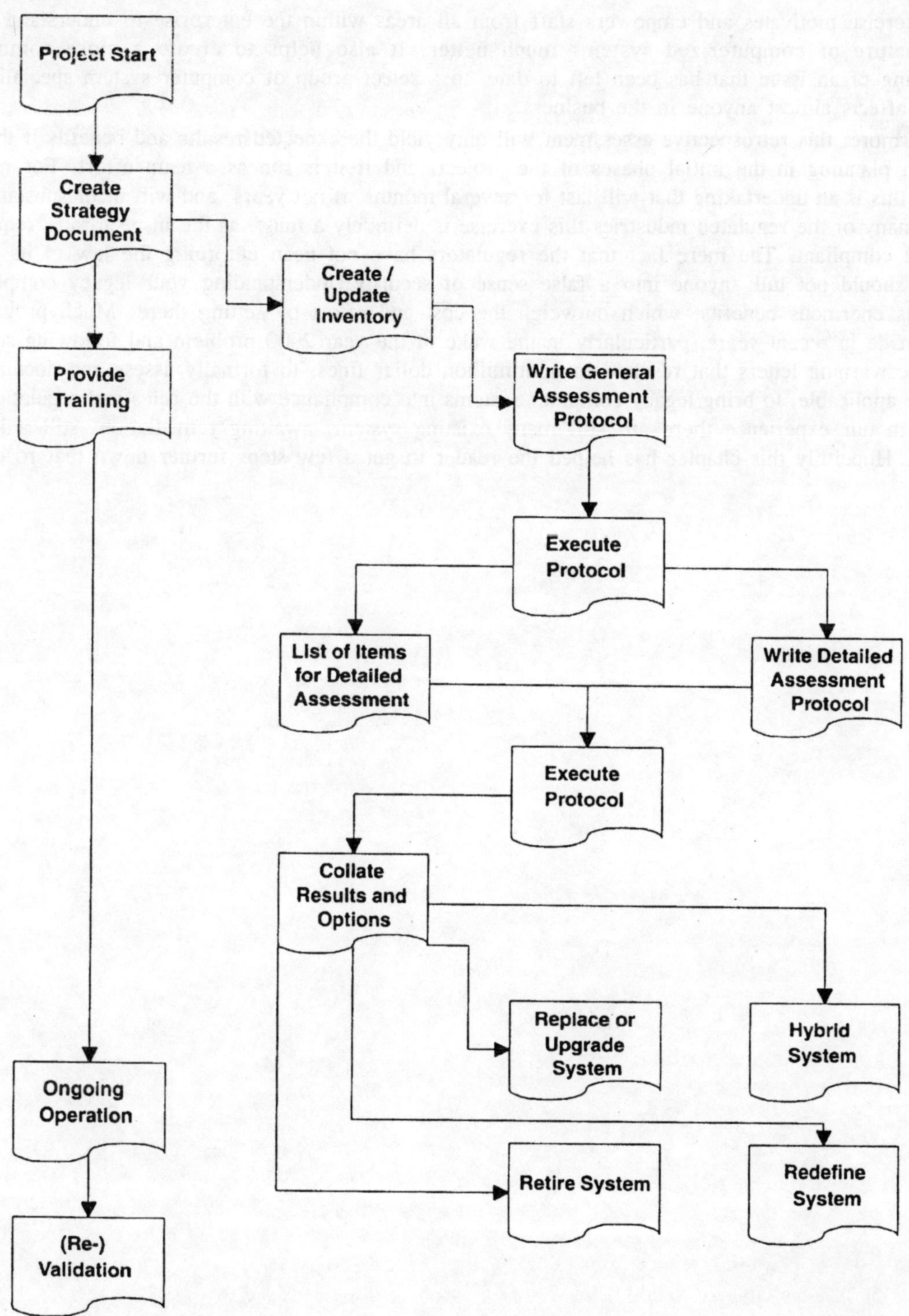

Fig. 14.1. Project flowchart.

building exercise motivates and empowers staff from all areas within the enterprise to understand the complex nature of computerized systems much better. It also helps to create a more common understanding of an issue that has been left to date, to a select group of computer system specialists, but which affects almost anyone in the business.

Furthermore, this retrospective assessment will only yield the expected results and benefits if there is thorough planning in the initial phases of the project, and if it is run as a team effort. For most companies this is an undertaking that will last for several months, if not years, and will incur substantial cost. For many of the regulated industries this exercise is definitely a must, as the inspectorates require them to be compliant. The mere fact that the regulators have not been enforcing the law to its full extent yet should not lull anyone into a false sense of security.Understanding your legacy computer systems has enormous benefits, which outweigh the cost and effort of getting there. Much progress has been made in recent years, particularly in the wake of the year 2000 problem and following some high profile warning letters that resulted in multimillion dollar fines, to formally assess and document and, where applicable, to bring legacy computer systems into compliance with the rules and regulations. However, in our experience there are still many existing systems awaiting remediation; still a long way to go. Hopefully this chapter has helped the reader to get a few steps further down that road.

15

QUALITY SYSTEMS MANAGEMENT

Managing for quality is and always has been a critical task of management no matter what the industry. In the pharmaceutical industry today, achieving quality of products, services, and processes is as important as it ever was; however, today we need to achieve it with reduced resources. We need to do more with less. We need to be as concerned with the quality system's efficiency as well as its effectiveness. Rising regulatory and customer requirements make this ever more challenging. In this article, we will define the components of the quality system. We will present the pros and cons of various models of a quality system—drug GMPs, the medical device quality system regulations, ISO 9000, and the Malcolm Baldrige award criteria. In addition to guidance on the design of the quality system, we will describe some techniques that we have found to be effective in managing it.

QUALITY SYSTEM

Traditionally in the pharmaceutical industry, the quality function is divided into two parts, quality control and quality assurance. Quality control centers on testing products to assure their compliance to specification. It is in general concerned with evaluating events from the past. FDA has recognized this deficiency with the often-quoted philosophy that "you cannot test quality into a product." Quality assurance is focused on building quality into a product through activities like validation, process and environmental control, and documentation. Quality assurance is in general concerned with events in the present. Only relatively recently has the pharmaceutical industry begun to emphasize a quality management accountability for continuous improvement of processes, people, and culture. Quality management is about the future, about prevention, and management's role in improving the quality system. A system is a group of parts, components, or processes that work together to achieve a common goal. For the quality system, the common goal is understanding and meeting customer's needs. The components of the quality system are processes, people, and culture. There are four types of processes that comprise the system:

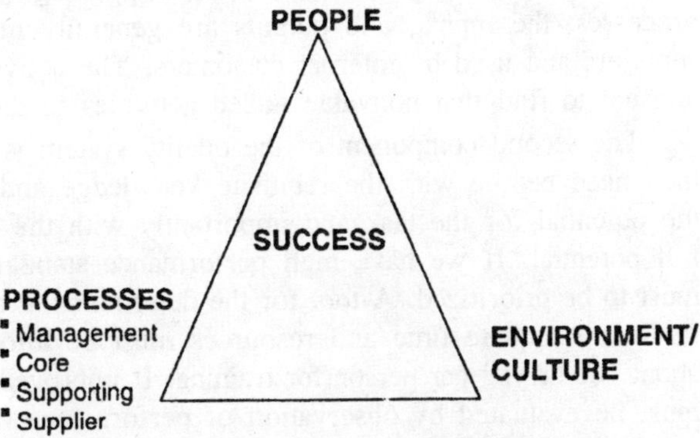

Fig. 15.1. Quality system components.

1. *Management*—the management processes are the most important. Some of the management processes that are critical to the quality system are: the communication of policy, standards, directions,

objectives, and priorities to the organization; periodic reviews of the quality system's health and need for improvement; creation of the quality culture; and ensuring the availability of adequate resources.

2. *Core*—the core processes are those that produce product for sale to a customer. For each step in the core process, the critical control points or variables and the acceptable ranges of these variables must be identified. The controls may be done in process by production or off-line in the QC labs. The quality of the core process depends principally on the design of the process and its validation; i.e., on its intrinsic capability.
3. *Supporting*—some of the key supporting processes in a GMP plant are: audits, change control, failure investigations, labeling (artwork generation, labeling use and control), maintenance, materials management, complaint handling, product release, stability/expiration dating, training, trend analysis, and validation. Supporting processes add value in proportion to their contribution to the core process.
4. *Supplier*—the supplier process is essential for the proper functioning of the core process. The quality of the core process depends to a large degree on the quality of incoming raw and packaging materials. The goal is supplier partnership. The quality of the supplier's own processes directly impacts the quality of your core process.

The focus on process quality is important because the work gets done through processes. The quality of the output depends on process quality and efficiency gains come from process improvements. It is also necessary to remember, "over the long haul, strong people cannot compensate for a weak process. All too often, management relies on individual or team heroics to overcome fundamentally flawed processes." The most important component is ownership; i.e., the process is actively managed. One generally finds that departments are managed but processes are not. For internal processes, the supporting processes, the inputs, and outputs are generally information; information that is supplied by internal suppliers and used by internal customers. The activities in the process should be value added. It is not unusual to find that nonvalue added activities in the pharmaceutical manufacturing plant exceed 25%.

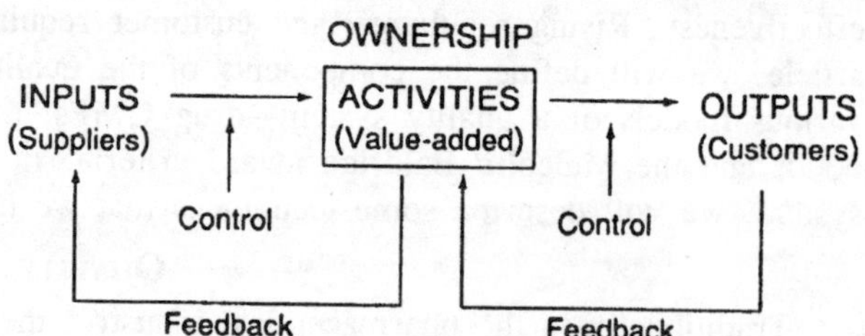

Fig. 15.2. Model of a process.

The second component of the quality system is people. Given that we have capable processes, we then need people with the requisite knowledge and skills. We have to hire and promote people with the potential for the task and importantly with the correct attitude. We need to develop them to their full potential. If we have high performance standards, all employees will have training needs. These must to be prioritized. A tool for the determination of training needs and their prioritization is described in Ref. Adequate time and resources must be allocated to training. World- class companies allocate about 100 hr yr^{-1} per person for training. If improved performance is the goal of training, its effectiveness must be evaluated by observation of performance or by improvement in business metrics.

The third component of the quality system is culture. Given capable processes and skilled employees, management needs to create a culture that fosters the desired behavior and that supports the natural motivation of employees to take pride in a job well done. Some aspects of the quality culture are:

1. There is a clear vision of the desired future and how to get there.
2. Management leads by example—if quality is number one, it is number one on management's agenda and decisions are made accordingly.
3. Performance standards are high, employees are held accountable for their actions and performance; feedback is frequent, with emphasis on positive feedback.

4. There is a lack of fear in the workplace, innovation/ improvements are encouraged with the understanding that sometimes mistakes will be made.
5. Individuals are respected and participate in the management of the organization to the extent of their capabilities.
6. Learning, individual and organizational, is valued.
7. Teamwork is fostered.
8. Adequate resources are provided.

Models of a Quality System

The Food and Drug Administration's (FDA) manufacturing regulations for drug products were published as Current Good Manufacturing Practice for Finished Pharmaceuticals in the Federal Register, Vol. 43, No. 190, September 29, 1978. These cGMPs along with various guidances published since 1978 provide the rules by which drug products to be sold in the United States must be manufactured. The cGMPs are not a good model of a quality system. They are not structured as a system, but are more a set of specific rules. In this limited sense, they define compliance but miss the mark in defining an adequate quality system. There are some significant flaws, vagaries, and omissions in them. The basic philosophy of these cGMPs is the philosophy of quality of the 1950s and 1960s—control, inspect, do not trust production, and the QC/QA department is responsible for quality. A good model of a quality system is provided by the FDA's Quality System Regulations for medical devices. It is based on the ISO 9000 standard. These regulations are based on a modern, up-to-date philosophy of quality. They view quality as a total system, hold management responsible for quality, and emphasize the importance of design and quality planning. Furthermore, FDA's inspections of medical device plants are system based.

Our recommended model of a quality system for a plant producing drug products is ISO 9000 : 2000, with the addition of the rules specific to drug products taken from the cGMPs. ISO gives the requirements for a quality management system, while the cGMPs gives the compliance requirements. The year 2000 version of ISO 9000 represents the current best thinking about quality and how to achieve it. Fig. 15.3 represents ISO's view of the quality system. ISO 9000 emphasizes the criticality of the role of top management for the achievement of quality products and processes. This role is described in detail in the document. Besides the emphasis on system and process, ISO highlights the importance of culture/ environment. "Through leadership and actions, top management can create an environment where people are fully involved and in which a quality management system can operate effectively." The Malcolm Baldrige quality award represents a still higher standard. It is very comprehensive, involving all aspects of the business. It's core values and concepts are similar to those of ISO 9000. Note the heavy weighting given to results. The winners of this award generally score in the 700's. It provides a useful tool for a self-assessment, a benchmarking tool, even if your organization does not want to go to the expense of applying for the award.

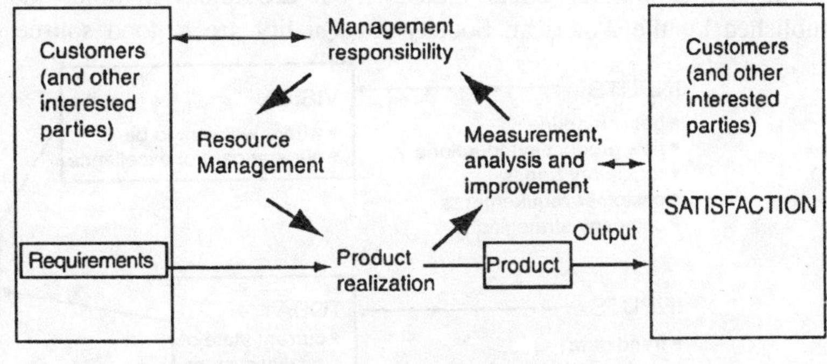

Fig. 15.3. Continual improvement of the quality management system.

After reviewing model quality systems like ISO, Malcolm Baldrige, or the European Quality Award, it is evident that cGMPs fall short of being a true quality system. They lack many elements common to these quality models such as leadership, planning, process orientation, and continuous improvement. A corollary concern is sometimes expressed that the pharmaceutical business is so regulated that a best practice quality system like ISO is not sufficient. However, a central tenant in all good quality systems is a customer focus, continuously evaluating customer needs/requirements and satisfaction. Companies that truly understand and put in practice these quality systems will have no trouble meeting regulatory customer requirements.

Quality Planning Process

In order to continuously improve the quality system, there must be in place a quality planning process. The purpose of this process is:

1. To evaluate the current quality system relative to the desired quality system, both short and long term.
2. To develop action plans and allocate resources so that the desired improvements in the quality system are achieved.
3. To monitor and measure performance against the plan.
4. To adjust the plan as needed.

This planning process represents the first four steps in the continuous improvement cycle, discussed in the section "The Quality Improvement Process."

The quality planning process begins with setting competitive standards, with creating the vision of excellence that ensures success and that focuses and motivates all employees. An important part of creating this picture of the desired future is benchmarking; both business and quality targets and the processes that enable the achievement of these targets. One can benchmark best internal performance and even other pharmaceutical plants/companies. However, some of the best quality practices are not found in the pharmaceutical industry, but are found in other industries. The books and magazines published by the American Society for Quality are a good source of best quality practices. One can

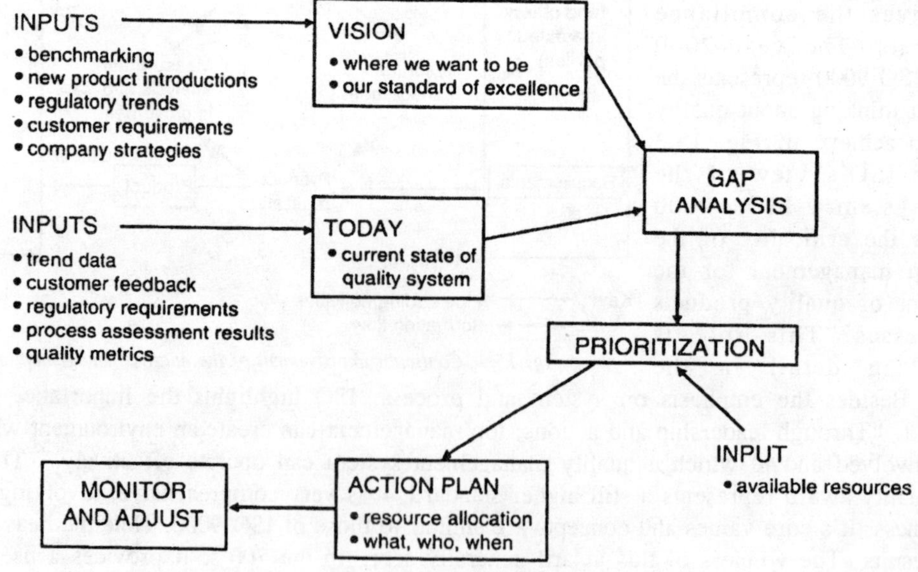

Fig. 15.4. The planning process.

also learn much from the Malcolm Baldrige winners. The second step is to honestly and accurately assess one's current state. The performance of process assessments has proven to be an effective tool for doing this. This method differs significantly from the traditional compliance audit. It focuses on efficiency as well as effectiveness in achieving standards. It looks beyond observations or symptoms for root causes. It focuses on the quality of the processes and their outputs. It borrows from the Malcolm Baldrige award the evaluation of:

1. Approach (process design and process ownership).
2. Deployment (training, resource allocation, and integration among departments and with other processes).
3. Results (continuous improvement of performance metrics).

Once the desired end-point is determined and the current situation is assessed, a gap analysis is completed and objectives are set to close the gaps. An important step in the process is the prioritization of objectives, based on balancing available resources with risks. The development of the plan is ideally a participative one, involving the maximum number of people. After the plan is developed, personal and team performance objectives need to be aligned with the goals of the plan. Finally, it is necessary to integrate the quality plan with the overall business plan. "What gets measured gets done." The health of the quality system and the effectiveness of the quality plan need to be monitored. Therefore selecting the right set of quality metrics is important. Traditionally quality costs are broken down into preventive, appraisal, internal failure, and external failure costs. A commonly used indirect measure of internal failure costs is not-right-first time. Cycle time is another useful indirect measure of quality. Process quality can be measured. Processes can be rated on a 1–5 scale where:

1. Process and ownership not defined, personnel are not trained, results show process is ineffective.
2. Process and ownership are defined, personnel are trained, process metrics are in place; but process is not always followed and results need improvement to meet minimum standards.
3. Process is consistently followed and results are satisfactory.
4. Process has been continuously improved in effectiveness, efficiency, and cycle time over the past 2 yr. It is appropriately fail-safe and mistake proof.
5. Based on benchmarking process is considered world class.

For each key process there should be a set of metrics. These process metrics could consist of process cost, effectiveness, right-first-time, and customer satisfaction. Examples of metrics for the change control process are:

1. Cycle time.
2. Changes made without an adverse product impact (%).
3. Number of changes successfully implemented per year.
4. Customer/employee satisfaction with change control process.
5. Completeness of documentation.

The quality metrics need to be reported to management so that they can determine the health of the quality system and take whatever action is necessary to improve it. The importance of metrics and their selection cannot be over emphasized. "People need an assessment of some kind to give them a sense of where they really are. They need to know the starting point from which they will proceed in improving the quality of their contribution."

Quality Improvement Process

The link between quality planning and quality improvement is execution. The continuous improvement cycle starts with benchmarking and internal assessment to arrive at a gap analysis. From the gap analysis an action plan with assigned leadership, resources, timelines, and metrics is developed. From this quality plan, the plant's human resources must successfully execute the plan for improvement to occur. It is the leadership's responsibility to assure that the plan is "do-able," appropriate and adequate resources are assigned, and that the culture of the plant supports change. This starts with the project leaders who must have not only the technical skills, but also the project management and people skills to accomplish the project. Training in the proper skills to lead a quality improvement project is available from many consulting firms promoting the concept of "Six-Sigma." People trained in these skills are often called "*Black Belts.*"

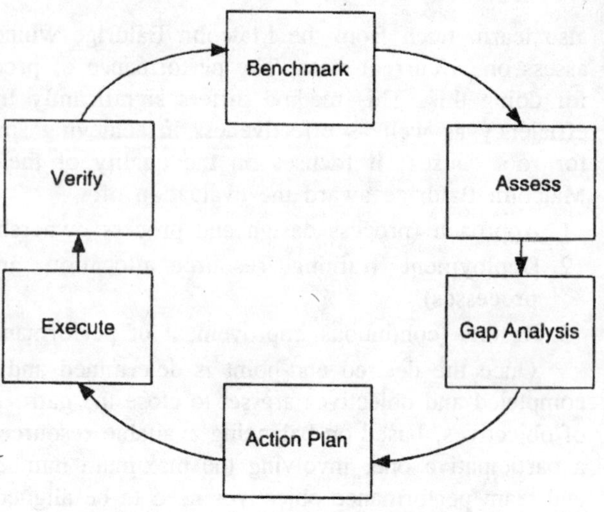

Fig. 15.5. The continuous improvement process.

Once the project has been completed and determined to be successful by appropriate metrics, it is time for management to reinforce the culture of continuous improvement through appropriate team rewards and recognition. It is best practice for the plant to reinvest some of the saving from any improvement in other improvement opportunities.

Responsibilities in the Quality System

Quality must be every employee's responsibility. The quality department will never succeed in forcing quality into products and processes. Instead, the plant's management team must, by their actions, hold each employee accountable for the quality of their work. Management must, in turn, assure that all employees understand the requirements, have the necessary skills, and have adequate time and resources to perform their job. The specific responsibilities of some key management personnel are:

1. Plant manager, the champion of quality
    - Establish the expectation that quality is everyone's responsibility by his leadership actions.
    - Establish in the total organization a quality culture of customer focus, continuous improvement, and accountability for quality.
    - Assure appropriate resources are provided for quality and compliance.
    - Make quality planning a prime component of the plant's planning process.
    - Recognize and reward quality performance.
2. Quality manager
    - Own the system/process assessment process.
    - Facilitate system/process design and improvement teams.
    - Assure the organization is adapting to changes in the external environment.
    - Develop the needed quality knowledge and skills within the organization.
    - Interpret the compliance and customer requirements.
    - Assure quality/compliance accountabilities are fulfilled by organization.
3. Production manager
    - Assure processes are performed, measured, controlled, and documented as designed.
    - Identify root causes of failures and implement preventive actions.

- Provide opportunity for the workforce to identify and implement quality and efficiency improvements of processes.

4. Engineering manager
   - Provide an infrastructure that is appropriate, calibrated, validated, controlled, documented, and maintained.
   - Provide technical support to the improvement process.
5. All employees
   - Focus on the customer, internal, and external.
   - Continuously improve one's process.

Leadership and Management

We have seen already that both ISO 9000 and the Malcolm Baldrige award criteria give prominence to the role of top management in establishing, maintaining, and improving the quality system. Visionary leadership according to the Malcolm Baldrige award:

1. Sets direction.
2. Creates customer focus.
3. Establishes clear and visible values.
4. Sets high expectations.
5. Creates strategies and systems to achieve excellence, stimulate innovation, build knowledge and capabilities.
6. Inspires and motivates the workforce.
7. Encourages all employees to contribute, to develop and learn, to be innovative, and to be creative.

To put these leadership goals into practice, we have established Quality Management Teams (QMT) in each of our plants. The QMT consists of the complete plant management team—quality, production, engineering, technical support, human resources, and finance. The plant managers chair the QMT to symbolize their responsibility for quality and because they have the power to assure all employees follow the quality principles. The purpose of the QMT is:

1. To provide plant management with a forum to exercise their responsibility for the establishment and maintenance of an adequate and effective quality system.
2. To foster a partnership to manage continuous improvement in quality by focusing on processes, people, and culture.
3. To jointly plan for improvement of the quality dimensions of business performance and to own the quality plan.

The QMTs meet monthly for at least an hour and quarterly for a more extended time to perform a complete review of the quality system and quality plan. Quality is fundamentally about customer focus. Both the pharmaceutical industry and the FDA have this in common; their customer is the patient. While quality control and quality assurance are important, best quality practice today emphasizes the management of the quality system. The quality system consists of important processes, highly skilled people, and an empowering/motivating culture. Training of personnel at all levels must be a priority for management. The recommended model of a quality system is ISO 9000 with the specific requirements of GMPs added. Continuous improvement of the quality system is assured by having an effective quality planning process. All employees must take responsibility for the quality of their work. A critical but difficult process is communication. Management must provide the direction (top–down), listen (bottom–up), and encourage cross-functional cooperation. It is clear that quality depends on the leadership of the organization.

16

Optimization Methods

Optimization of a formulation or process is finding the best possible composition or operating conditions. Determining such a composition or set of conditions is an enormous task, probably impossible, certainly unnecessary, and in practice, optimization may be considered as the search for a result that is satisfactory and at the same time the best possible within a limited field of search. Thus, the type and components of a formulation may be selected, according to previous experience, by expert knowledge (possibly using an expert system), or by systematic screening as described later. Then the relative and/or total proportions of the excipients are varied to obtain the best endpoint, or a process is chosen, and a study is carried out to determine the best operating conditions to obtain the desired formulation properties. Both of these are optimization studies. This article concentrates on statistical experimental design-based optimization.

Screening, Factor Studies, and Optimization

Systematic screening and factor influence studies are closely related to optimization, being often sequential stages in the development process and involving statistical experimental design methods. Screening methods are used to identify important and critical effects, for example, in the manufacturing process. Factor studies are quantitative studies of the effects of changing potentially critical process and formulation parameters. They involve factorial design and are also quite often referred to as screening studies; however, the resulting relationships have just as often been used for optimization.

The type of study carried out will depend on the stage of the project. In particular, experimental design may be carried out in stages, and the experiments of a factor study may be augmented by further experiments to a design giving the detailed information needed for true optimization. It cannot be stressed to highly that the quality of a statistically designed experiment depends on the choice of experimental run with respect to an a priori model, and this quality can and must be assessed before starting the experiments.

Brief Historical Review

Statistical methods for screening, factor studies, and optimization have been available for a long time: factorial designs since 1926; screening designs since 1946; and the central composite design for response surface optimization, was introduced by Box and Wilson, in 1951. Their use started to be described in the pharmaceutical literature from the early 1970s, but it was only from approximately 1988 that there was a sudden increase in the number of published articles, and the numbers have continued to rise. A conception or presupposition of the difficulty or complexity of experimental design had to be overcome. The change has been attributed of course to a great extent to the availability of computing power and of relatively inexpensive high-performance software that allows previously difficult or advanced methods to be applied. In particular, much attention is now being given to robust processes and formulation, and there are developments in treating non-linear and highly correlated responses.

Methods for Optimization

There are four primary methods. First, there is the statistically designed experiment, in which experiments are set up in a (normally regular) matrix to estimate the coefficients in a mathematical model that predicts responses within the limits of formulation or operating conditions being studied. This is generally the most powerful method, provided the experimentation zone has been correctly identified, and is the subject of most of this article. Second, the direct optimization method, the best known being the sequential simplex, is a rapid and powerful method for determining an experimental domain, best combined with experimental design for the optimization itself. Third, there is the one-factor-at-a-time method in which the experimenter varies first one factor to find the best value, then another. Its disadvantages are that it cannot be used for multiple responses and that it will not work when there are strong interactions between factors. Finally, the non-systematic approach in which the knowledge and intuition of the developer allow him to improve results, changing a number of factors at the same time is often surprisingly successful in the hands of a skilled worker. Where he is less skilled or less lucky, he can waste a remarkable amount of time and resources.

SCREENING

Obtaining a Formulation Suitable for Optimization

Once the dosage form has been selected, the excipients must be identified, their choice often limited by practical considerations of time and resources determined by patents, company practice, or according to expert knowledge. However, it may be possible or necessary to test a number of different excipients for each function, for example, several diluents, lubricants, binders. This approach has proved useful in drug–excipient compatibility testing in which protoformulations are set up according to a statistical screening design to assess stability and compatibility.

Here the *factor* is the excipient's function. This can be set at different levels, the level being the excipient itself. So the factor may be "binder," and the levels are, for example, HPMC, povidone, polyvinylacetate, and no disintegrant present. A mathematical model relates the response (in this case, degradation) to composition. It includes variables corresponding to each factor with (qualitative) levels corresponding to each excipient. Plackett and Burman described designs suitable for treating this kind of problem. Designs with the factors at only two levels are widely used. However, there are other designs at 3, 4, and 5 levels as well as asymmetric designs derived from them in which the various factors take a different number of levels.

It is assumed that there are no *interactions* between factors; that is to say, the effect of a given excipient on stability does not depend on what other excipients are found in the formulation. (The same reasoning applies to other kinds of factors or responses.) This can only be an approximation; however, if it should be necessary to take interactions into account, many more experiments would be needed, and it would probably be necessary to limit the number of levels for each factor to two for the number of experiments to be manageable.

The choice of excipients may be considered a qualitative optimization, their quantitative compositions not having yet been optimized. This and the fact that the process used will most likely be on a small laboratory scale may affect the affect the choice of excipients. However, it is in most circumstances an unavoidable limitation. This is an experimental design for testing the compatibilities of experimental drug (at two concentrations) with a number of number of excipients. The samples, which were wet granulated, were stored for 3 weeks at 50°C/50% relative humidity. The mean degradation level was high, at 6.2%, indicating a fairly unstable drug. The effects of each excipient were calculated by linear regression, or, because the design is orthogonal, by linear combinations of the responses. There, the degradation for each excipient is calculated in each excipient type (e.g., disintegrant), setting the excipients in the remaining type to a hypothetical mean value. Thus, the value for magnesium is the mean response for all mixtures containing magnesium stearate, and the effect of stearate on the response is the difference between this figure and the global mean.

Inspecting the results shows that the disintegrant and binder have major effects, and mixtures containing sodium starch glycolate and HPMC are more stable than those containing croscarmellose sodium and povidone, respectively. Diluents had only small effects here, however, these were much greater in the mixtures stored at low humidity, where mixtures containing microcrystalline cellulose or, especially, calcium phosphate were less stable than those containing lactose or mannitol. Thus, a capsule based on lactose, sodium starch glycolate, HPMC, and magnesium stearate (the last being selected for reasons of feasibility, there being no difference in stability between it and glyceryl behenate) was formulated and gave satisfactory stability.

Before Optimizing a Process

The major choice to be made here is that of equipment, and that will depend on what is available in the laboratory and also in the factory. There may be a very large number of factors to be studied, and it will probably be necessary to identify the critical factors before optimizing the process. This stage will probably be at the laboratory scale, whereas the optimization proper is carried out at pilot scale. Because process factors are usually quantitative and continuous, two levels only, at minimum and maximum values, are often tested in screening and factor influence studies. Thus, the highly efficient, two- level Plackett–Burman designs and two-level factorial designs may be used for screening. For example, in screening (assuming no interactions), up to 11 factors, (continuous or discrete or qualitative with two levels) may be tested by means of 12 experimental runs. The difference between minimum and maximum for each factor is generally quite large. Such a test clears the ground for optimization process.

Methods for screening factors

Because a large number of factors may need to be screened, the postulated model must be simple. It is usually assumed that the response(s) y depends only on the level (value or state) of each factor x_i separately and not on combinations of levels. The model is thus first-order, for example:

$$y = \beta_0 + \beta_1 x_1 + \beta_2 x_2 + \beta_3 x_3 + \beta_4 x_4 + \beta_5 x_5 + \varepsilon$$

If the factors are quantitative, they are set at their extreme values. Thus, if the factor is granulation time, and the possible range is 1.5–7 min, the normal values tested are 1.5 min and 7 min. They are expressed in terms of dimensionless *coded variables*, normally taking values –1 and +1. Thus, on transformation to the coded variable x_1, 1.5 min corresponds to $x_1 = -1$, and 7 min corresponds to $x_1 = +1$.

If the factors are quantitative, they may take any number of levels. Only two-level designs are described here. Qualitative levels are set arbitrarily at the coded levels. If, for example, the screening method was one of the factors tested, wet screening could be set at –1 and dry screening at +1 (or vice versa). Quite wide limits are generally chosen for screening quantitative factors. They are then often narrowed for more detailed quantitative study of the influence of factors where interactions between factors them are taken into account and for determining a predictive model for optimization. The designs, proposed by Plackett and Burman in 1946, comprise experiments in multiples of four. They will allow screening of up to one less factor than the number of experiments. Those with 2^n experiments (4, 8, 16, 32,...) are also fractional factorial designs. The non-factorial designs have particular properties and complex *aliasing*, which has been held to make their interpretation difficult but also gives them certain advantages over the fractional factorial designs. The 12-experiment design, shown in coded variables, is such a design, and is useful for about 7–11 factors.

The structure of the design is shown clearly in the table because the experiments are in their standard order. However, they should be carried out in a random order, as should all the designs described here, as much as is practicable. The coefficient β_i is the effect of the factor X_i, and is equal to half the average change in the response y when the level of the factor is changed from $x_i = -1$ to $x_i = +1$. It is estimated (as b_i) in the Plackett–Burman design by subtracting the sum of the responses for experiments for which $x_i = -1$ from those for which $x_i = +1$ and dividing by the number of experiments. Important and unimportant effects can then be identified according to their absolute values.

Use of results of a screening design

Estimation of the effects allows influential or possibly influential factors to be identified. Non-influential factors (small effects) will not require further study. They may be set at their midpoints, at their most economical values (e.g., a short mixing time), or at their apparently best value even if the measured effect is apparently non-significant. After elimination of these non-influential factors, there may still be too many factors to optimize in terms of the resources available (time, raw material, operators, availability of equipment, etc.).

Generally, these less influential factors are kept constant, equal to their best level and the remainder optimized. In more complex situations, it is advisable to carry out a more detailed study between the screening and optimization (response surface studies). This could be a completion of the screening study by means of a complementary foldover design or by a separate quantitative study to allow individual effects of the factors and/or their binary interactions to be calculated separately (shown in factorial designs, later). All these studies on the process are generally done after the optimization of the formulation. However, because the effects of formulation and process changes are not generally independent, it may become necessary to carry out some sort of process study at the same time as the formulation optimization.

Quantitative Process Studies Using Factorial Designs

Purpose

Whereas the purpose of a screening study is to determine which of a large number of factors have an influence on the formulation or process, that of a factor study is to determine quantitatively the influence of the different factors together on the response variables. The number of levels is usually again limited to two, but sufficient experiments are carried out to allow for *interactions* between factors.

Two-level full factorial designs

The simplest such designs are the 2^k full factorial designs, in which the experiments are all the 2^k possible combinations of two levels of k factors variables. Therefore, they consist of 4, 8, 16, 32, 64,... experiments for 2, 3, 4, 5, 6,... factors. Examples are given in Table 3 of the 2^2, 2^3, and 2^4 designs (each enclosed at the right and below by the solid lines). Thus, lines 1–4 of columns 1 and 2 show a 2^2 design for two factors, and lines 1–16 of columns 1–4 a 2^4 design for four factors. The design is transformed into an experimental plan (with the natural or experimental values of the factor variable at each level −/+ 1. The mathematical model associated with the design consists of the *main effects* of each variable plus all the possible *interaction effects*, interactions between two variables, but also between three and four factors and, in fact, between as many as there are in the model. However, although two-factor interactions are important, three factor interactions are normally far less so. Higher-order interactions are invariably ignored and the values determined for them attributed to the random variation of the experimental system.

Determining Active Factors from the Results of a Factorial Design

We take the four-factor model as an example. The complete synergistic mathematical model consists of the constant term, four main variables ($\beta_1 x_1 ... \beta_1 x_4$), six interactions between two factors ($\beta_{12} x_1 x_2$,...), four interactions between three factors ($\beta_{123} x_1 x_2 x_3$,...) and one between four factors. The last five of these are not generally expected to be important. The model is thus:

$$y = \beta_0 + \beta_1 x_1 \ ... + \ \beta_{12} x_1 x_2 \ ... \ + \ \beta_{123} x_1 x_2 x_3 \ ... \ + \beta_{1234} x_1 x_2 x_3 x_4 \ + \ \varepsilon$$

The effects (coefficients) β_i in the model are estimated, usually by multilinear regression. The values obtained b_i are estimates because of the random experimental error (represented by ε in the equation). The next step is to decide which of the 15 effects calculated are *active* or important.

The are a number of ways of doing this. If the experiments have been replicated, ANOVA will reveal which effects are statistically significant. Otherwise, we rely on the fact that most of the effects are probably small and distributed randomly about zero. Thus, we look for the effects with the largest absolute values that stand out from the others. Making a normal probability plot of the distribution of their values is a widely used method. The responses are usually treated separately; however, when there are a number of more or less correlated responses being studied, appropriate combinations (principal components) may be analyzed instead of the original responses. Once the important effects have been identified, a simplified model can be written. If an interaction term has been identified, the corresponding main effects should also be included in the model even if they are not all found active. Thus, if the interactions between the factors X_1 and X_2 and the main effect of the factor X_1 are active, $b_2 x_2$ should be included in the model as well as $b_1 x_1$ and $b_{12} x_1 x_2$.

Two-Level Fractional Factorial Designs

The number of experiments needed to study five or more factors in a full factorial design is large, and to determine the main effects and their interactions, a fraction of the full design is often sufficient. These are $2k—r$ fractional factorial designs, where $r = 1, 2, ...$ for the half, quarter, etc. fractions. Note that the first four columns are the same as the four factor, full-factorial design, and the column for the fifth factor is constructed by multiplying the first four columns together. Methods for constructing such designs and their limitations are described in many textbooks. Evidently, for the 2^{5-1} design, the 16 triple and higher interactions are not determined. In fact, they are confounded with the calculated effects. Thus, the estimate of the interaction between factors one and two includes the triple interaction between the other three factors. Because the latter is assumed negligible, this does not usually matter. Menon et al. studied the formation of pellets by fluid-bed granulation using this design. The five factors investigated were (X_1), the binder concentration; (X_2), the method of introducing it (dry or solution); (X_3), the atomization pressure; (X_4), the spray rate; and (X_5), the inlet temperature.

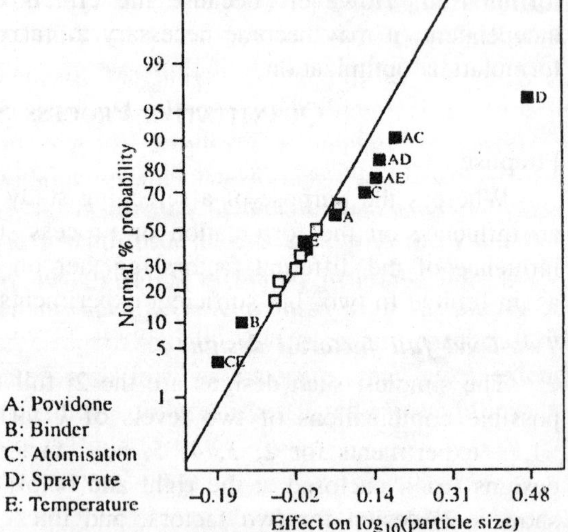

Fig. 16.1. Calculated effects form a two-level factorial design. Those to the left and right of the line are considered active.

The coefficients of the model are calculated by linear regression (the logarithm of the particle size was used here) and then plotted as a cumulative distribution of a normal plot. The important coefficients are those that are strongly positive or negative, for example, the spray rate b_4 and the interaction between atomization pressure and inlet temperature b_{35}. Others not identified on the diagram are not considered significant and could well be representative mainly of experimental error. The equation can thus be simplified to include only the important terms. However, if interactions are included, their main effects should be included also, even if they are small. Here, we have:

$$y = \beta_0 + \beta_1 x_1 + \beta_2 x_2 + \beta_3 x_3 + \beta_4 x_4 + \beta_5 x_5 + \beta_{13} x_1 x_3 + \beta_{14} x_1 x_4 + \beta_{15} x_1 x_5 + \beta_{35} x_3 x_5$$

Information that Can Be Obtained

The significant main effects are identified and also quantified. Thus, increasing the spray rate over the range studied will give an increase in the log(particle size) of twice 0.24, representing a more than threefold increase. However, it can be seen that there is an interaction with the binder concentration; that is, the effect of spray rate depends on the amount of binder in the formulation. The effects of increasing spray rate are shown for both high and low levels of binder; the effect of spray rate is much greater at high levels of binder. However, the effect of binder also interacts with two other factors, the atomization pressure and the inlet temperature. Thus, the individual variables cannot be considered separately. Note also that there is a great deal of information often hidden in large designs, and, in particular, indications on factors affecting the robustness of a process may sometimes be extracted.

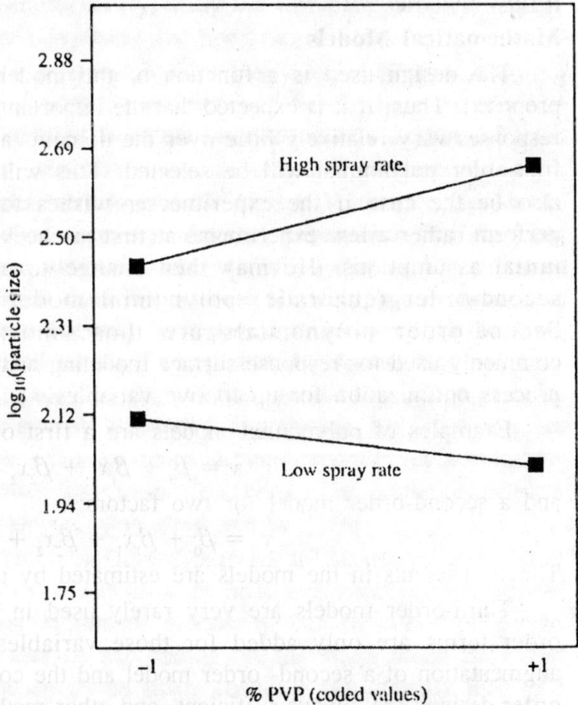

Fig. 16.2. Calculated effects from a two-level factorial design. Interaction diagram for spray rate and % povidone on particular size.

Use of Center Points

In both screening and factor-influence studies in which the factor is quantitative, it is tempting to interpolate between the upper and lower limits. This is useful if only to find a more restricted zone for further study. However, in the case of a screening study, the limits studied are often so wide that it would be most unlikely for the estimated model to be accurate enough for prediction, and there is also likely to be curvature of the response surface over the experimental domain. Such attempts are less risky for the more detailed factorial studies, but even then, they should be used with caution.

Adding center points (experiments at the center of the domain, coded co-ordinates 0, 0,...0 is useful for factorial and screening experiments), even though they do not enter into the calculation of the model equation because:

1. They are often a priori at or near the most interesting conditions;
2. They allow identification of curvature in the responses (by comparing calculated with measured responses);
3. If they are replicated, the experimental reproducibility may be assessed; and
4. They may allow extension of the experiment at a subsequent stage to a central composite design for modeling of response surfaces.

EXPERIMENTAL DESIGNS FOR PROCESS OPTIMIZATION (INDEPENDENT VARIABLES)

In this section, we look at methods of obtaining a mathematical model that can be used for qualitative predictions of a response over the whole of the experimental domain. If the model depends on two factors, the response may be considered a topographical surface, drawn as contours or in 3D. For more factors, we can visualize the surface by taking "slices" at constant values of all but two factors. These methods allow both process and formulation optimization.

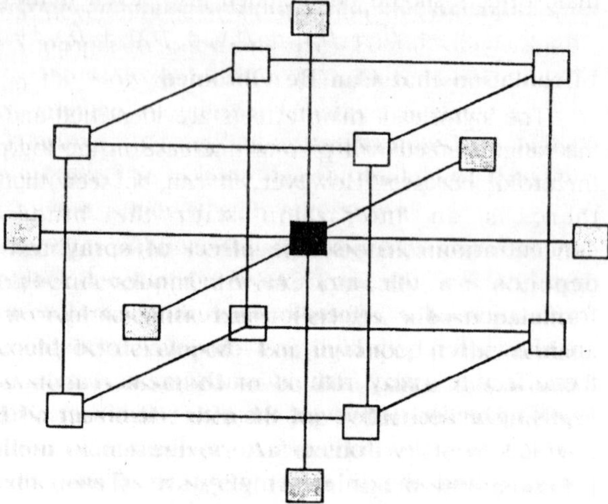

Fig. 16.3. Central composite design for three factors. The factorial points are shaded, the axial points unshaded, and the center point(s) filled.

Mathematical Models

The design used is a function of the model proposed. Thus, if it is expected that the important responses vary relatively little over the domain, a first-order polynomial will be selected. This will also be the case if the experimenter wishes to perform rather a few experiments at first to check initial assumptions. He may then change to a second-order (quadratic) polynomial model. Second-order polynomials are those most commonly used for response surface modeling and process optimization for up to five variables.

Examples of polynomial models are a first order model for five factors:

$$y = \beta_0 + \beta_1 x_1 + \beta_2 x_2 + \beta_3 x_3 + \beta_4 x_4 + \beta_5 x_5 + \varepsilon$$

and a second-order model for two factors:

$$y = \beta_0 + \beta_1 x_1 + \beta_2 x_2 + \beta_{12} x_1 x_2 + \beta_{11} x_1^2 + \beta_{22} x_2^2 + \varepsilon$$

The coefficients in the models are estimated by multi- linear least-squares regression of the data.

Third-order models are very rarely used in the case of process studies and, in any case, third-order terms are only added for those variables where they can be shown to be necessary (i.e., augmentation of a second- order model and the corresponding design). This does not mean that second-order designs are always sufficient, and other methods of constructing response surfaces may sometimes be useful.

Statistical Experimental Designs for First-Order Models

The design must enable estimation of the first-order effects, preferably free from interference by the interactions between factors other variables. It should also allow testing for the fit of the model and, in particular, for the existence of curvature of the response surface. Two-level factorial designs may be used for this.

Important points to note when using a first-order model, with or without interactions, are that:

1. Maximum and minimum values of responses are of necessity predicted at the edge of the experimental domain;
2. The first-order model should normally be used only in the absence of curvature of the response surface. If the experimental values of the center points are different from the calculate values (i.e., there is lack of fit), then the response surface is curved and a second-order design and model should be used; and
3. The experimenter should test for interaction terms between two factors in the model. If interactions seem to be important he should make sure that they are properly identified.

Statistical Experimental Designs for Second-Order Models

Central composite design (Box–Wilson design)

This is the design most often used for response surfaces. It is a combination of a factorial with an axial design with experiments at a distance of $\pm\alpha$ along each axis (thus, the name). It requires a relatively large number of experimental runs, which can be a disadvantage if resources are limited. However, it can be carried out in two stages: the factorial design first then the axial design if the results are satisfactory. If we wish to study the system by varying the parameters around a point of interest, the domain is a sphere, and the coordinates of axial experiments are outside those of the factorial ones. α is chosen to give the best statistical properties (e.g., constant prediction precision) and lies between 2 and approximately 2.4. Center-point experiments must be done as part of both stages. Another advantage is that each factor is at five levels, thus allowing testing of lack of fit and for the possible need for cubic terms in the model.

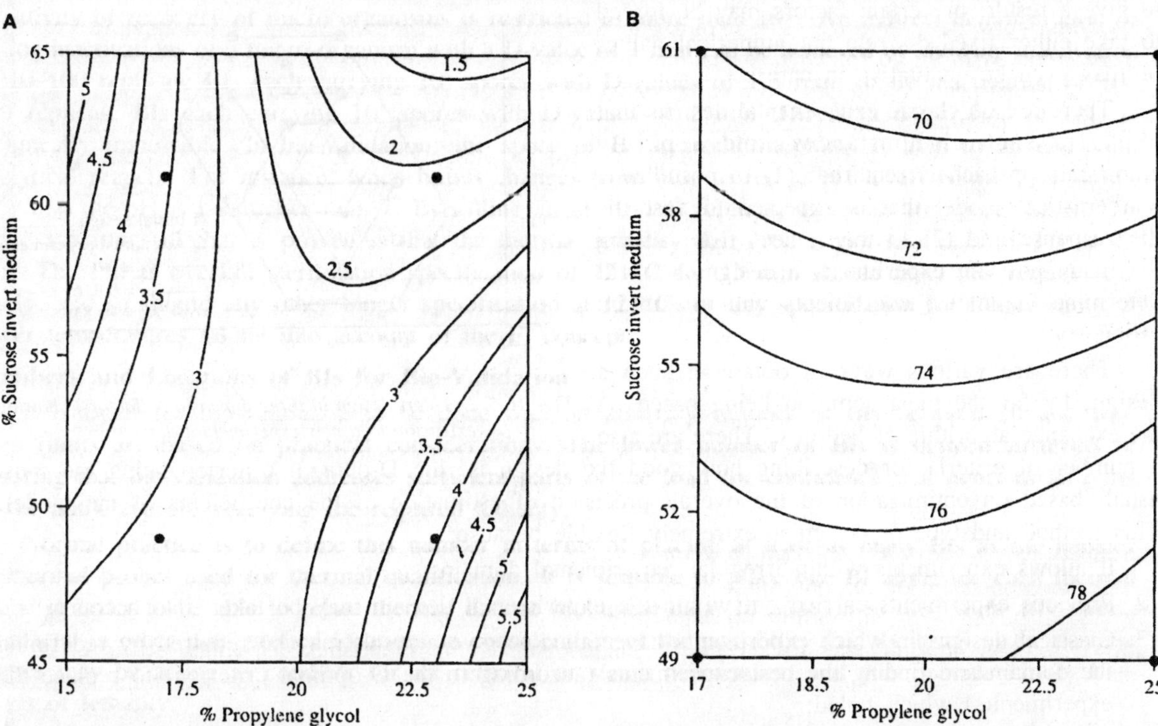

Fig. 16.4. Contour diagrams of (A) turbidity and (B) cloud point as function of % propylene glycol and source invert medium.

Other standard designs

The central composite design is most often used, however, there are others whose particular properties make them particularly useful. One of these is the Doehlert design, which is part of a continuous hexagonal network. It requires slightly fewer experiments than does the central composite design but cannot be set up by augmenting a factorial design.

It can be seen that the hexagonal design for two factors is the first seven rows and the first two columns. Thus, it possible to add a factor to a design. Another advantage is that because it is part of a continuous network, it allows the experimental domain to be shifted in any direction by adding experiments at one side of the domain and eliminating them at the other. Vojnovic et al. give an example of its use in granulation.

Hybrid designs are saturated or almost saturated designs; that is, they have only enough experimental runs to calculate the coefficients of the quadratic model (10 runs for 3 factors 16 runs, for 4 factors, and 28 runs, for 6 factors). They are useful when the responses are not expected to vary enormously but where the quadratic model is esteemed necessary and resources (in possible numbers of experiments) are low. If the experimental region is defined by maximum and minimum values of each factor, then the domain is "*cubic.*" The central composite design can be applied to such a situation, the axial points being set then at ± 1, coded values corresponding to the minimum and maximum allowed values.

Mixed and Irregular Domains—D-Optimal Designs

If the experimental domain is cubic and spherical or spherical, the standard experimental designs can normally be used. However, the domain may be irregular in shape as certain combinations of values variable may be excluded a priori for technical reasons or may even have been tried and failed to give a result, or certain factors may be forced to take either fixed discrete but numerical values or may even be qualitative in nature.

There are no classic experimental designs that exist for such circumstances, and a purely empirical approach is required: (1) to postulate a mathematical model that is expected to describe the response and (2) to then select from among the many possible experiments a design that will determine the model coefficients with maximum efficiency.

There are various ways of obtaining such a design, by far the most common being based on the exchange algorithm of Fedorov. There are also a number of criteria for describing how good the design is, the D-optimal criterion being the most usual, based on optimization of the overall precision of estimation of the coefficients of the model. This method and type of design is extremely flexible because:

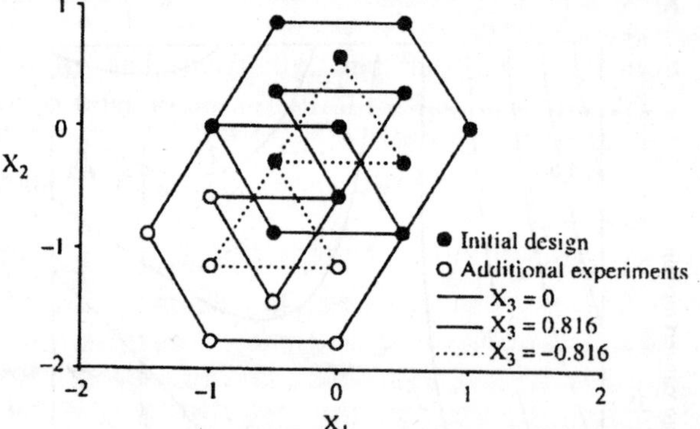

Fig. 16.5. Doehlert design in three dimensions (factors) showing extension to a new experimental domain.

1. It allows experiments within irregular experimental domains;
2. Previous experiments carried out within the experimental domain may be taken into account;
3. Classical designs in which experiments have failed to give a result may be repaired by redefining the domain and finding the best experiments (according to the D-optimal criterion) to replace the experiment(s) which failed;
4. The models may be polynomials with missing coefficients, or even non-polynomials;
5. The experiments may be carried out in two or more stages, with models of increasing complexity;
6. Further experiments may be added to a D- optimal design to validate the model (lack of fit); and
7. They can be used for mixture models with constraints.

In conclusion, a wide variety of experimental designs is available, allowing the design to be selected according to the problem in question, rather than adapting the experiment to the design.

Experimental Design for Formulation Optimization (Mixture Designs)

Formulations almost invariably consist of mixtures of a drug substance and excipients. Their properties usually depend not so much on the quantity of each substance present as on their proportions. The total comes to 100%, so the number of independent variables is one less than the number of components. This has the effect that the models and the designs have particular properties, and the designs described above (screening, factor studies, and response surfaces) normally cannot be used. The entire topic of mixture designs is fully described by Cornell.

Mathematical Models for Mixtures

Because there is one less independent variables than the number of components, the polynomials take a particular form. For example, for three components, where the response y has a first-order dependence on the fractions x_1, x_2, x_3, because $x_1 + x_2 + x_3 = 1$,

$$y = \alpha_0 + \alpha_1 x_1 + \alpha_2 x_2 + \alpha_3 x_3 + \varepsilon$$

becomes

$$y = \beta_1 x_1 + \beta_2 x_2 + \beta_3 x_3 + \varepsilon$$

The variables cannot be varied independently. If there are no upper and lower restraints on the proportions of the components, the domain for three factors can be described as a equilateral triangle whose apices represent the pure components. A four-component mixture is described by a regular tetrahedron. For five components, the equivalent 4D figure must be imagined.

Just as the first-order mixture model has a different form from that for independent variables, so does the second-order design:

$$y = \beta_0 + \beta_1 x_1 + \beta_2 x_2 + \beta_3 x_3 + \beta_{12} x_1 x_2 + \beta_{13} x_1 x_3 + \beta_{23} x_2 x_3 + \varepsilon$$

The special cubic model describes a certain third- order curvature in the response surface.

$$y = \beta_0 + \beta_1 x_1 + \beta_2 x_2 + \beta_3 x_3 + \beta_{12} x_1 x_2 + \beta_{13} x_1 x_3 + \beta_{23} x_2 x_3 + \beta_{123} x_1 x_2 x_3 + \varepsilon$$

Mixture Designs and the Simplex Experimental Domain

The equilateral triangle and regular tetrahedron are described above as the domain of a mixture where all possible compositions of the components are allowed for are regular simplexes. (In the remainder of the section, they are referred to as simplexes.) Such circumstances in which there are no composition restraints are rare in formulation. However, if each component is present at a minimum level, and no other constraints are imposed, then the domain is also a simplex. Designs in this case, primarily attributed to Scheffe, are derived very simply. That shown in Fig. 16.6 for three components is suitable for first-, second-, and partial third-order models. The latter is the central composite design and is quite commonly used. Test points for checking model fit are also shown.

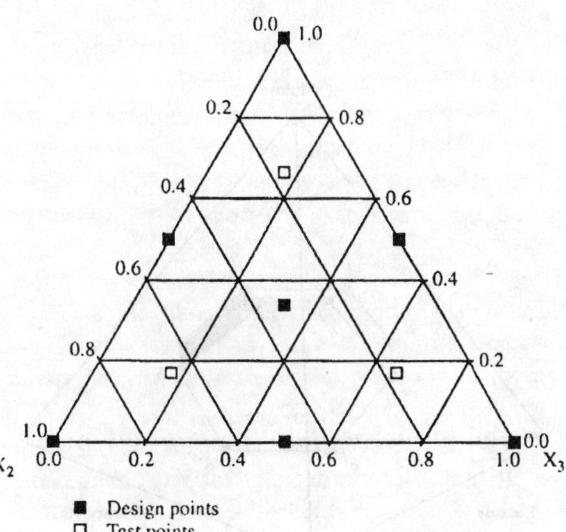

Fig. 16.6. Scheffe central composite design for three factors. Open squares are test points.

Constrained Systems and Pseudocomponents

Simplex designs are quite rarely used because such circumstances in which there are no composition restraints are rare in formulation. However, if each component is present at a minimum level, and no other constraints are imposed, then the domain is also a simplex. An example could be of the solubility of a drug being tested in ternary or quaternary mixtures of pharmaceutically acceptable solvents. The single constraint might be that a minimum percentage of water is required. In any case, the experimental domain would be a regular simplex, and standard designs may be used. In the case of solid dosage forms, simplex domains are rarer still. A possible example might be a study of the optimum composition of a diluent in a tablet formulation, the proportions of the active substance and other excipients being held constant. The diluent might consist of a mixture of lactose, microcrystalline cellulose, and starch, and its composition might then be adjusted to obtain optimum tableting properties as well as rapid disintegration and dissolution (for rapid action of the drug after the patient swallows the tablet). Again, standard experimental designs such as the simplex-centroid design may be used.

Constrained Systems and Non-Simplex Designs

Limits in the amounts of excipients present normally lead to the domain taking on an irregular shape. Each component must be present within a given concentration range to fulfill its function. For example, lactose or cellulose may make up most of the amount of a tablet or capsule, whereas magnesium stearate is limited to between 0.5 and 2%. In particular, when there are both upper and lower limits, the space is almost invariably non-simplex. Mixture models (such as those of Scheffe) are still useful, especially when there are three or more such excipients with fairly large ranges of variation. In solid formulations, this is often the case for diluents (or fillers) and also for the polymers or waxes incorporated into controlled-release tablets to form a matrix through which the drug diffuses slowly out when immersed in aqueous fluid, i.e., in the gastrointestinal tract.

The experimental designs of non-simplex experimental regions are D-optimal for the selected model, obtained by an exchange algorithm. Thus, we have the example of the optimization of a sustained-release tablet for which the release rate of a highly water-soluble drug was limited by its diffusion though a matrix. The matrix-forming substance is a cellulose derivative swelling in water (hydroxypropyl-methylcellulose) but the diluents microcrystalline cellulose, lactose, and calcium phosphate also have a role. These four components were varied as well as the percentage of drug substance (to have two doses at constant tablet mass), and the experimental domain defined. A D-optimal design was then

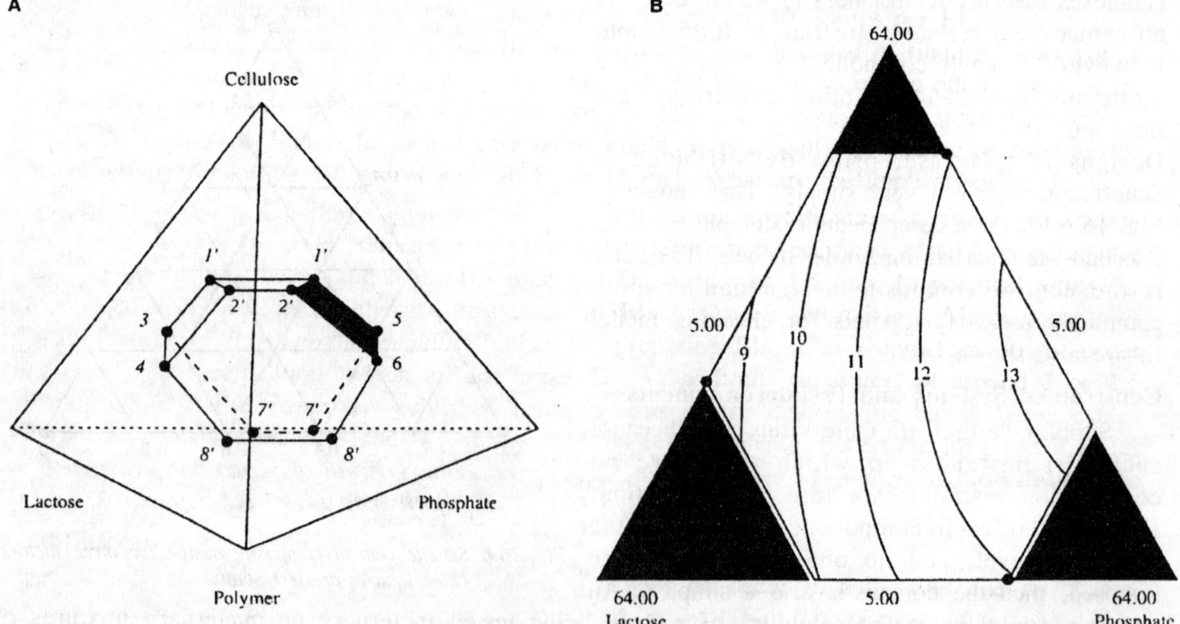

Fig. 16.7. D-optimal mixture design. (A) definition of the design space. (B) Contour plot of mean dissolution time at 25% polymer content.

obtained for a second-order mixture model (using an exchange algorithm), the experiments performed, and the results analyzed by multilinear regression to give response surfaces as contour plots. The formulation could thus be optimized to give the required drug release profile. It is interesting to note that the work was done in two stages. Initially, experiments were chosen for a first-order mathematical model from the projected second-order design. These were carried out first, to check that there was no problem and that the experimental domain was adequate, before doing the remaining experiments for a predictive model that could be used for optimizing.

Conditions for Independent Variable Designs

If one of the components (for example, a diluent or solvent) is in considerable excess, and the limits for all other components are narrow in comparison, then it can be eliminated from the analysis because its concentration changes little. The concentrations of the remaining components can then be treated as independent variables, and the methods described previously can be applied without using the special considerations for mixtures.

Optimization Methods Using Response Surface Methodology

Graphical Methods

It is usually relatively simple to find the optimum conditions for a single response that does not depend on more than four factors once the coefficients of the model equations have been estimated, provided, of course, that the model is correct. Real problems are usually more complex. In the case of pellet formation, it is not only the yield of pellets that is important but also their shape (how near to spherical), friability, smoothness, and ease of production. The optimum is a combination of all these. One possible approach is to select the most important response, the one that should be optimized, such as the yield of pellets. For the remaining responses, we can choose acceptable upper and lower limits. Response surfaces are plotted with only these limits, with unacceptable values shaded. The unshaded area is the acceptable zone. Within that acceptable zone, we may either select the center for maximum ruggedness of formulation or process or look for a maximum (or minimum or target value) of the key response.

Graphical Optimization of Two Opposing Responses

When there are only two independent factors (including the case of three mixture components), the responses may be plotted on a single graph. Graphics programs that allow plotting of upper and lower allowed limits of the responses, with portions of the diagram where there the responses are outside the limits shaded, are useful because they allow an acceptable zone to be identified very rapidly. The objective was to reduce the turbidity as much as possible and to obtain a solution with a cloud point less than 70°C. A level of invert sucrose as high as possible was preferred (in spite of its deleterious effect on the cloud point). Slices were taken in the propylene glycol, sucrose plane (X_2, X_3) at different levels of polysorbate. An optimum compromise formulation is found at approximately 58% sucrose medium, 4.3% polysorbate 80, and 23% polyethylene glycol. The method becomes difficult with four independent continuous factors, and for five or more variables, the method is totally impracticable despite its simplicity. The number of "slices" to be examined is simply too high—up to 125 diagrams to be displayed or plotted. Under such circumstances, the desirability method must be used.

Desirability

Derringer and Suich described a way of overcoming the difficulty of multiple, sometimes opposing, responses. Each response is associated with its own partial *desirability function*. If the value of the response is optimum, its desirability equals 1, and if it is totally unacceptable, its value is zero. Thus, the desirability for each response can be calculated at a given point in the experimental domain. An overall desirability function can be calculated by multiplying all of the r partial functions together and taking the rth root. Evidently, if the desirability for any response is zero at a point, the overall desirability there is also zero. The optimum is the point with the highest value for the desirability. The experimenter should study the contour plot of the desirability surface around the optimum and combine this with contour plots of the most important responses. A large area or volume of high desirability will indicate a robust formulation or set of processing conditions. A number of different forms, linear, convex, concave, unilateral, bilateral, are available for the dependence of the partial desirability on the value of the response. Weighting of responses is also possible. The method requires appropriate computer software, but it is a very powerful method of optimization, and with practice, it is relatively easy. It is especially appropriate for four or more factors. McLeod et al. gives an example.

Limitations of Response Surface Methodology

The approach of using a mathematical model to map responses predictively and then to use these models to optimize is limited to cases in which the relatively simple, normally quadratic model describes the phenomenon in the optimum region with sufficient accuracy. When this is not the case, one possibility is to reduce the size of the domain. Another is to use a more complex model or a non-polynomial model better suited to the phenomenon in question. The D-optimal designs and exchange algorithms are useful here as in all cases of change of experimental zone or mathematical model. In any case, response surface methodology in optimization is only applicable to continuous functions.

Lately, there has been a great deal of interest in the use of artificial neural networks in many fields, including that of prediction and expert systems, and they are of interest here for the description of response surfaces that have a non-linear relation to the factor variables. In such cases, the response surface may well fit the data better than that calculated from the model estimated by least-squares regression. However, the choice of experiments is still important for the artificial neural network approach, and it is best selected in a regular pattern. The central composite design, in which each factor takes five levels, is a generally a good compromise. Great care must be taken not to "overfit," and, in general, more experiments are required than for the classic RSM approach.

Searching for a New Domain

Steepest Ascent Method and Optimum Path Methods

Screening and factor studies will sometimes indicate whether, and if so, where we should search for an optimum within the domain being studied. However, if the optimum (we are considering a single "key" variable here) lies outside the present experiment, then the steepest ascent method comes into its own. The direction of steepest increase of the response in terms of the coded variables is determined, and then experiments are carried out along this line. If a maximum or minimum value (according to the target) is found along this line, the point at which it is found could be the center of a new experimental design for optimization. The optimum path method is similar and is used for extrapolating from a second-order design along a curved trajectory.

Sequential Simplex Optimization

Unlike the other optimization methods described here, the sequential simplex method for optimization neither assumes nor determines a mathematical model for the phenomena studied. A simplex is a convex geometric figure of $k+1$ non-planar vertices in k dimensional space, the number of dimensions corresponding to the number of independent factors. Thus, for two factors, it is a triangle, and for three factors, it is a tetrahedron. The method is sequential because the experiments are analyzed one by one as each is carried out. The basic method used a constant step size, allowing the region of experimentation to move at a constant rate toward the optimum. However, a modification that allows the simplex to expand and contract, proposed by Nelder and Mead in 1965, is more generally used. It has been reviewed recently by Waters.

Optimization by the extended simplex method

Assume that we wish to optimize a response depending on three to five factors without assuming any model for the dependence other than the domain being continuous. We choose an initial domain and place a regular simplex in it. The experiments for the initial simplex are then carried out and the response measured. In the basic simplex method, an experiment is done outside the simplex in a direction directly opposite to the "worst" point of the simplex. The worst point is discarded, and a new simplex is obtained, the process being repeated. The simplex therefore moves away from the "poor" regions toward the optimum. In the extended simplex method, if the optimum is outside the initial experimental domain, we may leave it rapidly while expanding the simplex for a region with an improved response. As the simplex approaches the optimum, it is contracted rapidly. Of the experiments of a given simplex let *W*, *N*, and *B* be the "worst" (*W*), "next worst" (*N*), and "best" (*B*) points of the initial simplex. A new experiment *R* is carried out opposite point *W* to give a new simplex reflecting the original one. Depending on the value of the response at *R* relative to that at *W*, *N*, and *B*, the step size may be expanded to arrive quickly at the region of the optimum, and then be contracted around the optimum. "$R > W$" means that point *R* is better than point W, etc.

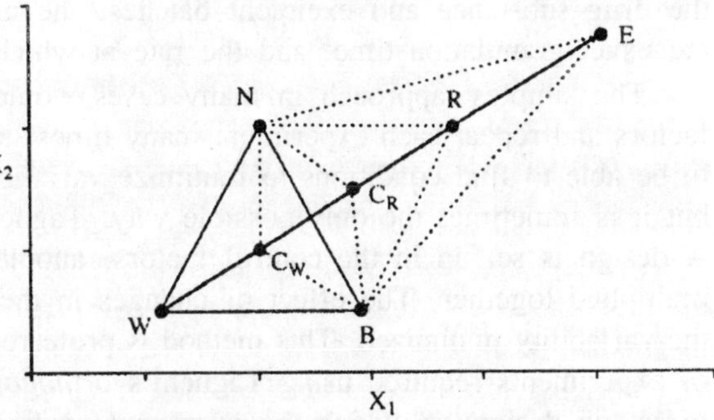

Fig. 16.8. Summary of the expanded simplex method of Nelder and Mead.

R replaces *W*	if:	$N \leq R \leq B$	Reflection
	or:	$R > B$ and $E \leq B$	
E replaces *W*	if:	$R > B$ and $E \leq B$	Expansion
C_R replaces *W*	if:	$W < R \leq N$	Contraction (exterior)
C_W replaces *W*	if:	$W > R$	Contraction (interior)

At the end of the sequential simplex, if more detailed information is needed, the experimenter may carry out a response surface study around the supposed optimum.

Designing Robust Processes and Formulations

Until now, optimization and improvement have been taken as being equal or closer to what is considered most desirable with respect to the mean responses. However, it is also necessary that all units of all batches manufactured fall within those specifications. Apart from variation in the measurement method, all variation is attributed to the manufacturing process and the manufacturing and storage environment.

Taking the traditional quality control approach, any product that is within the specifications will pass and is considered equally good. However, one might still normally consider that the nearer the response to the target, the better the product. Therefore, the key is to choose a formulation and/or condition that gives a product not only as close as possible to the target, but with as little variability as possible. The basic concepts and seminal work in this field are from Taguchi, who stated that any product whose performance characteristics are different from the target values suffers a loss in quality, which he quantified by a parabolic function. He then classified factors as: (1) *control factors*, which can be controlled under normal operating conditions and (2) *noise factors*, which are difficult, impossible, or very expensive to control. The effects and interactions of control and noise factors could be measured by means of an experimental design, and then settings of the control factors would be determined that would minimize the effects of the noise factors. One problem in such an approach, apart from the difficulty of controlling noise factors, is to know what they are. Examples of possible noise factors are the drug substance and excipient batches, the ambient temperature and humidity, the machine used, the exact granulation time, and the rate at which liquid is added.

The simplest approach in many cases would be to set up an experimental design in the control factors and repeat each experiment many times, hoping for enough natural variation in the noise factors to be able to find conditions to minimize variation. This requires a very large number of experiments, but it is sometimes the only possible way. Taguchi's solution was to vary the noise factors artificially. A design is set up in the control factors, another (factorial) design in the noise factors, and the two multiplied together. The effect of changes in the noise factors can thus be assessed at each point and the variability minimized. This method is preferred to the previous method, but non-etheless, the number of experiments required using Taguchi's *orthogonal networks* is extremely high. Now it is more usual to set up designs in which the number of experiments, although still high, is minimized and to find regions where the response is equal to the target value and is at the same time highly insensitive to the noise factors. The design must allow interactions among noise factors, and not only the control factors themselves, but preferably all the terms in the control factor model. It should be noted that there is a great deal of information "hidden" in large factorial designs (n = 16). When analysis shows that only a few factors are significant, the residuals (differences between calculated and measured values) may be analyzed. A small spread of residuals under certain conditions as opposed to others may indicates better reproducibility of the process or formulation under these conditions.

Lead Optimization

Sensible lead candidate selection for preclinical development and registration should reduce the high rate of drug attrition, the cost of which increases with the distance that the failed drug candidate has proceeded down the research and development pipeline. It is estimated that "adverse" toxicokinetic and safety factors encountered during animal and human exposures in drug development account for approximately 60% of the reasons for termination during development. Of this 60%, a combination of undesirable animal and human toxic events account for 21% of the total factors involved. Rates of attrition are high, especially during the early regulatory toxicology and clinical phases of testing. Not surprisingly, because of the large number of hits identified from primary high-throughput screens, lead candidate optimization has, therefore, emerged as a critical decision-making milestone from both ethical and commercial perspectives. Essentially, the "old" or, in many cases, current, strategy is to take several lead candidate compounds through early small-scale clinical pharmacological/toxicokinetic/safety studies in vivo before a final selection is made following 1 month toxicology exposures on the lead development drug candidate for clinical exposure. Any later problems with the compound may then facilitate the design of a lead optimization "screen" at an earlier stage for possible follow-up compounds. A more modern and desirable approach would be (and is used in many cases now) to insert a mandatory in vitro ADME-Tox "screen" at the stage before the preliminary in vivo ADME-Tox exposures, which would then produce a "clean" lead development candidate (LDC) for full regulatory testing. In short, there is a need for early rapid and robust screening assays which that will allow a lead series of compounds to be ranked for desirable or undesirable characteristics.

These preclinical lead optimization technologies (PLOT' S), must be sufficiently rapid to interface with high-throughput screens without creating a further pipeline bottleneck, be predictive of drug failure,

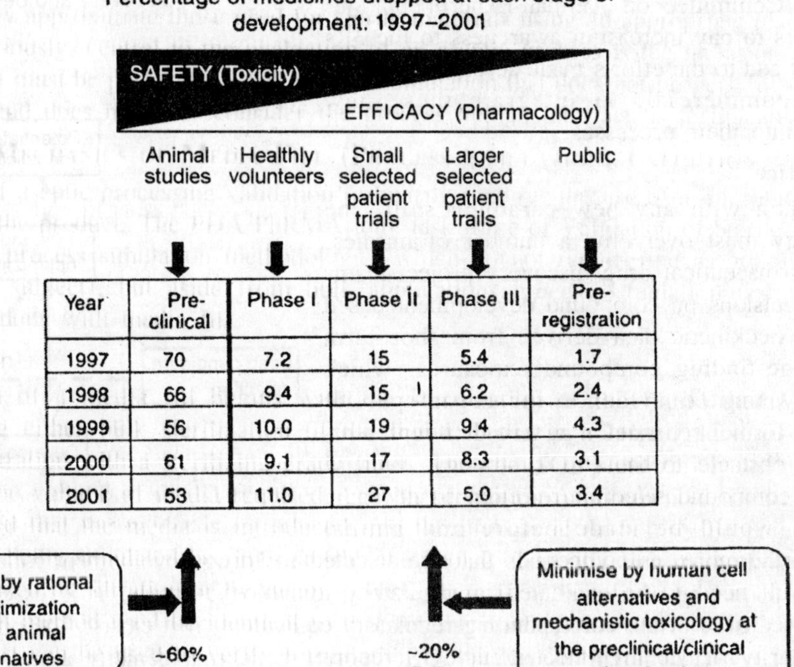

Year	Pre-clinical	Phase I	Phase II	Phase III	Pre-registration
1997	70	7.2	15	5.4	1.7
1998	66	9.4	15	6.2	2.4
1999	56	10.0	19	9.4	4.3
2000	61	9.1	17	8.3	3.1
2001	53	11.0	27	5.0	3.4

Fig. 16.9. Tabular representation of preclinical and clinical testing phases of drug development at which new compounds have been shown to fail for toxicokinetic and safety reasons.

and be highly cost-effective. The assays which constituting the PLOT platform are typically in vitro systems, miniaturized and amenable to automation, thereby achieving the required throughput with minimal compound use, another crucial and limiting factor for facilitating the process of lead optimization. Industry recognition of the Three Rs (3Rs) of *reduction*, *refinement*, and *replacement*, through the implementation of ethical review processes (ERP), have been partly instrumental in the increasing acceptance and incorporation of alternative in vitro models in early drug development. Additionally,

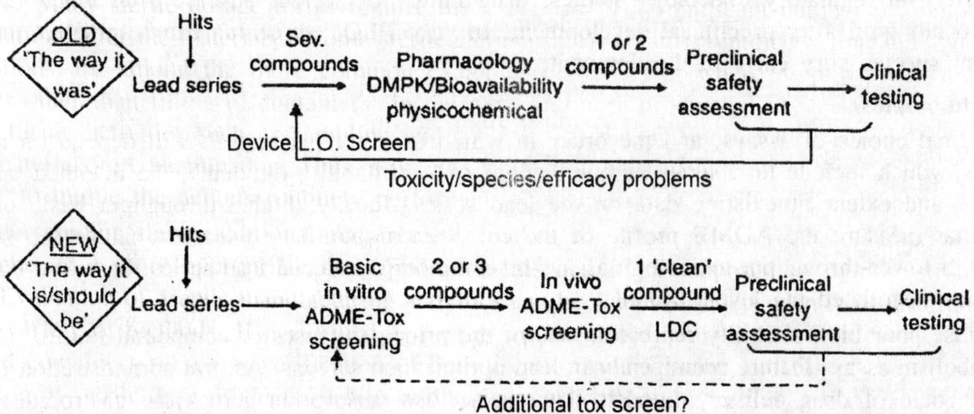

Fig. 16.10. Diagramatic representation of old and new strategies for lead optimization of new pharmaceutical molecules.

pressure from other bodies such as the UK House of Lords Select Committee on Animal Experimentation, for researchers to pay increasing awareness to the 3Rs will hopefully add to the efforts made across all sectors, public and commercial, to integrate these new technologies into their processes.

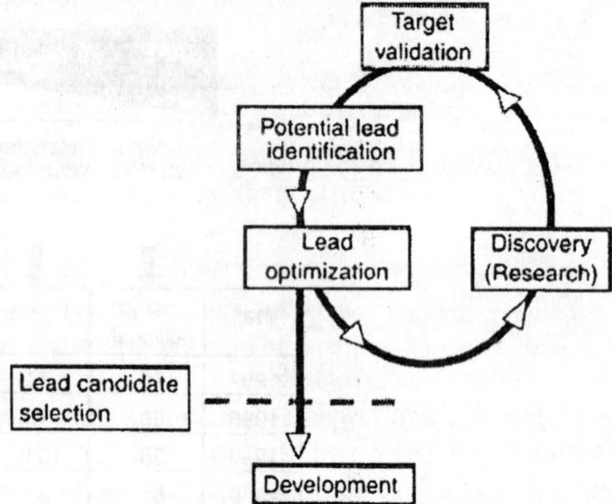

Fig. 16.11. The R&D "pipeline" in modern drug development.

Plot in Practice

In common with any new paradigm shift, the PLOT strategy must overcome a number of hurdles. Hitherto, pharmaceutical drug discovery project teams have made decisions on compound development based largely on toxicokinetic data derived from short-term in vivo, range-finding compound exposures, which provide very limited evidence for organ-specific toxicity. This former reliance on in vivo data represents a significant obstacle to the PLOT strategy, because decisions on compound selection/rejection based on in vitro PLOT would be made before any animal exposure. Furthermore, as compounds that are selected for drug development following assessment by PLOT will still need to be evaluated in regulatory toxicology studies, it is essential that the PLOT screens are predictive of the corresponding regulatory equivalent, if it exists. The point is well illustrated by the popularity of the high-throughput SOS reporter gene mutagenicity assay, which gives results that correlate well with the regulatory gold-standard Ames assay, and requires one-tenth of the amount of compound compared with the micro-Ames assay.

There are many individual reasons for preclinical/clinical drug failure. These include mutagenicity, target organ toxicity, and poor bioavailability, the last being a result of a number of factors including poor absorption across the gastrointestinal tract, rapid clearance, or metabolism. A major factor for preclinical/clinical failure is the lack of suitable, practical, and/or sensitive biomarkers for target organ toxicity from which hazard and risk prediction can be extrapolated cross-species. It is anticipated that the advent of Molecular Toxicology (i.e., toxicogenomics and proteomics—see later sections) will add considerable impetus to the toxicology biomarker area and incorporation into clinical pathology test batteries during drug development. Finally, unless the correct non-rodent species is selected for predicting human safety in regulatory toxicology studies, drug failure or serious adverse drug reactions (ADRs) may not occur until after preclinical development. In vitro PLOT screening can help select the correct non-rodent species very early in development.

Plot Technologies

The final choice of assays, and the order in which they are performed, will depend on a number of factors, which include lead series number, compound availability (amount), the intended target, and the nature and extent of existing data on the lead series. Ideally, higher-throughput basic or level 1 screens that measure the ADME profile of the compounds should be used to analyze the large lead series, with lower-throughput toxicology assays reserved for a reduced lead series, based on compounds which have negotiated the level 1 filter.

Because poor bioavailability represents one of the principal causes of compound failure, absorption and metabolism assays feature prominently in lead optimization screens. As oral administration represents the ideal route of drug delivery, models that predict low absorption across the gastrointestinal (GI) tract are commonly employed. Caco-2 cell assays have been widely used to predict drug uptake across the GI track, and a good correlation between in vitro and clinical data certainly exists for certain drugs. This assay can also predict compounds that are substrates for the P-gp transporter, which leads to the undesirable efflux of an absorbed drug back into the lumen of the gut, resulting in its excretion. One draw back of the Caco-2 is its relatively low throughput, and so the parallel artificial membrane permeability assay (PAMPA) is increasingly used as a higher-throughput assay for the cost cost-effective assessment of passive drug absorption. Because these artificial membrane lack the cellular proteins associated with the active transport/efflux, or indeed metabolism, Caco-2 assays or cell lines transfected with specific drug transporters and human P450s may be used as a second and third tier for compounds with high permeability in the PAMPA assay.

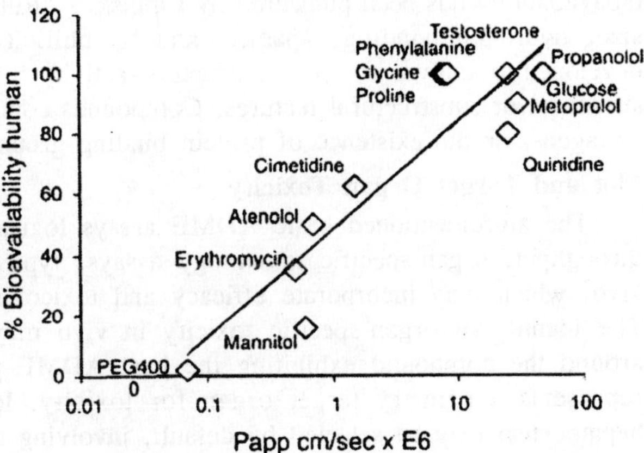

Fig. 16.12. Graphical representation of correlation between human bioavailability data for a series of known drugs and Caco-2 cellular permeability data.

This principle of offering minimal core assays to screen large lead series applies well to the assessment of metabolism, which would be included as a level 1 assay. In vitro metabolism assays might initially concentrate on compound stability in the presence of hepatocytes, microsomes, or an S9 extract, but extend to drug interactions on a more restricted series because apparent metabolic stability may be a result of inhibition of P450 function. As CYP3A4 accounts for ×40% of the total cytochrome P450 in man, and is responsible for the metabolism of ×50% of clinically used drugs, it makes sense to screen the inhibition or induction of this enzyme. Modulation of CYP3A4 activity is traditionally investigated by measuring enzyme function, i.e., testosterone metabolism or looking at enzyme levels by polymerase chain reaction (PCR) or Western blot, which may not be a cost-effective approach for large series lead optimization.

However, recent advances in our understanding of the molecular basis for CYP3A4 induction have identified the PXR (pregnane X receptor) as being important in drug- induced expression of this and other CYPs. Consequently, PXR reporter gene assays are being used to screen drugs with the potential to induce CYP3A4, with positive results justifying a more intensive investigation. Other enzymes worth consideration are those where the existence of functional polymorphisms could limit the geographical market for a drug.

Mutagenicity testing is normally performed fairly late in compound development; however, as regulatory genetic toxicology testing in our laboratories consistently produces 20–25% in vitro positive results each year—which at best results in significant delays while further investigations are conducted or, at worst results, in compound failure—a faster and earlier screen is required. As described above, there now exist high-throughput reporter gene assays for mutagenicity, such as the SOS/umu assay. This has low compound requirements, and is suitable for inclusion in the PLOT platform. The basis for this microassay, originally developed by Oda et al. and adapted by Reifferscheid et al., is that *Salmonella typhimurium*, carrying the SOS DNA repair gene fused to a reporter, respond to DNA damage by transcribing the fusion gene whose expression is correlated with the extent of DNA damage. A mammalian reporter assay, in which the human DNA repair genes are fused with a reporter, is currently unavailable and eagerly awaited.

In Silico Plot

Because compound availability will typically be limiting in terms of compound use, there is clearly an advantage in being able to perform computational physiochemical predictions of compound partition coefficients, isoelectric points, and solubility, based on structure. The computational prediction of drug bioavailability has been pioneered by Lipinski's "Rule of Five," which is based on compound molecular size, hydrogen bonding capacity, and lipophilicity. Increasingly sophisticated packages are being developed to analyze compound structure–activity relationships (SAR), i.e., ascribing toxicity to certain structures or substructural features. Compounds containing aromatic amines will be flagged as potential mutagens, or the existence of protein binding groups will be used to identify potential sensitizers.

Plot and Target Organ Toxicity

The aforementioned basic ADME assays logically precede compound investigation in the lower-throughput, organ-specific toxicology assays, typically selected on the basis of single exposures in vivo, which may incorporate efficacy and toxicokinetic endpoints, subject to compound availability. The identity of organ-specific toxicity in vivo may stimulate the synthesis of a further lead series around the compound exhibiting the best ADME profile in the level 1 screens. Because the liver represents a primary target organ for toxicity, level 2 screening for hepatotoxicity (e.g., using hepatocytes) may be selected by default, involving measuring enzyme release or metabolic activity by using primary hepatocytes in vitro. Although access to fresh human hepatocytes is always likely to remain problematic, it is anticipated that technical improvements will overcome current shortcomings in the quality of cryopreserved cells. The increasing acceptance of in vitro assays by the regulatory bodies may also influence the choice of organ cultures. The ICH S7B Safety Pharmacology guideline, for instance, recommends cardiac toxicity to be evaluated on all new pharmaceuticals by investigating their potential to cause a delayed ventricular response in vitro in isolated cardiac Purkinje fibers and/or human cell lines transfected with HERG channels, alongside measurements in conscious animals.

An alternative rationale for the selection of level 2 assays can be based around the intended target tissue; thus, drugs designed to target the central nervous system or immune system would warrant the use of level 2 assays to screen for, e.g., neurotoxicity or immunotoxicity, respectively. A second area where immunotoxicicity screening would be especially important are clinical indications involving immunocompromized patients, where a functional assessment of the immune system is required as part of the preclinical development. These would include HIV and transplantation patients, who would be especially vulnerable to compounds with even minimal immunotoxic side effects. The in vitro assessment of reprotoxicity and teratogenicity have typically employed the low-throughput mouse whole-embryo, micromass, or xenopus assay. However, recent progress has been made in this area with the validation of an in vitro embryotoxicity assay employing a stem cell line, which is amenable to higher throughput and represents a genuine level 2 in vitro assay. In summary, level 2 in vitro assays are employed to select, from lead compounds associated with the least target-organ toxicity, by using an appropriate in vitro screen. This process of in vitro screening, alternated with in vivo exposure, may even extend beyond lead candidate selection in situations where lead candidate failure necessitates a lead follow-up series to be synthesized and screened in vitro by using PLOT platform.

Irritancy, Corrosivity, Sensitization, and Phototoxicity

This is an area of significant advancement for industrial chemical notification and registration where several in vitro techniques have been legislated in favor of animal tests in certain scenarios or take their place in tier-testing strategies. The European Medicines Evaluation Agency (EMEA) has also taken a positive stand on the replacement of animal studies by in vitro methods. There is not a widespread use of primary in vitro screening assays by pharmaceutical companies to detect potential skin and eye toxicity in the lead optimization process. However, as some of these assays will be required as part of the worker safety/transportation/preclinical regulatory package, there are instances when these tests should perhaps be considered as part of the selection process. In vitro assays exist that may be suitable for the assessment of skin and eye toxicity, some of which have received recent acceptance of by the EU regulatory authorities under the 27th Adaptation to Technical Progress following their successful validation by ECVAM. Accepted tests currently include measurement of skin corrosivity (i.e., EpiDerm or rat skin transcutaneous electrical resistance) and phototoxicity (3T3 cells). Other assays undergoing validation may already be acceptable to the regulatory authorities on a case by case basis (i.e., eye irritancy); however, in the absence of a positive result, an animal test would still be required. In addition to corrosivity and phototoxicity, it is anticipated that in vitro assays will ultimately allow irritancy and sensitization to be predicted.

In addition, when considering pharmaceutical compounds requiring intravenous, ocular or topical routes of administration as a strategic part of their development plan, then the same consideration for early in vitro screening should be made. In fact, if the final development plan for a particular therapeutic class indeed required such routes, then the lead optimization process (or some later preclinical selection step) could screen for these eventualities at an early stage.

Molecular Toxicology and Plot

It has been stated that there are no toxicologically relevant outcomes in vitro or in vivo, with the possible exception of rapid necrosis, that do not require differential gene expression arising through mRNA transcription or stabilization. These "stress" gene responses constitute an evolutionary developmental means by which an organism can protect itself from a hostile external environment, and activate survival or "*self-destruct*" processes through apoptosis. Thus, the use of microarray technology [gene expression microarrays (GEMs or ToxChips)] to establish gene expression "*fingerprints*" or expression patterns following compound exposure, and thus to develop screening systems for in vitro lead optimization processes, has become attractive to preclinical scientists interested in drug safety. For more in-depth information on the type and extent of stress genes and their expression patterns, the reader is referred to Refs. In addition to the measurement of gene expression, it is now possible to perform high-throughput proteomic profiling on cell extracts or body fluids by using platforms such as Ciphergen' s protein chips or specific protein profiles using antibody arrays. The analysis of protein vs.versus RNA may be preferable where the correlation between gene expression and protein is poor, where there is a low dynamic range for RNA upregulation, or in situations where protein function is post-translationally regulated (e.g., by phosphorylation) for instance. Furthermore, because biomarkers may be readily found in blood and urine, they provide a non-invasive source of starting material for proteomic analysis. Ultimately, this process will identify a lead development candidate molecule (lead candidate selection), by virtue of its failure to switch on "patterns" of stress genes or toxicity genes. The type of logistics potentially involved in preclinical toxicogenomics, where lead candidates are tested in organotypic cultures or in vivo to look for evidence of toxicity using molecular endpoints in conjunction with traditional methodologies. Comparison with existing in vivo and emerging in vitro databases will increasingly allow the prediction of compound toxicity, allowing further rounds of lead optimization to be performed in vitro to find cleaner drugs. This toxicological PLOT screen would, then, allow lead development candidate molecule selection by employing higher-throughput molecular technologies.

Cellular and Molecular "Tools in Regulatory Toxicology

Following lead candidate selection and progression to the regulatory safety assessment program, toxicogenomics can be once more used, to complete various aspects of the preclinical and clinical hazard and risk assessment process: this involves applying the same basic technologies as described

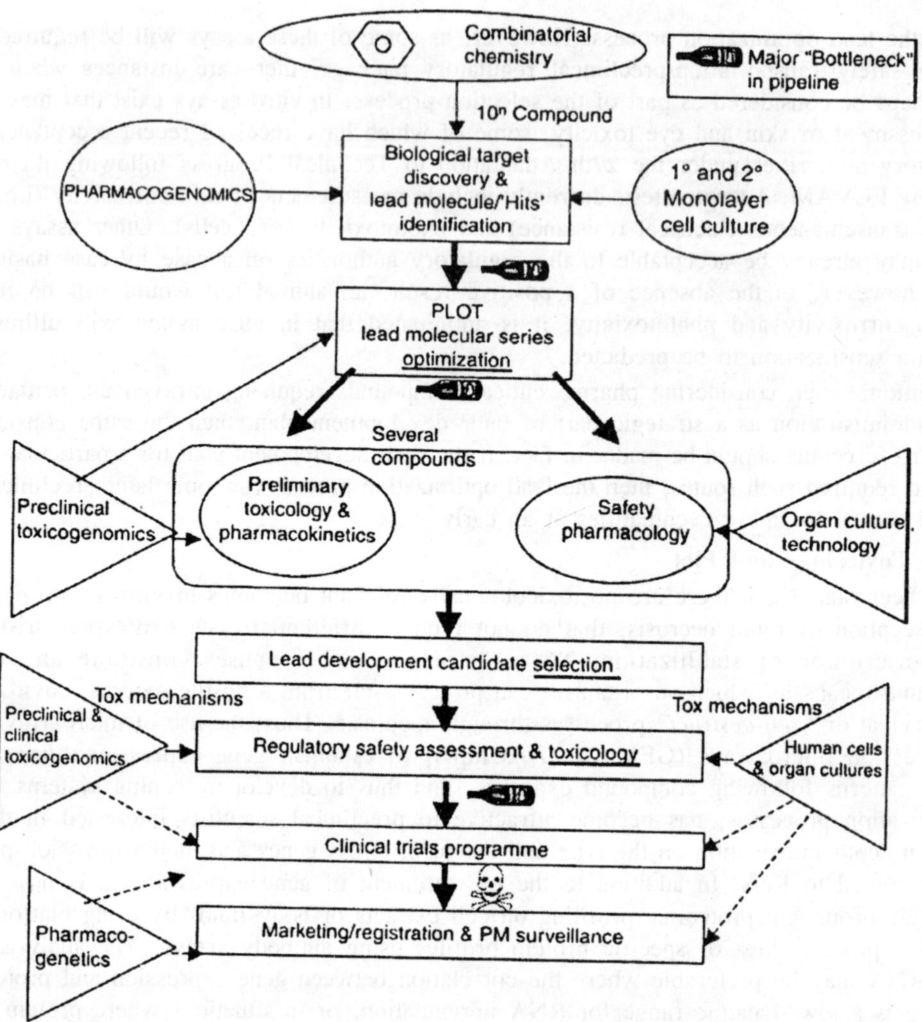

Fig. 16.13. Diagrammatic representation of the different stages in drug discovery and development showing where pharmacogenomics, toxicogenomics, and pharmacogenetics can be applied to a more "sophisticated" paradigm in tandem with the use of various cell culture technologies.

above. However, there may be differences in interpretation of data, and more emphasis may be placed on the use of cells (*in vitro* or *ex vivo*) from non-rodent (e.g., dog or primate) species and humans. This would help to facilitate risk assessment as one moves from animal to human safety and Phase I clinical trials, as well as the administrative and regulatory processes associated with new drug development.

Single nucleotide polymorphisms (SNPs) are single nucleotide differences present throughout the genome, which differ between unrelated individuals. Where they result in changes to the coding region of genes, the cSNPs may affect protein efficiency or specificity, which may ultimately result in adverse drug reactions (ADRs), as in the case of some of the P450 polymorphisms. This problem is well illustrated by certain CYP2C9 polymorphisms and warfarin-associated haemorrhaging. The availability of SNP databases will increasingly permit pharmacogenetics to reduce the uncertainty in predicting an individual's response to new medicines by SNP profiling. Pharmacotoxicogenetic analysis of such SNPs will add information and enable a better selection to be made of volunteers or patients, and will ensure optimal safety/efficacy assessment for drug-tailored trials and therapies with the registered drug. The importance of pharmacotoxicogenetics has not been lost on the regulatory bodies, and there is already an ongoing dialogue between the European Medicines Evaluation Agency and the pharmaceutical industry, to discuss the implications of this technology for the design of clinical trials.

Hurdles and the Way Forward

It is of paramount importance to bear in mind that applying preclinical and molecular clinical technologies to regulatory drug development toxicology and human risk assessment, as described above, may preclude some pharmaceutical organizations from take-up on this strategy until the regulatory perspective is more clearly defined. Toxicology bioinformatics databases (containing gene expression data) are evolving that also contain conventional histopathology, hematology, and clinical chemistry data, in attempts to link these new molecular technologies with those biomarkers already established and familiar to regulatory toxicologists. Commercial organizations, as well as academic and governmental

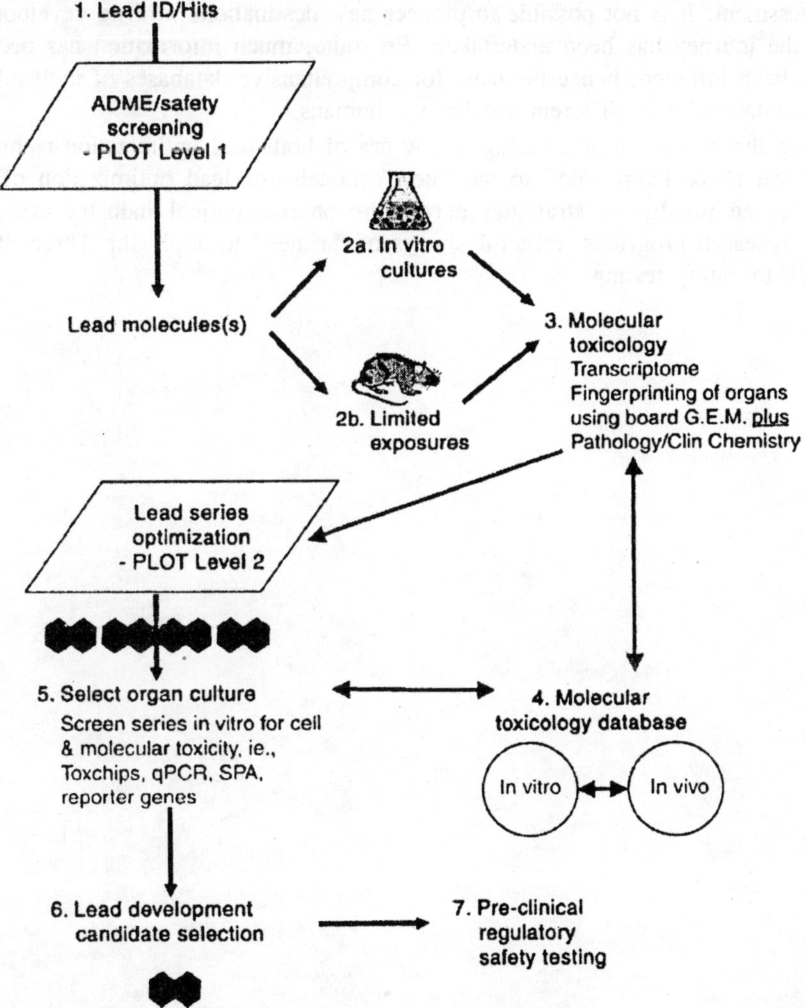

Fig. 16.14. A potential strategy for the selection of a lead development candidate molecule using toxicogenomic technology.

regulatory agencies, are now mindful of this need and are using both in vivo and in vitro exposure data to this end for both pharmaceuticals and industrial chemicals. In particular, human and rat hepatocytes have recently been extensively used for such validation studies and toxicogenomic data incorporated into databases alongside in vivo animal exposure data. In addition, (and from a pragmatic perspective), there may be the need to redefine the formal risk-assessment process (from a quantitative standpoint) in progressing from animal to first human exposure in terms of these new and relatively unknown "sets" of sensitive molecular biomarkers which may result in different no-observed effect levels/lowest observed effect levels, from the classical toxicopathological endpoints, and thus in potentially different levels of safety margin factoring in risk assessment.

In this paper, we have attempted to describe how basic ADME level 1 and organ toxicology level 2 PLOT platform assays can interface with high- throughput screens to help make decisions on selection of a lead development candidate. It is envisaged that histopathology will increasingly be used in parallel with more-sensitive open gene array or proteomic analysis of tissues following in vivo exposures, as a means of identifying new "batteries" of toxicopathological biomarkers for preclinical toxicology and human safety assessment. It is not possible to pioneer new destinations in drug development and safety assessment until the journey has been undertaken. En route, much information has been collected and "casualties" have been inflicted, hence the need for comprehensive databases of molecular toxicological informatics to be established in different species vs. humans.

It is clear then that we are now entering a new era of both lead optimization technology and drug development. As we move from "old" to the "new" models for lead optimization of pharmaceutical molecules, harmonized preclinical strategies across the pharmaceutical industry are gradually being incorporated into research programs, mindful always of the need to apply the Three 3Rs principles of Russell and Burch to safety testing.

17

VALIDATION OF A LIMS SYSTEM

LIMS systems are computerized information management systems. These have been increasingly widespread since the 1980s onwards not only in the pharmaceutical world, but also in the forensic, food, medical devices, clinical trials, academic and research and development arenas; and in general in all sectors of industry that have, as a common characteristic, a need for a source of laboratory information organized in a such a manner that it allows easy handling. A minimum workflow for a typical laboratory can be the following:

1. Creation of a sample.
2. Analysis.
3. Calculations of physical or chemical parameters.
4. Analysis report.

To reproduce these minimum tasks electronically, the main reasons for which a company or institution has LIMS are:

1. Organized storage and retrieval of information generated in the laboratory, either across a site or a corporation.
2. Dedicated chain of custody of information.
3. Reporting.

The above-mentioned features may be performed either automatically or manually, but other secondary desirable features are now increasingly becoming more important.

1. Automated data collection.
2. Automatic reporting.
3. Interfacing with other business systems.

That means that the industry is adopting the available technology very quickly, particularly as the cost–benefit ratio is more attractive now than previously. For example, the features available today for servers, workstations, storage devices, and network hardware make the systems more and more complex in structure not only in terms of the hardware involved but also in terms of the software features available, while the costs have not increased at the same rate.

Regarding the software, LIMS can be seen as a client–server application that stores data in a centralized database, composed of many tables. There are several database models available, but nowadays the most important, from the LIMS perspective, is the relational model, which allows for easier design and use of customized databases. There are, though, some points in which the use of these systems differ between industries. In particular, and because of the regulations affecting the pharmaceutical and medical devices industries, the design, use, and features of any LIMS system will be different from those in other industries where there are fewer regulatory restrictions.

LIMS Software Development Lifecycle and Validation

Validation in a software context means "confirmation by examination and provision of objective evidence that software specifications conform to user needs and intended uses, and that the particular requirements implemented through software can be consistently fulfilled." In the case of a LIMS system, validation starts from the same moment of gathering the business and regulatory requirements for such a system. Whatever the requirements may be, there are a number of basic areas to consider in a LIMS application, whether bespoke or standard-off-the-shelf software. These are the database and its tables. If the system is a standard commercial one, it will be supplied with a set of minimum database tables in order to run as supplied. That can be enough for some laboratory needs, although it is almost always necessary to customize the number and layout of the tables composing the database. In the case of full-bespoke systems, that task will be carried out from scratch, designing the whole set of tables (and their corresponding relations).

There are two important types of tables composing a database. One group is formed by the so-called *dictionaries*, which store "*static*" or support data composed of product specifications, tests, calculations, users, in short, all the information not directly associated with a sample. The other group of tables is related to information associated with sample results, which means values entered either manually or automatically as a result of performing tests on samples using laboratory instruments. The most important of all the tables in a typical sample-oriented LIMS is the samples table, which stores all the sample-related information by means of indices. The key index is normally the sample number, which is automatically generated by the application.

There are two scenarios for the development and customization of the LIMS database and its tables (also called the "*back end*" of the LIMS). The LIMS might rely on its own proprietary-developed database or on a widely available, non-proprietary database management environment. Use of open or well-known models such as SQL, My-SQL is recommended, otherwise a very well-tested and documented model, instead of starting with a new model for databases. This is for reliability, support, and maintainability of the system itself. The LIMS team must decide to which model the database will adhere. Normally LIMS supplier companies also provide database support for their products for both design and maintenance. Where the LIMS design will rely on an open database, there are several tools available to accomplish those tasks.

The front-end of any LIMS system is composed of the user interface and its elements (macros, scripts, routines, etc.), and outputs (data tables, reports, exported files, etc.). Again, a commercial-off-the-shelf application will be supplied with a minimum set of screens and elements to facilitate the interaction with both the end- user and the database, while in a custom-built application all the screens must be built from the ground up. It will be very unlikely that two laboratories, even as part of the same company, could ever use the same front-end application layout, since the screens and their associated elements are related to each particular laboratory's needs, tasks, and products or materials for analysis. In the case of a commercial application, it will come supplied with developer tools for screen customization, report creation, script editing, and whatever is necessary to set up a system from the front-end side. If the system is going to be built from scratch it is advisable to use well-known, supported, and documented applications for its development. In particular, it is good engineering practice to use code writers, compilers, and profilers that have been broadly tested and are well-known in the industry.

The remaining area that requires detailed attention is the interfacing of the LIMS with instruments for automatic data collection, and with other systems for data exchange. This is a relatively new area in industry but due to the availability of cheaper, more reliable and higher capability hardware is growing steadily. Interfacing to instruments is a business decision that may require very different levels of work, depending on the nature of the instruments to be connected. In general, the LIMS can be interfaced either directly or indirectly to the instruments: in the first case this is done by means of a commercially available or company developed interface. Such a bespoke interface requires detailed knowledge of both the instrument electronics and software and the LIMS end, but nonetheless it is not normally a huge task. Indirect interfacing is found when an instrument (or a series of them) is connected to the LIMS application by another software system acting as signal collector and digitizer, which then parses the data into LIMS. This is normally the case found in chromatography equipment, for instance, when specialized software such as chromatography data systems act as instrument data controllers, sending the sample-related data onto the LIMS application afterwards. The amount of work done by the LIMS team is, therefore, variable.

Interface with other business systems comes from the need of two or more business users to share of the same piece of information. This concept should be borne in mind when buying a LIMS or when starting to develop a new one, regardless of the timescale. Every LIMS design should keep open the options of exchanging data with other business systems. It is clear now that the amount of work necessary on development, customization and validation, once the LIMS project and its philosophy have been agreed by the user company or institution, will depend upon the end-users, business and regulatory needs, and on the decision to develop a fully bespoke system or to customize an existing commercial one.

Validation Roadmap — Requirements for a New or Existing System

The main "user" of the LIMS will be the quality assurance department. It will use the LIMS to organize its laboratory duties and to store and report the information for the analyses generated. That information will be represented in several ways, and decisions will be made using this information that will impact on the business itself. Also, inputs and outputs to and from the system might have an impact on other departments' operations. Hence, whether the need is for a new application or an existing one is judged to be insufficient for the business, at the outset, the LIMS team must gather all the requirements from the different departments and affected users of the system. Typical requirements specify:

1. All inputs the system will receive.
2. All outputs the system will produce.
3. All functions the system will perform.
4. All performance requirements the system will meet (data throughput, reliability, timing, etc.).
5. Definition of all internal, external, and user interfaces.
6. Operating environment for the software (hardware and operating system).
7. All ranges, limits, defaults, and specific values the system will accept.

There are many techniques available to actually gather the requirements for a solution. In the pharmaceutical industry the best way to effectively carry out this exercise successfully is to determine the requirements for each concerned area separately. This is based on the nature of the different areas present within the typical pharmaceutical manufacturing company, but it should also allow for the different backgrounds, education, and experience of the individuals involved in different tasks. The better and the clearer the requirements, the more chances for success in any project. The LIMS team should categorize the requirements into at least two categories, depending on the current and prospective needs for the system.

1. Mandatory requirements: ones that the system needs to meet, otherwise it will not be fit for its intended purpose.

2. "Nice to have" requirements: Those ones that it would be desirable for the system, but not of immediate need. In a LIMS these might include barcode readers and label printers, or a module for interfacing with certain types of instruments, for instance.

These requirements are gathered in a document which states the expectations for that system at a high level. That document will be the "guideline" for the analysis of the different options available to the LIMS team — can all the requirements be satisfied with a commercially available system, or it is necessary to develop a tailored one? The team will then go a step further in this process. Once the user requirements for this application have been gathered, the LIMS team will need to produce a high level document called software requirements specification. This describes, at high level, the requirements for the software application as a whole, a system or subsystem, or simply a "bolt on" to the existing system, depending on the case.

With all these requirements on the new or existing system, the LIMS team will start to survey the different options. Typically, the team will translate the user requirements into a request for proposal (RFP) document, that will set the basic criteria to be met by either the software developer contractor, the internal software developer group, or the off-the-shelf software supplier. The solution for any particular need will be agreed and then analyzed; it might be either for a entirely new system or subsystem. The extent of the documentation produced will depend on how bespoke or standard the solution is, and its technical complexity.

Risk Management and Traceability Matrix

Risk management is a necessary activity not only in a regulated environment, but in all the activities related to software conceptualization, design, implementation, and ongoing operation. In this context a business and regulatory risks analysis must be made, with flexibility to be adapted to changes. As with any other activity related to software there is a high probability that the risks will change during the software development life cycle process due to redefinitions of requirements, changes of the design philosophy, or other parallel changes not originally taken into account. There are many published frameworks for risk management, one of the most widespread is that proposed in GAMP 4, which provides a good methodology for identification and measurement of risks associated with the system under analysis. The complexity of project management of this nature, regardless of whether a new or existing application, grows along with the progress of the project itself. It is good business and engineering practice to keep tracking the requirements to the specifications and then to the design and build of the software, as well as taking the same approach with the associated risks and their mitigating actions. Some risks may be mitigated by putting written procedures in place, in other cases the developer or whoever configures the system should be aware of the risks that require remediation or mitigation in the system itself. Whatever the case, the evaluation of risks throughout the entire lifecycle of the project should be traceable.

Considerations within a LIMS Environment

The U.S. 21 CFR Part 11 rule is related to the use of electronic records and electronic signatures in a regulated environment. This U.S. FDA rule, as well as other equivalents worldwide, means to promote technology to reduce the amount of paperwork typically generated within a quality assurance structure, and therefore to speed up and streamline the process of batch approval. The rule sets the minimum criteria that any system* should meet to consider the electronic records generated by it as equivalent to paper records, and the electronic signatures applied to these electronic records as equivalent to the handwritten signatures. Broadly speaking, the system must ensure:

1. "Data accuracy, reliability, consistent intended performance and the ability to discern between invalid or altered records." Requirement met by design and validation of the system.

2. "The ability to generate accurate and complete copies of records in both human readable and electronic form suitable for inspection, review, and copying by the agency." Requirement met by the design of the system.
3. "Protection of records to enable their accurate and ready retrieval throughout the records retention period." Requirements regarding data backup, disaster recovery, and archiving.
4. "Limiting system access to authorized individuals." Requirement met by design and configuration of the system. Most (probably all) of the commercial LIMS applications allow different access levels, and the configuration of different privileges for each chosen access level. That means in practice that a particular individual within the organization should have access to perform actions and to read or write data, according to that individual's job description and responsibility.
5. "Use of secure, computer-generated, time-stamped audit trails to independently record the date and time of operator entries and actions that create, modify, or delete electronic records...." Requirement met by the design and configuration of the system. The fact that the LIMS systems core is the database tables does facilitate compliance with this aspect of the rule. Special care, however, has to be taken during the configuration of the audit trail before going live since the data generated by the use of this feature adds data to the data tables and therefore the whole system's performance may decay as a result of too much data added to the database. Also, this data is necessary for review and auditing purposes; it is not data that will normally be used externally. Therefore, special effort should be made at the time of configuring other tools or interfaces needed within the system to avoid creating this information if the process does not require it.

   It is also expected that static or support data will be at least version- controlled. The system must allow the storage of previously entered information for specifications, calculations, test specifications, and other support data that could be required for auditing or regulatory purposes.
6. "Use of operational system checks to enforce permitted sequencing of steps and events, as appropriate." Requirement met by design and configuration of the system.
7. "Use of device checks to determine, as appropriate, the validity of source data input or operational instructions." Requirement met by design of the system.

Another part of the rule requires that the users of the system shall be made aware of their accountability in using electronic signatures. In fact, this aspect relies on the procedures and practices across the company or division actually using the system, according to the FDA's applicable predicate rules. In this context, the LIMS team should map the actual paper process and establish when the paper signatures are required, and translate the conclusions of this exercise to the developer or eventually the system administrator, who will actually implement the electronic signatures as required. This ensures that the quality assurance department will provide a rationale whenever a signature is required. All the decisions made by the LIMS team should be documented and archived, since they are subject to future changes, as any other aspect of the LIMS system itself.

The developer or customizer of the LIMS application should be aware also of the fact that the definition for electronic signature is "... a computer data compilation of any symbol or series of symbols executed, adopted or authorized by an individual to be legally binding equivalent to the individual's handwritten signature," and that even biometric methods can be applied for the identification of any individual executing an action on a record contained in the LIMS system. The manifestation of an electronic or biometric signature, nonetheless, has to adhere to the following.

1. It must have the name of the individual executing the signature.
2. It must have the date and time when that signature has been applied.
3. It must also contain the meaning of the signature (approval, reviewing, for instance).

It is important to take this into account when configuring reporting tools, or for review purposes when creating a screen showing the workflow on a given sample.

Building or Customizing the System — Giving Shape to the Application

Once all the requirements have been gathered, the supplier's ability to deliver a quality and reliable product assessed (or assembled by the developer team), the risks determined and all regulatory requirements have been taken into account, the next step is to build the system or to buy the most appropriate off-the-shelf option offered to the company's LIMS team. Requests for proposal are matched against the different solutions offered. The cost–benefit analysis is made, a potential provider (or more than one in the case of very complex systems) is selected and audited for compliance with the company's own quality systems, all concerns about business continuity are resolved (availability of technical support, local helpdesk, and other related issues), and then the developer's group within the LIMS team will embark on customizing the application and making it suitable for the business, according to the requirements set previously. The customization of an entire LIMS application comprises several related tasks, which can be divided in layers:

1. User interface.
2. Interfaces with "external" systems.
3. Database tables and core program settings.

System Database

The most extensive work to be done in the whole LIMS system is on the database, in customizing the system tables. This in turn will determine how the system and user data will be stored. The behavior and features of that set of tables depends greatly on the available technology. In the past most systems used commercial proprietary databases, whereas today the model and technology supplied by Oracle has been more broadly accepted. This is becoming the *de facto* industry standard for many reasons:

1. Ability to handle data transactions very effectively.
2. Ability to easily interact with other commercial systems (or bespoke ones) for reporting.
3. Use of well-known database languages such as SQL in a user-friendly environment, among other reasons such as worldwide customer post-sales support.

The LIMS system will be supplied with a minimum set of tables and a configuration that will make the application operate once installed, but nonetheless the company must adapt the system to its needs. To achieve this, the database developer must "map" all the data that will need to be stored and their inter-relationships, define data types, define all the attributes for every single piece of information to be handled by the database's tables. Then the prerelease test plan must be developed, which can constitute the basis of the operational qualification testing phase during the validation exercise.

Interfacing with other business systems

Very rarely will a LIMS system operate without interacting with other business or laboratory systems. In most cases it will be necessary to develop or configure either bespoke or commercial interfaces. For extensive and complex interfaces, the LIMS team may well define the need to treat this aspect as part of another separate project, since some interfaces at instrument level might involve extensive programing tasks, as in the case of software used to control hardware such as chromatography or spectroscopy equipment, for instance. In other cases, the interfaces may consist of a simple series of scripts using some features of the operating system underlying the application. The LIMS team will decide and prioritize according to the business needs of the systems to interface initially, and dedicate more effort to those. In any case, extensive testing must be planned for these interfaces, which can also be used as part of the operational qualification for the whole application.

When choosing commercial off-the-shelf interfaces for laboratory instrumentation or other business system interfacing, part of the problem has been already defined. It is already known that the interface has been designed to operate with both systems to be interfaced, and therefore the LIMS team should only be concerned with the interface settings and other constraints, such as network hardware and overall performance. The LIMS team must make sure that the interfaces have been thoroughly challenged and tested to ensure that they will perform as desired; again, these tests can be part of the operational qualification of the entire application.

User interface

The layout of the user interface will begin to be defined within the software requirements specifications and the functional specifications as provided by the system supplier or the developer's team. At this stage the system will consist, in a minimum configuration, of screens at user level, which need to be adapted to the business needs. The developer must "map" the end user needs and define:

1. The type of screens needed.
2. The sub screens.
3. All the elements required to successfully make the system operate in a clear and safe manner.
4. How the screen elements will interact with the database fields.
5. What the general behaviour will be, paying particular care of the regulatory requirements.

The more the constraints on the data analyst, the less the possibilities of making errors afterwards, so whenever possible the developer should base its strategy on limiting the choices of making decisions or entering information by the end user. The use of pull-down or option lists instead of free text input fields will make the data more consistent across the system and minimize the probability of error. The design of queries is an activity to which special care should be given. The entire functionality of a screen may depend on the use of such queries, therefore the developer must ensure that the information retrieved matches exactly with the intent of each individual query. A slight difference in the criteria applied to sort the information out from the database may deliver undesirable results.

The allocation of privileges and permissions to different levels of authorized personnel is sensitive to the configuration of the access levels, so the developer must pay particular attention to the configuration of the requirements in this area. Another special requirement is introduced by electronic signatures. The developer must base the implementation of e-signatures based on the rationale provided by the quality assurance department. At this stage, the planning of the testing of the whole should commence. This will constitute another element for the basis of operational and installation qualification.

Pre- "Cut Over" Testing and "Go or No Go" Decision

Exhaustive testing must be carried out on all the components that will form the system to be delivered to the business. Modules will be tested by using normal cases, boundary limits and worse case scenarios, the code will be inspected, and integration tests done. When the final release is ready, the developer's team should have already planned the necessary installation qualification tests, which will verify that the application is installed according to its design specifications. All the tables, modules, scripts, routines, user interface elements, scripts, and other files for both the server application and the terminal clients must meet these specifications for naming, versioning, length, location, operating system, and the hardware should be qualified so that it meets the application's needs.

The system as a whole must be challenged against the operational situations it was designed for. Operational qualification must include both functional testing (the functionality meets the requirements) as well as boundary and worse case scenarios (the functionality is still performing without showing failure outside its normal value range). The team may decide which functions are more important and prioritize them (producing a rationale), and test these more important functions more thoroughly than the others, saving time and effort.

The test plan should be created during the software development phase. The methodologies used to identify test cases should be independent of programming personnel, but they should take account of the technology of the application and the software and programming concerns related to testing. The methodology for testing typically will consist of:

1. *Module testing*. This focuses on the examination of subprogram functionality and ensures that functionality not visible at system level is examined. This should be done before the integration of the entire system.
2. *Functional testing*. Tests to expose program behavior in response to the normal case and in response to worst-case conditions. The application will be challenged against the domains of input and output, responses to invalid, unexpected and special inputs. This type of testing should be applied at the module, integration, and system levels of testing.
3. Integration-level testing focuses on the transfer of data and control across a program's internal and external interfaces. If the LIMS contains a large number of modules this type of testing should be conducted to demonstrate that the added modules do not affect the behavior of the existing ones.

These activities must be carefully documented, test scripts must be followed in full, and any rationale for not doing so must be documented. Deviations (internal to the project) will be raised if a test does not match with its expected outcome. At the end of this exercise the team must review the results of this activity and if errors are found they should be categorized, in order to make the "go or no go" decision of implementing the system in the "live" environment.

1. Irrelevant errors, such as typographical errors at the time of writing the test scripts.
2. Minor errors, such as the use of upper- or lowercase letter in fields not constructed for them.
3. Tolerable errors that must be communicated to the supplier.
4. Severe errors, such as algorithms performing wrongly, that must be communicated to the QA department, which lead to the failure of the validation exercise until resolution.
5. Disastrous errors, such as database integrity. Impossible to go any further with the validation effort.

Test scripts should be written in such a manner that do not allow ambiguity of interpretation. This aims to achieve two objectives:

1. The scripts will be executed without leaving the tester to follow paths other than stated.
2. The review process will be aligned with the same level of criticality as when the test has executed them.

The minimum content of test scripts are as follows:

1. Test script identifier — unique identifier of the test script.
2. Purpose — description of the feature to be tested.
3. Special requirements and prerequisites (other subsystem running and providing data input, for instance).
4. Test procedure steps.
5. Cross-reference with documents, such as the user manual, whenever applicable.
6. Test log — expected outcomes and observed results.
7. Unexpected events.
8. Resolution of unexpected events.
9. Pass or fail criteria: State the criteria to successfully pass the test. Does the test pass or fail?
10. Sign off by tester and peer reviewer.

Post "Cut Over" Testing — Performance Qualification

Once it has been decided to release the final candidate version of the system, it will be installed in the live environment. At that stage, some of the errors found in the previous tests may have been already resolved, and the system will be tested to assess that it meets the user requirements specifications. The system will be tested as to how it will operate in "live" business conditions, therefore the ability of the system to transport data among the other different systems by means of the interfaces will also be tested. Standard operating procedures for all the instances of operation of the system must have been produced or updated, whichever is applicable.

Special Considerations

Data Archiving and Migration

Whenever the quality assurance department has previously had a LIMS system, existing data will need to be migrated between the existing system and the new one; between database tables and other system components. Migration or archiving should be carried out using qualified tools and the necessary precautions taken for not losing any data during this exercise. The quality assurance department will decide the cut-off point from where the sample results data needs to be in the new system. Among the data that must be migrated are the static data which belongs to the dictionaries: material specifications, tests, calculations, for instance, as well as other data that was on the preceding system, such as database queries, report definitions, and operating system settings files, for example. All these activities will need to be fully documented to ensure future traceability and maintenance.

Archiving of records is a business sensitive task: keeping only as many records that have to be on-line in the system prevents the system losing performance and therefore saves users' time. Also, as the database grows considerably, the risk of suffering system crash also rises considerably. It is advisable, therefore, to carry out this activity at time periods according to the company's schedule declared in a SOP. This is, technically, an activity not exempt from threats. Very powerful hardware will be needed to roll the database over and rebuild the new tables whenever deleting records from a table and rebuilding it. Failure to achieve this successfully may lead to data loss. Today's available hardware creates options when choosing a strategy for data archiving. The prices for data storage solutions are much cheaper than in the past, thus allowing more data to be stored at lower cost. A possible strategy might consist, then, of making duplicate replicas of the system database from time to time and placing the files on an archiving storage drive, keeping them ready for connection when needed, thus minimizing the time needed to have the old data ready for either business or regulatory purposes.

Reporting and Query Tools

Reporting tools are used to retrieve and show the information stored in the database for specific purposes tracking of in-process samples and batches, planning of an analyst's daily tasks, and at a higher level in the organization, for trend analysis, quality-based decisions on a product or process, and certificates of analysis and release. Whatever the case, the developer must make sure that the reports, whether using electronic signatures or not, respond to a precise design, in order to retrieve the information as required in each case, and make the logical decisions matching the results obtained with specified criteria. Queries shall be validated, as well as the templates used for preparing each report, since quality decisions will be made on them. Also, when an external application is used to retrieve data from the database, it has to be made clear that the application should have read-only access to the system tables, and that the use of such information shall be documented.

It is advisable then, to use qualified and reliable tools for querying the system and producing reports, with frozen queries as much as possible and authority control for accessing these templates. If the records have to be submitted electronically, the use of electronic signatures is mandatory. In this context, if the report needs to travel across an open network (where the company does not exercise any control on the system access, such as the Internet, for instance), then encryption of that data becomes a requirement, according to the regulatory expectations.

Disaster Recovery and Business Continuity

Another aspect of the implementation and validation of a LIMS system regards disaster recovery measures to ensure business continuity. Here, the solution to be adopted depends on the nature of the risk analyzed. In case of a power supply shutdown it may be appropriate that the system will use an emergency alterative power source, such as an uninterruptible power supply system (UPS) or even by a separate mains power supply, that will allow enough time to successfully shut the system down, thus avoiding the risk of data loss or further damage to the system.

In other high complexity scenarios, the company must evaluate the potential impact of data loss, and other solutions can be adopted. In some cases the solution might be the use of two-mirror servers, one running locally and other remotely, to reduce the risk of losing data to a very low level, since only the last transactions will be vulnerable. In any case, it is up to the company to evaluate how much risk of data loss is acceptable. This assessment is made with the following elements:

1. Maximum period the system can be inoperative because of automatic data loading or external access to the system (other company sites need to have access to the local LIMS).
2. Time needed to upload the handwritten recorded information.
3. Maintenance costs of backup or mirror systems.
4. Availability of local technical support for backup systems.
5. Likelihood of all given disaster scenarios to occur.

Assuming that the company has made the decision for the most cost-effective and technically sound solution, it will be necessary to test the disaster recovery plan periodically. This not only includes testing the technical system recovery, but also the existence of accurate and up-to-date procedures. Normally the related tests will be run when the system is not needed for normal operation, e.g., during an annual manufacturing shutdown period.

Maintenance

As with any other computerized system, maintenance of a LIMS comprises a series of operations destined to ensure the proper ongoing operation of the system, as specified. This is achieved by a series of activities such as change control management, procedural controls, ongoing performance evaluation (in order to detect system slowdowns or database overload), maintenance of user access controls (logical and procedural), SOP reviews, and system log reviews. All such activities are carried out in order to keep the system in a validated state. Criteria for revalidation should be based on a careful evaluation on the change to be implemented and the impact on the data accuracy, security, and integrity. This will allow for targeting of revalidation efforts.

Examples of changes to a system include hardware maintenance and upgrade, upgrade of the operating system, and evolution of the LIMS application overtime. Configuration management will ensure adequate identification, control visibility and security of any changes made to hardware, firmware, network, program source code, or any specialized equipment associated with the LIMS.

The ultimate responsibility for ensuring that the system is still under a validated state relies upon the local IS/IT and quality assurance departments: As demonstrated until now, the IS/IT department will have the primary responsibility for the technical aspects related to the system, including the execution of some revalidation work, periodic retesting of some features according to internal procedures (e.g., backup and restore), and the updating of technical documentation whenever needed. The QA department however, will monitor that all the procedures and working instructions are in place and up to date, and maintain a good liaison with IS/IT for all the user-related maintenance activities, including maintenance of user accounts and system access, assignation of system access levels, identification of new business requirements and user training.

CASE STUDY: A LIMS IN ASTRAZENECA

This case study considers the validation of a LIMS at one of AstraZeneca's manufacturing sites. The site carries out formulation and packing operations for products for the U.S.A. and other countries, and so is subject to FDA regulation. There are both chemical and microbiological laboratories, and all of the samples are managed using a common LIMS. This section deals with the project management and technical approaches adopted for the LIMS validation.

The topics discussed include:

1. Background and resource issues.
2. Project planning and start-up.
3. Document development and management.
4. Project monitoring.
5. Risk assessment.
6. Conclusions.

Background and Resource Issues

The site has around 450 employees and systems validation expertise is provided by a two-person systems quality group. Due to the range of systems validation and quality aspects managed across the site, this group was unable to provide sufficient resource for the preparation of lifecycle documents for the validation project. Similarly, the system administrator in the IS department, although having the technical expertise to carry out some of this task, did not have sufficient time available. It was decided to employ an external validation consultancy company to assist in this task.

Generation of Proposals

Based on the knowledge within the systems quality group and others in the factory, a shortlist of four consultancy companies was drawn up. The first step in the selection process was to meet with each consultancy company in turn to discuss AZ's requirements and expectations. Before doing this, internal meetings were held to agree these requirements and expectations, and a summary of these was provided to each company prior to the meetings. This summary was not in the form of a user requirements specification, since the contract to be awarded was not for the supply of a system but for the supply of services. Instead it included a description of the scope of the system, and statements of AZ's expectations around the scope of supply for the company. It was indicated to each consultancy company that it should recommend methods and approaches for the work as well as suitably-skilled people. Each company was given between half and one day, depending on mutual availability, to discuss the project requirements, at the AstraZeneca site. To maximize the common understanding, AZ ensured that a cross-section of people from systems quality, IS and QC departments were available for these discussions. The agenda for each meeting was similar. The company was given time to present its background, experience, and approach to validation. AZ then presented the general scope of the project, and time was allowed for the company to ask further questions to enable it to develop a proposal for the work.

Assessment of Proposals

Within three weeks of the conclusion of these meetings, all the relevant proposals had been received by AZ, and the assessment of the proposals began. The key stakeholders from systems quality, IS,

QA, and QC were invited to a meeting where a structured decision-making technique was used. After a brief review of the status of the project and the proposals, the following steps were carried out.

1. A brainstorm of factors that would influence the decision (selection criteria).
2. Grouping and filtering of the factors to produce a final list of criteria.
3. Relative weighting of the criteria.
4. Scoring of each proposal against the criteria.
5. Multiplication of scores by weights and totalling of weighted scores.
6. Discussion of, and conclusions from, the results.

From the first two steps, the following criteria were identified (*not* in order of importance).

1. Validation expertise.
2. Knowledge of LIMS in general.
3. Knowledge of Beckman LIMS in particular.
4. "Confidence" level in the consultant to deliver.
5. Availability and location.
6. Quality of presentation during proposal discussions.
7. Cost.

For commercial reasons it is not possible to state the relative weights given to each criterion by AZ, in any case, these would vary from project to project, depending on constraints such as regulatory risk and budget. The criteria included measurable factors as well those requiring judgement to assess. The purpose of using the technique was to give these varying factors the correct relative weighting and therefore reach the optimum choice. The method of allocating weight was agreement on which criterion was the most important, and give it a weight of 10. All the other criteria were then judged in relative importance against this, giving a range of weights from 10 down to three. Once weights were allocated, the proposals were judged against each criterion in turn. Again, the proposal scoring best for a particular criterion was given 10, and the other proposals were scored relative to this. In both the weighting and scoring processes, there was no constraint on giving the same weight or score more than once. Once the scoring process was concluded, one proposal was provisionally selected, but before this decision was finally agreed, all the key stakeholders were given the opportunity to raise and discuss any concerns. In any structured decision- making process like this, it is vital that this chance is given, to ensure that buy-in has been achieved from all the people present. In this case, no concerns were raised which altered the provisional decision, and the choice of consultant was confirmed.

Project Planning and Start-Up

Once the consultancy company was chosen, the next major step was to conduct a project kick-off meeting, at which the final scope of the project would be agreed. The other major objective of this meeting was to make a positive start to the process of building the project team who would carry out the work. It was agreed with the consultancy that its resource would be based primarily on-site for the duration of the project, to maximize the integration of its people into the AZ project team.

Prior to the kick-off meeting, it was agreed with the consultancy that an initial period of a week would be used for the consultancy to perform its own assessment of the project in more detail. The aim of this was to provide further information on the time and resource planning stage, thereby reducing the risk of inaccurate estimates. During this and the succeeding stages, the availability of the system administrator and the key users from QC was vital, to ensure the consultancy was given the support it needed. At the kick-off meeting, a team-building exercise was used to help create a sense of team unity. The consultants on the project were included in this process from the outset, as the intention was to integrate them into the working environment on-site as much as possible.

In agreeing the final scope of the project a brainstorm was held to list all the possible activities that could be included in the project. Having reviewed the primary objectives of the project, this list was then assessed and the detailed scope agreed. One area where there were options on scope was the interface to SAP R/3. This interface is used to automatically transfer data about batches and required samples from SAP to LIMS, and to pass back the status results of the samples after completion. Since this interface uses bespoke code in both systems to carry out the data transfers, but operates and is tested as one entity, it was decided to designate the interface as a separate "system," and document and test it independently of the main LIMS. The validation of this interface was carried out in parallel with the LIMS validation but was carried out entirely by AZ personnel, with the exception of the technical code review carried out by the consultants.

The development environment for the site LIMS includes a development and test machine in addition to the production machine. It was decided that from the time of the kick-off meeting, further changes in system requirements would not be introduced, so that the documentation could be developed against a frozen version of the system requirements, implemented on the development machine. Building on discussions during the proposal phase, the scope of supply for the consultants had to be finalized in addition to the technical scope of the project. AZ on site, in their systems quality group, have people experienced in systems validation, and so the scope of supply for the consultants was not to deliver the entire validation package as a turnkey job. Rather, their scope was to provide expertise in particular phases of the validation. Using the standard validation lifecycle described in the local validation SOP, based on GAMP, the following documents were planned, with the prime responsibility for the preparation of each indicated.

Document	*Prime responsibility*
Validation plan	AZ
Functional specification	Consultants
Hardware design specification	AZ
Software design specification	Consultants
Code review report	Consultants
Protocol (test specification)	Consultants/AZ
Validation report	AZ
Maintenance and operation procedures	AZ

Documentation Development and Management

Validation plan

The validation plan was prepared by the systems quality group and approved internally. The validation approach documented in this plan was shared and discussed with the consultants during the revision phase of the document.

Functional specification

The functional specification (FS) was prepared by the consultants, working primarily with the AZ system administrator and a number of key users in order to verify the functionality. Due to the use of many standard functions of the core system, the document was written with the emphasis on the structure of the configuration for AZ's use.

Hardware design specification

The hardware design specification (HDS) was written by AZ in line with local SOPs, following the style and level of other recent projects.

Software design specification

The FS included all the configuration detail for AZ's application, but excluded the design for bespoke areas of code. The main function that required further design detail was that of reporting, where fixed reports had been written in a standard report generating language (a tool provided by the system supplier). Since these reports could be said to be implemented using code rather than simple configuration of standard functions, the detail design was taken out of the FS and included in a software design specification (SDS). Again, this document was prepared by the consultants. As described earlier, the bespoke code for the SAP interface was documented and validated separately.

Protocol

The protocol document included the hardware acceptance testing (IQ), the system acceptance testing (OQ), and the performance testing (PQ). This document was primarily prepared by the consultants, although the hardware test scripts for the IQ were prepared by AZ, due to the fact that the consultants had not been involved in the preparation of the BIDS. This document required the most iterations and discussion of all those produced, because of the need to reach a common understanding of the testing approach, the depth of testing, and the style of preparation of the test scripts. There were significant differences in the "normal" approaches adopted by AZ and the consultancy company. While these differences were not fundamental in the ability to qualify the system successfully, they were significant enough to cause a degree of rework to meet AZ's preferred style. It is recommended that existing protocols are used as examples and time is spent discussing in detail the structure of the test scripts with any consultant prior to the preparation of such a document, in order to reduce the leadtime for preparation. One example of these differences was in the use of generic test scripts which could be used and re-used to test the application of a similar function with different instances or parameters. AZ preferred to adopt a generic style where possible, to minimize the size of the protocol. The alternative is to include in the protocol all the necessary steps, with instances and parameters specified therein, to allow full testing without looping back to steps previously conducted. Both approaches are equally acceptable, but they have different advantages and disadvantages.

Generic test script	*Linear test script*
One per function, execution repeated for each instance.	All instances specified sequentially in script.
Instance-specific parameters excluded from script: reference made to design specifications.	Instance-specific parameters included in script: reference to design specifications unnecessary.
Lack of specific parameters reduces the chance of discrepancy with design specifications.	Repetition of specific parameters from design specifications increases the chance of discrepancy.
One script for all instances can be a problem if a subset of instances have slightly different functionality.	Differences in functionality between instances can be accommodated.
Preparation and review time reduced.	Preparation and review time increased.
Execution more complex due to continual cross-referencing to design documentation.	More simple execution.
More experienced testers needed.	Less experienced testers may be sufficient.

Validation report

The documentation stage following testing was the preparation of the validation report. At the AZ site concerned, this is carried out in two steps: the first report summarizes each test and confirms the completion of the qualification. The second and final report summarizes the completion of all the steps outlined in the validation plan, and justifies any excursions from that plan.

Procedures

In parallel with the validation life cycle activities, maintenance, operating and change control procedures for the system were prepared and approved internally where appropriate.

Project Monitoring

The timescale of the project meant that close monitoring of progress against plan was required. The production schedule on the site is such that there are only two normal shutdowns of any length during the year. Although the IQ and OQ testing could be performed offline on the development or test machine, the PQ could only be performed on the production machine after the transfer of the completed application from the development environment. This meant that the project had to be completed in a little over three months to meet the next planned shutdown. The only other alternative would have been to create another shutdown later or wait a further 7 months until the following shutdown. Neither of these alternatives were desirable from a business perspective.

To this end, a detailed project plan was drawn up by the consultants with AZ's input, detailing all the activities, milestones, and responsibilities. Several review meetings were then held to monitor progress against this plan, and new versions issued when appropriate. The most important progress meeting was held just before the start of the agreed shutdown. This was a final progress review to confirm the go or no go decision to implement the validated system in the production environment during the shutdown. Based on the progress made, the decision was go.

During the shutdown, the version of the system held on the development or test machine was loaded onto the production machine and the PQ tests were conducted. The validation report, which had been drafted earlier, was finalized and made ready for approval on the first morning of start-up following the shutdown. This meant that approval of the completion of the validation exercise could be given quickly to avoid any unnecessary delay in the use of the system in the laboratories. The end result was a project which was concluded on time, within the budget, and met its regulatory objectives.

Risk Assessment

An additional activity carried out for the LIMS was a process known within AZ as threats and controls analysis (TCA). This process uses a checklist to discuss key areas of system functionality, to identify potential threats to the proper performance of the system or the integrity of its data, and to recommend controls which should be put in place to meet these threats. Such controls are normally either system controls (i.e., the system design needs to be reviewed or changed) or procedural (i.e., included in the SOPs for the system operation and maintenance). This analysis ideally takes place when the functional specification is substantially complete (caution must be used to ensure any changes to the functional specification after the original TCA do not affect the recommendations from the analysis). The closure of the actions from the TCA is then reported in the validation report, although it is recommended that a status review of the actions is undertaken prior to the formal testing and qualification phase.

The standard checklist on site, which was used for the LIMS system, is:

General aspects	*Automated equipment*
1. Security and access.	17. Impact of equipment environment.
2. Hardware and software alarms.	18. Interfaces with equipment and processes.
3. User or operator interfaces.	*Information systems*
4. Interfaces with other systems.	19. Coding and identification.
5. System hardware.	20. Change of status of controlled items.
6. Operating system hardware.	21. Traceability of information.

7. Application software.
8. Data input (including initial data take-on).
9. Maintenance, services, and suppliers.
10. Change control (at all levels).
11. Loss of electricity.
12. Audit trail and maintenance of data.
13. Backup and restore.
14. Startup and shutdown.
15. Disaster recovery.
16. Operating procedures.
22. Management of data and material parameters.
23. Allocation, reconciliation, and returns.

The analysis was led by the systems quality group, to provide experience in the use of the checklist. An open question approach was used (how, which, why, when, etc.), rather than using closed questions which only require yes or no answers. IS, technical and user representatives were present to minimize the chance of unanswered questions. As a result of the analysis, a number of improvements and changes were made to the specifications, test coverage, and the procedures. At the conclusion of the validation project, it is considered that the key factors in its success have been:

1. Involvement of key stakeholders at the outset.
2. Close involvement of the consultant company in the scoping and estimating process.
3. Involvement of the key users at an early stage.
4. Detailed review of the specifications and protocol by key users as well as technical and validation staff.
5. Involvement of the key users in the OQ and PQ testing.
6. Use of knowledgable, experienced consultants.
7. On-site presence of the consultants.
8. Use of standard project management techniques.
9. Freezing of change: no additional requirements were introduced during the project.
10. Commitment of all people involved in the project.

The site now has a firm baseline for the validated status of its LIMS, and the experience of the project has shown that it is possible to achieve such positive results by clearly managing scope and the working relationships and responsibilities within the whole project team, including the consultants.

18

Medication Errors

A report issued by the Institute of Medicine in November 1999 has drawn unprecedented national attention to the prevalence of medical error, including medication error. The issues and complexities surrounding this problem are compounded by the array of players and solutions that must address it for the public health and safety of the U.S. population. Medical products and their manufacturers are reported not only as part of the problem but also as part of the solution. Ongoing national efforts in medication error reporting and prevention place the pharmaceutical industry far ahead of other medical product manufacturers. These efforts, headed by the United States Pharmacopeia (USP), have involved the industry since 1991 by sharing reports received from healthcare practitioners and documenting industry actions to the reported problems. The Institute of Medicine fosters a systems approach to error analysis that focuses on identifying the root cause of error within the system and not on blame of the individual. The report postulates that individuals who commit errors are often well trained, experienced, well intentioned individuals whose misfortune is a result of the unsafe systems in which they operate. With the advent of new technologies and the healthcare-delivery processes surrounding them, new problems are likely to surface, particularly as health systems are redesigned in response to this national call to action. The challenge to the pharmaceutical industry is to learn from its own experiences and the USP national database of errors. The industry will be expected to be knowledgeable of the medication use process for the health setting in which its products are used and to anticipate misuse by designing error out of products.

Scope of the Problem

Incidence of Medication Errors and Related Morbidity and Mortality

That medication errors occur frequently in U.S. hospitals has been well documented. In observation studies carried out between 1962 and 1995 on the rate of administration errors in a variety of inpatient settings, rates ranged from 0 to 59%. Estimates that medication errors occur in almost 7% of hospitalized patients have been reported. One study found that the frequency of medication errors was 1.4 per admission. When approximately 290,000 medication orders were analyzed, Lesar et al. estimated that there were almost two serious errors for every 1000 orders written. Based on a review of death certificates, it was estimated that nearly 8000 people died from medication errors in 1993 compared with almost 3000 people in 1983. Researchers found an error rate at two children's hospitals of 4.7 per 1000 orders.

A variety of error rates for different aspects of the medication use process have been reported. Researchers use different methodologies and definitions of "medication error" and study different aspects of the medication use process (i.e., prescribing, dispensing, and administering). Because there is no national standardization for the denominator used to report medication error rates, the denominator can vary among several: doses dispensed, doses administered, doses ordered, patient days. Therefore, the rates reported in the literature are limited in their use for comparative purposes. Research supports a systems approach to error prevention as well as to investigation of errors. This means that all aspects of the medication use process, including characteristics of the products themselves, should be explored for ways to improve safety in use.

Cost of Medication Errors

Medication errors are costly to both the patient (direct costs such as additional treatment and increased hospital stay) and to society (indirect costs such as decreased employment, costs of litigation). The cost of medication errors in a 700-bed teaching hospital, based on a study in 11 medical and surgical units in two hospitals over a 6 month period, was estimated at $2.8 million annually. The increased length of stay associated with a medication error was estimated at 4.6 days. In a 4 year study of the costs of adverse drug events (ADEs) in a tertiary care center, 1% of these events were classified as medication errors. The excess hospital costs for ADEs over the study period were almost $4,500,000, with nearly 4000 days of increased hospital stay. Harm attributable to drugs is a major reason for malpractice claims associated with medical procedures. The average compensation for medication errors between 1985 and 1992 was almost $100,000. Most compensation for medication errors is for larger amounts that are agreed on in out-of-court settlements. None of the costs cited above include the cost of patient harm or subsequent hospital admissions.

USP's Efforts to Standardize Medication Errors

History of USP and Its Involvement in Medication Errors

The USP is a private, not-for-profit organization whose mission is to promote public health through the creation of standards and authoritative information for the use of medicines and related technologies. The USP's authority to set standards is established by the Pure Food and Drug Act and by the Federal Food, Drug and Cosmetic Act. These standards include those for quality, strength, purity, packaging, labeling, and storage of drug products. The USP also creates the official name for drug products and is a member of the United States Adopted Names (USAN) Council that sets the non-proprietary name for drugs in the United States. The USP has been involved in reporting programs for health professionals for nearly 30 years through its USP Practitioners' Reporting Network (USP PRN). These programs support the standards-setting activity by providing practitioner- based experiences about the quality and safe use of medicines in the marketplace.

Nearly a decade ago, the USP agreed to coordinate the medication errors reporting program for the Institute for Safe Medication Practices. The Institute was seeking a home for its grass-roots program and believed the program could have greater impact on the national level. Through the program, the USP hoped to learn of those circumstances in which the product labeling, packaging, or name of product caused or contributed to an error. Then, the USP envisioned setting standards to address the issues and thereby to prevent future errors. In 1994, the USP signed an agreement to purchase the program from the Institute, established the USP Medication Errors Reporting (MER) Program, and began its long-term commitment to the program as an important part of the USP's standards-setting process. As a condition of the agreement, the ISMP continues to receive copies of reports submitted to this program for its education and advocacy work.

Healthcare professionals report errors in which they are involved as well as errors that they observe or are party to. Reported information forms a database used by the USP to identify problematic situations, to heighten practitioners' awareness of these situations, and to make appropriate interventions regarding issues with drug products.

USP Medication Errors Reporting Program

The prevention of medication errors is the primary objective of the USP MER Program. It collects and analyzes potential and actual medication errors submitted by healthcare practitioners. The program affords healthcare professionals the opportunity to report medication errors and thereby to contribute to improving patient safety by sharing their experiences. To report an error, practitioners may phone USP toll-free at 1-800-23ERROR. A voice-mail system allows a report to be left 24 hr a day, 7 days a week. Reporters may submit reports anonymously or speak directly to one of USP' s health professional staff. Alternatively, a report may be submitted to USP in writing. Report forms may be obtained by calling the USP directly or via an on-demand fax- back system. Practitioners may also access the form online on the USP's website. Medication error information submitted to the USP is entered into a nationally recognized repository for medication error reporting. This database serves to track, monitor, and analyze medication errors from a systems-based perspective. The USP develops educational resources and materials to disseminate best- practice solutions and error-avoidance strategies to students and practitioners.

The MER Program is presented in cooperation with the Institute for Safe Medication Practices and is a partner in MED WATCH, the FDA's medical products reporting program. Although the FDA does not usually assert jurisdiction over practice issues, which are often involved in medication errors, it is concerned with issues relevant to product quality such as labeling and packaging, and product names, both trade and generic. When medication errors concerning product labeling and packaging are reported through the MER Program, pharmaceutical manufacturers are notified. They respond frequently and voluntarily make changes in labeling and packaging. Depending on the nature of the medication error, the MER Program reports provide material for ongoing discussions between the FDA and manufacturers and, if warranted, for regulatory action. Furthermore, reported information identifies broader issues that may become the basis for instituting industry-wide changes. The reported concerns of practitioners have prompted the USP, FDA, and various drug manufacturers to institute numerous changes and improvements to drug products and have contributed to safer medication prescribing and use.

Facility-Based Reporting May Help Define Denominator of Errors

Because of its leadership and experience in the prevention of medication errors, the USP began to receive inquiries from hospitals seeking a nationally standardized database that would help them meet its accreditation requirements and also to compare rates of medication errors among hospitals. Hospitals were willing to share their adverse experiences with other participating hospitals but only if the report could be shared on an anonymous basis. In 1998, the USP developed MedMARx, an Internet-accessible database of medication errors for hospitals. Reports submitted to the system are anonymous so that participating hospitals will share information openly. The database is structured to become part of the hospital's internal quality-improvement program and captures not only errors but prevention strategies taken by each hospital in response to errors. This valuable aspect of the national database enables hospitals to practice risk prevention, not just risk management, by learning from the unfortunate experiences of others. It is expected that this database will become a rich repository of information not only for hospitals but for the pharmaceutical industry as well.

USP's First Advisory Panel on Medication Errors

In 1996, the USP created an ad hoc Advisory Panel on Medication Errors. The mission of the Panel was to provide practitioner review of reports received through the USP MER Program and to make recommendations relative to USP's standards-setting, information, and reporting programs. The Panel chairperson also has a unique opportunity to make broader recommendations through its seat on the National Coordinating Council for Medication Error Reporting and Prevention (NCC MERP). The chairperson of the Advisory Panel on Medication Errors is an ex-officio non-voting member of the NCC MERP. The USP Advisory Panel on Medication Errors is a unique and unprecedented opportunity for healthcare professionals to provide peer review of medication errors occurring nationally and to recommend far- reaching strategies for medication error prevention. The Panel consists of 12 actively practicing volunteers representing medicine, nursing, and pharmacy. This year a Safe Medication Use Expert Committee will be elected to replace the Panel. For the first time, with the formation of this committee, a formal mechanism will be in place in the standards-development process for the purpose of providing direct practitioner input to standards development for the safer use of pharmaceuticals.

A National Coordinating Council Is Initiated

After a few years operating the MER Program, the USP realized that the solutions addressing the myriad issues identified through the program were beyond the mission of its standards-setting capacity. Indeed, errors proved to be multidisciplinary in origin and multi- factorial in cause. These other practice-related and process-related aspects surrounding medication errors needed to be addressed. In 1995, the USP spearheaded the formation of the NCC MERP. The NCC MERP promotes the reporting, understanding, and prevention of medication errors relative to professional practice, healthcare products, procedures, and systems. The Council is composed of 20 national organizations and agencies, representative of health professions, licensing boards, healthcare facilities, pharmaceutical manufacturers, regulators, standards- setters, and others. The USP is a founding member of and Secretariat to the Council.

Since the Council's formation, it has produced several important work products. Among them are the standardization definition of the "*medication error*," the development of a series of recommendations designed to reduce errors in the medication use process, and the adoption of a severity index for categorizing the outcome of medication errors. The "Recommendations to Correct Error-Prone Aspects of Prescription Writing," the first set of suggestions issued by the Council, included a list of "*Dangerous Abbreviations*," abbreviations that are frequently misunderstood or have often been implicated in medication errors and should never be used. In addition to being used in prescription writing, these abbreviations can be found in proprietary product names, on manufacturers' product labels, and in advertising by pharmaceutical manufacturers. The pharmaceutical industry can support this effort by avoiding the use of these abbreviations. The Council also produced an extensive set of recommendations to reduce errors attributable to labeling and packaging. The recommendations are targeted to regulators and standards-setters, healthcare organizations and professionals, and the industry. The practical importance of the Council's recommendations lies in a joint endorsement by a diverse group of organizations ranging from experts in safety issues to manufacturers of drug products to regulators. The importance of achieving consensus through a collaborative effort by these national leading healthcare and consumer organizations furthers the adoption of non-punitive, systems-based approaches to reduce medication errors.

Error Avoidance Strategies for the Industry–Designing Error Out of Products

The USP's medication error-reporting programs have uncovered a number of reported error-prone situations that could help industry consider the problems that should be addressed in advance, starting with the selection of a drug name and including the development of labeling, packaging, and dosing devices. Some of these cases are presented here. In many, the manufacturer corrected design flaws immediately and successfully. These should be considered showcase examples of industry responsiveness. The cases should also serve to teach certain designs in labels or packaging that should be avoided. And finally, the cases demonstrate how products can be misused because of the systems with which they interface.

Characteristics of Product Errors

Keep in mind that the medication use process is a complex continuum that requires the successful interaction of multiple allied health professionals, technology, and the patient. It can be described as a succession of joined, but distinct processes, known as *nodes*. Each node in the medication use process is, in actuality, a discrete system and presents an opportunity for the occurrence and prevention of medication errors. Medication errors have been defined in many ways depending on research methodologies, incident reporting systems, risk management, or total quality-improvement systems. The USP uses the broad definition of medication error from the NCC MERP. "A medication error is any preventable event that may- cause or lead to inappropriate medication use or patient harm, while the medication is in the control of the healthcare professional, patient, or consumer. Such events may be related to professional practice, healthcare products, procedures, and systems including: prescribing; order communication; product labeling, packaging, and nomenclature; compounding; dispensing; distribution; administration; education;- monitoring; and use."

Thorough documentation of medication errors provides information about the severity of the error as it relates to the outcome of the patient, the product(s) involved, the level of staff handling the product or processing the order, any contributing factors that may predispose a product to misuse, and the suspected root cause of the error. The USP adds certain codes to MER Program data to characterize the error as it was reported. These codes include the type of error and the possible cause(s) of error.

The pharmaceutical industry should pay close attention to these items in the earliest stages of product development, including clinical stages. Several years ago the drug zidovudine (an antiviral) was referred to as "AZT" in clinical trials. The abbreviation was brought along as the product was marketed. However, "AZT" had been a common abbreviation for azathioprine (an immunosuppressant), and several errors were made. The Institute of Medicine report suggests that the FDA develop and enforce standards for the design of drug packaging and labeling that will maximize safe product use. Table 9 should serve as a starting gate of areas to examine.

Case 051133: Poor label design; confusing or incomplete label information; packaging

A pediatric patient was presented to the emergency room (ER) experiencing seizures for which 150 mg of I.V. Cerebyx (fosphenytoin, an anticonvulsant) was ordered. The pharmacy technician took the call for Cerebyx and delivered three 10 ml vials of Cerebyx 50 mg PE (phenytoin sodium equivalents) per milliliter to the ER as a "*floor stock*" transaction. A nurse then misread the 50 mg PE/ml on the 10 ml container label, making the assumption that the entire vial contained 50 mg PE. The contents of all three vials were prepared for administration. Instead of 150 mg PE, the patient was administered 10 times the intended dose, or 1500 mg of PE. The patient later died. ER staff only discovered the error after the patient's blood phenytoin levels were returned from the laboratory.

Discussion

Serious medication errors, including some leading to death, have resulted from the interpretation of the Cerebyx product labeling. The terminology on the label, which previously indicated the concentration as being 50 mg of PE per milliliter, was misinterpreted as the total number of PEs per vial. Also, health professionals were reportedly confused by the use of "*phenytoin equivalents*," a prodrug concept introduced for this product. As a result, massive fosphenytoin overdoses were mistakenly administered. Fosphenytoin is a prodrug, a compound that undergoes chemical conversion in the body to become the therapeutically active compound phenytoin. Cerebyx dosage will continue to be expressed in PEs. This terminology was adopted in an effort to simplify therapeutic conversions between phenytoin sodium and fosphenytoin sodium (i.e., 500 mg of phenytoin sodium injection is equal to 500 mg PE of fosphenytoin sodium injection). The manufacturer pointed out that by using PEs, prescribers will not have to make dosing adjustments when converting from phenytoin sodium to Cerebyx or vice versa. To reduce the risk of incorrect dosing, all healthcare providers should prescribe and dispense Cerebyx in PEs. Parke-Davis has taken action to prevent future errors. The labeling for Cerebyx vials and packaging has been changed to further reinforce the total amount of drug in each vial. This is effective for both the 2 and 10 ml vials of the product. Although the new labeling further clarifies the total quantity of drug contained in the vial, the concentration of Cerebyx will remain 50 mg PE/ml.

Case 51832, 51845: Line extension creates confusion

Muro Pharmaceutical, Inc., introduced a new line extension, Prelone Syrup 5 mg/5 ml (prednisolone, a steroid), to the existing product, Prelone 15 mg/5 ml. Because only one strength of Prelone had been available for many years, it was a general practice for prescribers to write for "Prelone Syrup" without indicating the strength.

Discussion

Manufacturers need to consider the transition time needed by practitioners to become familiar with the existence of a new strength. Confusion of this type is also seen when "*long-acting*" versions of a product are added to a product line, thereby changing the dosing regime to less frequent intervals. The product name is prescribed without the "*long-acting*" designation, and a medication error results. In similar cases, suffixes also cause errors when the product line extension adds a second strength and places a suffix such as XL" after the product name to indicate long-acting release. Prescribers omit the suffix out of habit (for the initial formulation), and the patient receives the shorter-acting medication at the long-acting interval.

Muro Pharmaceutical, Inc., anticipated that a new concentration of an established product could indeed cause confusion and developed new packaging for both concentrations. Muro also sent mailers that announced the availability of two concentrations of Prelone to 32,000 pediatricians and 65,000 pharmacies, wholesalers, HMOs, and PPOs.

Cases 50446, 50499, 50519, 50534, 50736, 50820, 50918: Poor contrast compromises readability

The unit-dose packaging of the quinolone Levaquin (levofloxacin, an antibacterial) is silver foil with black letters. The dose is reverse shaded. A reporter noted that the packages have to be held at just the right angle to be able to read the label. It was reported to be especially difficult to differentiate between the 250 and 500 mg strengths because the numbers were so difficult to read.

Discussion

Ortho-McNeil is redesigning the packaging for Levaquin to improve readability. Manufacturers should be aware that practitioners often operate in areas that have poor lighting. This makes double-checking the label to prevent errors even more difficult. For some products, there may not be adequate time to read the label carefully the first time without having to look again because of poor contrast. The use of embossed printing on plastic containers has also been reported to be difficult to read because there is no contrast and no paper label to aid in distinguishing the products visually or identifying them properly.

Total volume is the key

Eight reports received from pharmacists expressed concern about the labeling on the Bentyl (dicyclomine hydrochloride, an antispasmodic) 2 ml ampul. Practitioners reported that the label indicates only the drug concentration, 10 mg/ml, and not the total volume. Some practitioners believe the label information is incomplete. In one report, a 20 mg dose was ordered, but two ampuls were administered (4 ml total instead of 2 ml), leading to an overdose. This happened because the reporter mistook 10 mg as the total contents of one vial.

Discussion

Reports received by Hoechst Marion Roussel have prompted the company to return to the old-style labeling that includes the product's total volume data. According to the firm, this change will be implemented as quickly as possible. Reports to the USP have identified the need for three items of information to appear on the vial or ampule: (1) the total volume; (2) the strength per milligram; and (3) the total strength per total volume. Although some manufacturers feel it would be unreasonable to include this amount of information on the container (especially containers of 1 and 2 ml sizes), this information would assure little chance of misinterpreting the contents or strength.

Cases 040925, 050419, 041485: Wholesaler errs due to label similarity

A pharmacist reported that vials of Marsam' s cefazolin sodium 1 g and 10 g appear identical in shape and have the same color flip-top closures. The pharmacy ordered the 1 g product from the wholesaler. Instead, the wholesaler sent 10 g bulk vials of cefazolin sodium along with stickers for the 1 g vial The pharmacy, which does not normally stock the 10 g vials, interspersed the 10 g vials with the 1 g vials in their stock. Several vials were reconstituted in error. Fortunately, no patients received the wrong dose of cefazolin sodium. In another reported incident, a pharmacist ordered the 10 g vials of cefazolin sodium but received the 1 g vials in error. Intending to reconstitute and then divide the 10 g vials into 1 g doses, a pharmacy technician inadvertently reconstituted the 1 g vials and proceeded to divide the total solution of each vial into ten 100 mg doses. Some of the prepared 100 mg doses of cefazolin sodium were administered to patients instead of their scheduled 1 g doses. No adverse effects to the patients were reported. The pharmacist felt the error occurred, in part, because the vials are identical in size and have similar labels.

Discussion

The pharmacist suggested that the color of the flip-top of the 10 g vial be changed. The company replied that although it is common practice to use color-coded labels and flip-tops to differentiate product lines or strengths, it tries to indicate the individual products in other ways, e.g., by varying the style and format of the label. Marsam revised the labeling of the cefazolin sodium 10g bulk vial to help distinguish it from the 1 g, single-dose vial. The newly revised labeling included the following:

1. The word "BULK" added in two places on the side panel
2. Screened color added to the box surrounding the product name
3. "10 grams" printed in color
4. The product name and strength on the back of the label printed in color

The use of color-differentiation is favored, whereas the use of color-coding is controversial because of the limited number of colors, color-blindness in our population, and inapproriate reliance on color in lieu of reading the label.

Case 042031: Packaged measuring devices

An order was written for 30 mg of Cyclosporine (an immunosuppressant) oral solution to be administered to a pediatric patient. However, for several days, the nurse administered 300 mg, believing that the syringe was calibrated in milligrams, not in milliliters. The oral solution is available as 100 mg/ml. As the pharmacist reviewed the error, he noted that the syringes accompanying the medication were never designed with pediatric patients in mind. It is not possible to calculate any dose less than 50 mg It is understandable how the nurse assumed that the "3" mark was for 30 mg—it is positioned between "2,5" and "3,5"(which are European expressions for the decimals 2.5 and 3.5). To harmonize products in the global market, the manufacturer chose to follow European convention for expressing numbers, which uses commas and decimals in the reverse manner as that as in the United States.

Discussion

This error is unusual because it involves a global trade issue. Manufacturers would prefer to harmonize products used in the United States with those available in other markets. If dose preparation was centralized in the pharmacy, this error might have been avoided. Other medication errors involving medication- dispensing devices reported to the USP have included the interchange of devices supplied with specific products. Each device packaged with a medication is calibrated for that medication based on the viscosity and concentration of the specific liquid it delivers. These devices are not calibrated in any standardized way; some are measured in milligrams (mg), others in milliliters (ml), and others in cubic centimeters (cc). Still others have calibrations for the strength per drop or per teaspoonful. Policies should be in place so that the dispensing or use of droppers or calibrated cups provided with specific medications is restricted to those medications.

Manufacturers that supply droppers with a stock bottle should supply enough droppers to enable breakdown of the liquid to usable volumes. For example, one company supplied only one dropper with its 8 oz bottle of morphine sulfate, even though the more common quantities dispensed are 2 and 4 oz. Alternatively, manufacturers should package medication in the volume expected to be dispensed per medication order.

Case 52348: Abbreviations

The USP received a medication error report involving the products Neumega (oprelvekin) and Proleukin (aldesleukin). Oprelvekin, a recombinant human interleukin-eleven product used to stimulate platelet production in selected patients undergoing chemotherapy, is sometimes abbreviated as IL-11. Aldesleukin, a recombinant human interleukin-two derivative indicated in designated patient populations for the treatment of metastatic renal cell carcinoma, is sometimes abbreviated as IL-2. In the reported error, a physician used the abbreviation "IL-11" when ordering oprelvekin for a patient. Unfortunately, the order was misinterpreted to be interleukin-two (i.e., the number eleven was perceived to be the Roman numeral two). Five or more healthcare professionals, including pharmacists and nurses, mistook the order to be aldesleukin. The error went undetected for 4 days, until it was noted that the inventory of aldesleukin was nearly depleted.

Discussion

Practitioners should be especially vigilant when orders for these interleukin products are received. If abbreviations have been used in an order, the order should be clarified to ensure that patients receive the intended medication. This medication error exemplifies the value of implementing prescribing guidelines, such as the recommendations adopted by the NCC MERP. Specifically, when writing an order, prescribers should avoid the use of abbreviations, including those for drug names. Drugs names should not have accepted abbreviations. Reference materials sometimes refer to these abbreviations as synomyns for the approved drug names. Manufacturers should discourage the use of abbreviations because of the potential to cause medication errors. The following cases demonstrate how products can be misused because of the systems with which they interface.

Case 052718: Electronic drug reference products

A pharmacist asked one of the clinical pharmacists for information about Cartia. Because an electronic drug reference listed the active ingredient as aspirin, the pharmacist was prepared to substitute an aspirin product for Cartia. The clinical pharmacist recognized the new product as Cartia XT (diltiazem, a calcium channel blocker) and prevented the error.

Discussion

The manufacturer of Cartia XT shared the reporter's concern and contacted the electronic reference source to investigate the matter. The publisher of the electronic reference stated that a salicylate product called "Cartia" is manufactured by Lusofarmaco in Portugal and Smithkline Beecham in Australia. Both Cartia products were verified as active current products by the publisher. The publisher said it has no way of excluding the foreign marketed Cartia because it is an active product imported from a master database that contains many foreign drug products. The electronic reference is published quarterly. "Cartia XT" was entered into the database that is currently being shipped to customers, who will now be able to choose between "Cartia" and "Cartia XT". This should reduce confusion between the products.

As with many hard copy drug reference books, electronic drug references have lag time between production and the customer's receipt of the reference databases. Unfortunately, this may result in inaccurate/outdated information and omission of current drug information, causing confusion and misinterpretation of drug information by the users. Healthcare providers should realize that reference sources, including electronic reference databases, are not infallible, and that they are only good as their contents of updated information. As a safeguard, the healthcare providers should make it a practice to check at least two different drug information sources to confirm information.

Case 52125: Computers and processing software

A pharmacist entered an order for Diflucan (an anti- fungal) for a patient who had been receiving Propulsid (a gastrointestinal emptying adjunct), which is a documented drug interaction. The pharmacy computer system had multiple drug interaction screens. The pharmacist passed these screens by pressing "next screen" without any resistance by the system for this dangerous drug interaction. The patient received two doses of Diflucan. On the second day, the patient coded and later died.

Case 51088

A patient died after 12 mg of I.V. Colchicine (an antigout medication) was given instead of 2 mg I.V. "*until diarrhea*," as ordered. The physician was contacted by the pharmacist but the physician insisted on the dose. The computer program did not warn about the dangerous dose, and nurses had no idea they were giving an overdose.

Case 50908

Amoxicillin was prescribed and dispensed to a patient with a penicillin allergy. The front of the patient's chart was not marked for an allergy, and the problem list indicating the allergy was covered with a misfiled document. The pharmacy software program does not screen for allergies, and the pharmacy profile was not marked with any allergies.

Digoxin pediatric elixir

Because the computer in one facility was limited to entering doses in milligrams, a neonate patient's 20 microgram dose of digoxin first had to be converted to the equivalent milligram dose before it could be entered into the computer. A pharmacist incorrectly converted the 20 mcg dose and then entered it into the computer as 0.2 mg (instead of 0.02 mg). Consequently, the patient received four 200 microgram doses of digoxin instead of the 20 microgram dose as ordered. The patient experienced digoxin toxicity before the error was discovered.

Teaspoonful vs. ml

By default, a certain software program printed "teaspoonful" for any syrup preparation when a numerical figure was not followed by a specific measure, such as ml, for the dose. A prescription for 1/2 ml albuterol syrup every 6 h for a 9 week-old infant was presented to the pharmacy, and the pharmacist entered "1 2" into the computer but did not enter ml. Therefore, by default, the label printed 1/2 teaspoonful every 6 h if needed for wheezing. The child was administered the overdose and was consequently admitted to the hospital emergency room for observation. Fortunately, the child was released with no permanent damage.

One vs. one-half

New computer software was used to enter the directions for a cough medicine with a dose of "1-2 teaspoonsful." Instead, the new software printed the label as 1/2 teaspoonful. The pharmacist did not check the label against the prescription and dispensed the product with the incorrect directions on the label.

Discussion

Computerized systems have become important tools in today's pharmacy settings. Computers have made prescription processing faster, easier, and more efficient. Computers have also provided for patient information to be readily available. However, as reliance on computers systems grows, care should be taken not to become totally dependent on these systems as the sole check in preventing medication errors.

Similar drug names

Confusion over similarity of drug names, either written or spoken, accounts for approximately one-quarter of all reports to the USP MER Program. Such confusion is compounded by illegible handwriting, incomplete knowledge of drug names, newly available products, similar packaging or labeling, and incorrect selection of a similar name from a computerized product list. The USP has produced a list of more than 1000 drug name pairs that have been reported as confusing. Manufacturers should refer to this list when selecting drug names. Recently, the USP voted to change Amrinone to Inamrinone when it was being confused with Amiodarone and caused fatal errors. This type of change is expensive to the industry and can be avoided by considering the potential for similarity in advance. Technologies and testing protocols, including voice and handwriting recognition, are available to help determine whether a drug name looks or sounds like another. The ability to predict error and thus avoid it is the focus of the science of human factors engineering. The adaptation of this science to the medication use process can help to predict the chances that a medication error will occur. Pharmaceutical manufacturers should design products including their names, labeling, and packaging so that errors can be avoided and safer systems and healthcare delivery result.

19

New Strategies for Target Identification

The essentiality of any given gene in a microorganism depends on the genetic background of the strain and the outside environment. Thus, distinct environments can modify the essentiality of a gene; for example beta lactamase genes are needed for bacterial survival in the presence of beta-lactams but not in their absence. By changing the environment, for instance, by adding an antibiotic to a medium or using *in vivo* models, one can expand the number of known essential genes of a given strain. All antibiotics in clinical use inhibit essential bacterial functions *in vivo*. Genes that are essential for growth, or required to develop an infection, or to confer resistance to antibiotics, are potential targets for drug discovery. Despite the large amount of literature available on putative bacterial essential genes, only a few published reports provide conclusive evidence. Most experiments are based on negative data, such as the inability to knock out a specific gene or use of conditional lethal mutants. Both approaches suggest, but do not demonstrate, essentiality of a wild-type nonmutated target. Target-based antibiotic discovery programs are effort-intensive and require a solid foundation of the quality of the target. Methods that firmly establish the essential nature of a large number of genes are needed for target discovery and evaluation.

Enzymes are attractive targets for new antibacterial discovery. Some of the most successful antibiotics, such as beta-lactams or quinolones, inactivate the transpeptidation reaction of penicillin-binding proteins and DNA topoisomerases, respectively; these enzymes catalyze essential reactions for bacterial growth. New enzyme inhibitors can be identified through mechanism-based drug design. This strategy has been successfully applied to the discovery of drugs such as HIV protease inhibitors but is more difficult to implement in antibacterial discovery programs. Inhibition of bacterial growth is a multifactorial process; this complexity limits the application of rational drug design to antibiotic discovery. An active compound has to cross membranes, avoid being effluxed, face hydrolysis or modification by a myriad of enzymes, and reach its bacterial target at concentrations sufficient to have a significant impact on cell growth. A better drug discovery approach is to increase the probability of finding novel inhibitors by combining a mechanism-based pharmacophore, designed to inhibit a specific target, or set of targets sharing a common feature, with large structural diversity. Purified targets and bacterial strains are screened with compound collections or combinatorial chemical libraries that are made of transition-state analogs, or other rationally designed analogs, and are biased to inhibit these targets. Metallohydrolases or Mur ligases are well suited for this discovery strategy. Biased libraries can be set up even when there is little information on a specific target. For instance, a putative metallo-enzyme identified through motif or homology searches can be screened for inhibitors using highly diverse combinatorial chemical libraries synthesized around a chelator moiety, such as hydroxamic acid or sulfhydroxyl groups, even when the function of the target remains unknown. The chelator moiety adds a strong bias to the library toward metallo-enzymes that other random compound collections do not have.

Enzyme-based screens will identify hits that inactivate the target but do not necessarily stop cell growth. Compounds that inhibit both enzyme activity and cell growth are of obvious interest. However, these activities may not be related. It is necessary to establish whether there is a causative relation between inactivation of the target of interest and inhibition of bacterial growth. Otherwise the discovery program may be pursuing two unrelated activities that more often than not reflect underlying toxicity problems. Thus, at least two kinds of assays are needed: one that measures the inhibition of the purified target and another that indicates whether inhibition of cell growth occurs through the expected mechanism of action.

This chapter focuses on a novel antibiotic discovery paradigm. Metallohydrolases and Mur ligases are used to illustrate this approach. New methods to identify and prioritize targets, develop screens, and evaluate new inhibitors are discussed. New developments in enzyme-based assays, such as pathway assays, are also presented. This new approach is opening new venues for screening targets that are difficult to screen because substrates are not easily available.

Metallo-Hydrolases: A Family of Targets for Novel Antibiotic Discovery

Evaluation of Candidate Metallo-Hydrolases and Construction of Screening Strains

A large number of metallo-hydrolases are present in bacteria. However, only a few are known to be essential for growth or involved in resistance. None of them is the target of antibiotics in clinical use. Candidate metallo-hydrolases for new antibiotic discovery were identified from public genomes searching for homologs of known metal-enzymes or identifying open reading frames (ORFs) that have defined motifs of metallo-binding sites. Multiple alignment tools were used to identify orthologs or paralogs from the retrieved sequences. The distribution in key bacterial pathogens and eukaryotes was determined. Genetic evaluation of the candidate ORFs provides evidence of the essentiality of the target.

Targets are evaluated using gene-to-screen (GTS) technology. This technology provides conclusive data on the essentiality of a gene and screening strains. GTS strains have a specific chromosomal gene under regulatable promoter control. If the gene is essential, then the strain is inducer-dependent for growth. Transcriptional control is chosen to modulate the level of a given target in *Escherichia coli* because of the extensive information available on promoter regulation. The positively regulated P_{BAD} promoter is an ideal regulatory system for modulating gene expression for several reasons: (1) the expression of an essential gene can be down-regulated to a level that does not support growth, an event similar to antibiotic action; (2) P_{BAD} can be induced to high levels of expression; and (3) the promoter is titratable over a range of arabinose concentrations. GTS strains have only a single copy of the target gene in the chromosome in a monocistronic operon under regulatable promoter control. The original gene is deleted in all constructs to eliminate any potential polar effect on downstream genes.

GTS strains have been constructed for a number of genes that code for metallo-hydrolases and used to evaluate these target candidates. GTS constructs have demonstrated essentiality of most of these genes with the exception of *ftsH*, coding for a zinc-containing protease. Temperature-sensitive mutants in the *ftsH* gene have been reported, and this gene was assumed to be essential. However, the lack of arabinose dependence of the *ftsH*-GTS strain, and the ability to knock out this gene, show that this gene is not essential in *E. coli*. These results illustrate the need for demonstrating essentiality with conclusive experiments for all candidate targets.

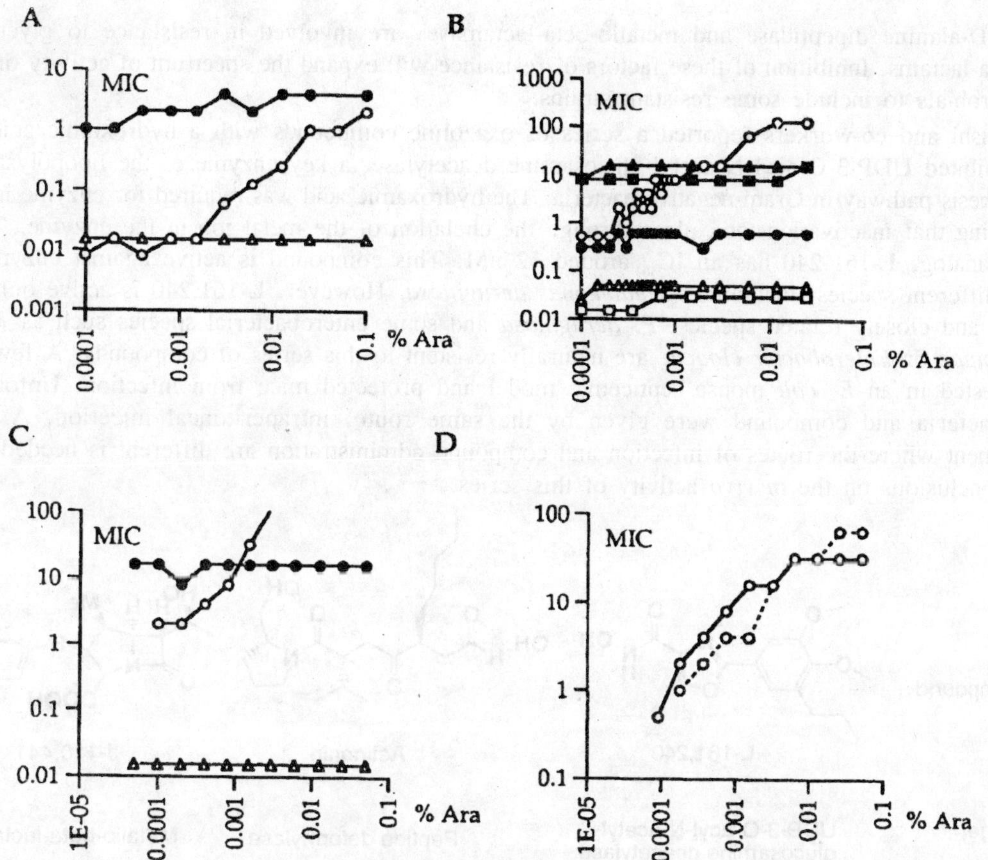

Fig. 19.1. Susceptibility of strains with a target under arabinose promoter control to specific inhibitions of the regulated target (open circles), and to other antibiotics, at a range of a arabinose concentration (MICs in μg/ml).

GTS constructs are also used for screening and establishing mechanism of action of enzyme inhibitors in bacterial cells. The intracellular concentration of the target under P_{BAD} control is modulated by the amount of inducer in the growth medium. At low arabinose concentrations, the strain becomes hypersusceptible to compounds that inhibit the down-regulated target. On the other hand, at high arabinose concentrations, the susceptibility to the specific inhibitor is much lower. This association does not exist for compounds that inhibit other targets. The selective hypersusceptible nature of these strains is used to screen for inhibitors of the down-regulated target and to determine the mechanism of action of inhibitors identified in screens that use purified enzyme. The method is independent of the function of the target, can be applied to any essential gene, and can be implemented with minimal effort to a large number of targets.

New Inhibitors of Metallo-Hydrolases

All the essential metallo-enzymes can be the starting point for a novel antibiotic discovery program. Peptide deformylase (PDF) and UDP-3- O-acyl-N-acetyl-glucosamine deacetylase are attractive because these enzymatic activities are absent in human cells. Methionine aminopeptidase (MAP) is present in both bacteria and eukaryotes. The latter have two isozymes, one of which is closely related to the bacterial enzyme, and the other resembling that of Archea. Despite the high homology between the bacterial and human enzymes, it is conceivable to discover a selective inhibitor of bacterial MAP. D-

Alanyl-D-alanine dipeptidase and metallo-beta-lactamases are involved in resistance to glycopeptides and beta-lactams. Inhibition of these factors of resistance will expand the spectrum of activity of existing antimicrobials to include some resistant strains.

Onishi and co-workers reported a series of oxazoline compounds with a hydroxamic acid moiety that inhibited UDP-3-O-acyl-N-acetyl-glucosamine deacetylase, a key enzyme of the lipopolysaccharide biosynthesis pathway in Gram-negative bacteria. The hydroxamic acid was required for enzyme inhibition, suggesting that inactivation took place through the chelation of the metal ion in the enzyme. The most potent analog, L-161,240 has an IC_{50} around 12 nM. This compound is active against enzymes from many different species, including *Pseudomonas aeruginosa*. However, L-161,240 is active only against *E. coli* and closely related species; *P. aeruginosa* and some enterobacterial species such as *Klebsiella pneumoniae* or *Enterobacter cloacae* are naturally resistant to this series of compounds. A few analogs were tested in an *E. coli* mouse septicemic model and protected mice from infection. Unfortunately, both bacteria and compound were given by the same route, intraperitoneal injection. A different experiment where the routes of infection and compound administration are different is needed to reach firm conclusions on the *in vivo* activity of this series.

Compound	L-161,240	Actinonin	J-110,441
Target	UDP-3-O-acyl-N-acetyl-glucosamine deacetylase	Peptide deformylase	Metallo-beta-lactamases
IC_{50} (nM)	12	0.8	<100
MIC (μg/ml)			
E. coli	1	>100	NA
S. aureus	>100	4	NA

Fig. 19.2. Antimicrobial compounds that inhibit metallo-hydrolases.

Chromosomal metallo-beta-lactamases that hydrolyze carbapenem antibiotics, such as imipenem, meropenem, or biapenem, are present in some *Stenotrophomonas*, *Bacteroides*, and *Aeromonas* strains. Some clinical *P. aeruginosa* and *Serratia marcescens* isolates have a plasmid that carries metallo-beta-lactamase genes. These enzymes are not inactivated by inhibitors of serine-based beta-lactamases such as clavulanic acid or sulbactam analogs. Enzyme-based screens have identified several compounds (methylcarbapenems, biphenyl tetrazoles, and several thioester derivatives) that inhibit members of this class of beta-lactamases. These compounds potentiate the activity of imipenem against carbapenem-resistant strains, and could be administered in combination with a carbapenem to extend the spectrum of activity.

Peptide deformylase is an iron-containing bacterial enzyme that removes the formyl moiety from nascent peptides. The gene that encodes for this activity, *def*, is essential in bacteria and is present in all public bacterial genomes where the sequence is complete. The active center of the enzyme is similar to thermolysin and matrilysin, well-known metallo-hydrolases. A hydroxamic acid-containing deformylase inhibitor, actinonin, was discovered by screening a biased compound collection. This compound strongly inhibits deformylase from *E. coli* and *Staphylococcus aureus*, and is active against Gram-positive bacteria and fastidious Gram-negative organisms. The compound is actively effluxed in *E. coli*, as shown by high susceptibility of efflux pump *E. coli* mutants; this is most likely the reason for the natural resistance of most Gram-negative bacteria.

A *def*-GTS construct was used to show that cell growth inhibition happens through the inhibition of PDF rather than another target. The intracellular concentration of deformylase is modulated by the amount of inducer in the growth medium. At low arabinose concentrations the strain became hypersusceptible to compounds that inhibit the down-regulated target. On the other hand, at high arabinose concentrations the susceptibility to the specific inhibitor was much lower. This association does not exist for compounds that inhibit other targets. The susceptibility of a *def*-GTS strain to actinonin was strongly associated with the concentration of inducer, thus demonstrating that the major target of actinonin in *E. coli* is deformylase.

Pathway Assays: A New Approach for Enzyme-based Screening

Mur ligases catalyze the consecutive addition of amino acids and dipeptide to UDP-N-acetylmuramic acid, a building block of the bacterial peptidoglycan. Arabinose-dependent GTS strains show that ligase genes are essential in *E. coli*. A fifth ligase, *mpl*, is not essential and is involved in the recycling of the peptidoglycan. This enzyme is present only in enterobacteria and catalyses the addition of the tripeptide to UDP-N-acetylmuramic acid. Mur ligase assays are cumbersome to run in high-throughput mode because of the lack of UDP-derived substrates. These compounds are not commercially available and have to be purified from cells, synthesized chemically or enzymatically. Two independent groups have recently developed ligase pathway assays. These assays use six enzymes of the cytoplasmic steps of murein synthesis (MurA through MurF). MurA and MurB enzymes are involved in the synthesis of UDP-N-acetylmuramic acid; MurC, MurD, MurE, and MurF ligases catalyze the consecutive addition of amino acids and D-alanyl-D-alanine dipeptide to this substrate. All six steps can be monitored in a single test vessel starting with the commercially available MurA substrate UDP-N-acetylglucosamine, required amino acids, and ATP, without the need to produce complex UDP-containing substrates for the intermediate steps.

Pathway screens require that the concentrations of enzymes and substrates are optimized so the rate of final product formation is linearly dependent on all enzyme concentrations. The concentration of each enzyme is chosen within the sensitive range at which any decrease of the enzyme concentration will cause a proportional signal decrease. In addition, the reaction signal is reduced to back-ground if the concentration of any one of the enzymes or substrates is not included. High-throughput screening requires detection methods that are amenable to the large number of samples tested. Formation of product can be monitored by high-performance liquid chromatography (HPLC) or by direct absorption scintillation assay (DASA). The latter is based on the binding properties of a positively charged scintillant-containing solid surface that will selectively absorb the UDP-containing products, but not the amino acids, under proper binding conditions. Tritiated D-Ala-D-Ala, which itself does not bind to the plate, is used to monitor the production of the final reaction product. It is possible to follow the reaction progress of any individual ligase by using different radiolabeled amino acids. This detection method is significantly more efficient for high-throughput mode than the HPLC-based method.

Several hits with IC_{50} less than 10 μg/ml were identified using this DASA-pathway assay, including one compound with an IC_{50} of 0.08 μg/ml. To deconvolute the effects of potential inhibitors in the pathway, inhibition of individual enzymes is tested for hits identified in the primary screening. For example, VRC374 was identified as an inhibitor for the pathway assay with IC_{50} of 25 μg/ml. It is apparent from these data that the inhibition observed in the pathway assay is due to the specific inhibition of MurA. This molecule inhibited a GTS strain carrying MurA under P_{BAD} control in an inducer concentration-dependent fashion, as expected for a MurA inhibitor. Pathway assays have several advantages: (1) individual assays can be combined into one, saving labor and reagents; (2) the reaction product of a previous step is the substrate for the subsequent reaction and avoids the need to obtain the individual substrates; (3) a pathway assay can detect "*dead-end*" substrates, compounds that are capable of being incorporated into the product of previous reaction but prevent the further elongation of the pathway.

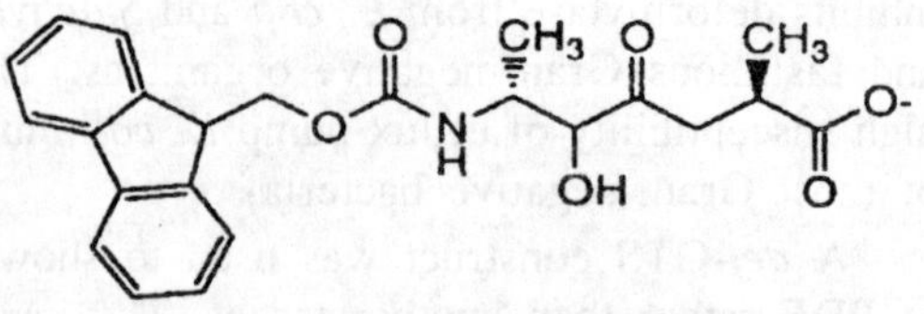

Fig. 19.3. Chemical structure of MurA inhibitor VRC374 identified with DASA screen.

Conclusions and Future Directions

The ultimate goal of any target identification and evaluation program is to select targets that have higher chances for success in the discovery of novel antibiotics. Enzymes that perform functions essential for cell growth, virulence, or resistance to antibiotics are good choices for novel antibiotic drug-discovery projects. GTS technology demonstrates the essentiality of a target and provides screening strains. In addition, the same constructs are used to determine the mechanism of action of new enzyme inhibitors active against whole cells. This powerful technology has been developed in *E. coli* and is under development in other key pathogens. Evidence on the essentiality of a gene obtained in *E. coli* cannot always be extrapolated to other species. For example, lipoprotein leader peptidase is essential in *E. coli*; on the other hand, the *lsp* homolog can be disrupted in *S. aureus*. The major target of an antibiotic can also be different. The primary target of ciprofloxacin in *E. coli* is gyrase, while topoisomerase IV is a secondary target. In *S. aureus* the order is inverted and topoisomerase IV is the major target. GTS can be developed in other bacterial species. The key feature of GTS technology is the use of a regulatable promoter. P*BAD* and other promoters regulated by members of the AraC/Xy1 S family of positive transcriptional regulators have been successfully used in other Gram-negative bacteria, and are natural choices to develop GTS strains in this group of organisms. The use of this technology in Gram-positive bacterial pathogens is more difficult because of the limited number of known regulatable promoters. The *tet* regulon has been used in *S. aureus* and a positively regulated promoter, P_A, has been reported in *S. pneumoniae*. These promoters are good starting points for applying GTS technology in Gram-positive bacteria.

Enzymes that are amenable to mechanism-based drug discovery are better choices for novel antibiotic discovery than targets that do not have any feature that can be used for designing an inhibitor. The combination of a family of targets, such as the metallo-enzyme family, and a biased compound collection based on molecules that have the potential to inactivate these targets, dramatically increases the chances of identifying novel inhibitors. The discovery of actinonin as a potent PDF inhibitor illustrates the success of this approach. The number of members of the metallo-enzyme family will increase as new motifs that define metal-binding sites are identified. There are many other families of targets, for example, Mur ligases or transferases, where the same approach can be applied. The different classes of proteases are particularly promising; a few of them, such as serine- or aspartyl-protease families, have well-defined inhibitor pharmacophores. A few bacterial proteases, such as leader peptidase I or HtrA protease, are essential for growth or play a major role in the processing of virulence factors and are the target of novel antimicrobial programs. A large number of chemical entities derived from protease inhibitor projects of therapeutic areas other than bacterial infectious diseases are available for screening. This universe of existing biased compounds makes protease targets very attractive for the discovery of novel antibacterials.

The large number of targets available requires the development of screens that save time, reagents, and test compounds. Pathway screens allow the testing of several targets at once, and use fewer resources than screens based on individual enzymes. In fact, Mur ligases can only be screened effectively in HTS format using this approach. Other pathways, such as the postranslational modification steps of initiation of protein synthesis or fatty acid synthesis in bacteria, are also amenable to pathway screening. The increasing application of rational drug-design strategies, which are often target driven, emphasizes the need to develop assays that address other major issues involved in the susceptibility of bacteria to any given antibiotic. Screens that address the role of factors involved in natural resistance are needed. The role of efflux pumps and the permeability barrier of the outer membrane is well documented in *E. coli* and other Gram- negative bacteria, and hypersusceptible strains have been constructed. Factors involved in natural resistance in Gram-positive bacteria remain largely unknown. Most of the research on this group of organisms is focused on acquired resistance or on pathogens that are naturally resistant to most antibiotics in clinical use, such as *Mycobacterium* species. A set of hypersusceptible mutants in Gram-negative and Gram-positive bacteria would increase the sensitivity of screens for HTS and help mechanism-based medicinal chemistry programs to improve the whole-cell activity of enzyme inhibitors.

20

METABONOMICS

Metabonomics is a branch of "omics" technologies focused on the analysis and measurement of endogenous metabolites. The workhorse of metabonomic applications has been nuclear magnetic resonance (NMR) spectroscopy, but applications and approaches incorporating separation techniques such as high performance liquid chromatography (HPLC), gas chromatography (GC), and mass spectrometry (MS) are being used with increasing frequency. Metabonomic approaches have been applied broadly in botanical sciences and biomedical studies, including both diagnostic medicine and basic research. To date, some of the most significant efforts and advances in metabonomics have been made relative to plant science. This review will focus on the technological aspects of metabonomic platforms, data collection and analysis, and will emphasize the use of metabonomics in understanding the pathophysiological changes associated with toxicological responses.

TERMINOLOGY: METABONOMICS OR METABOLOMICS

In reviewing the literature related to this field, two terms, namely *metabonomics* and *metabolomics* have been used by investigators. Originally, the field was described as metabonomics and defined as the "quantitative measurement of time-related multiparametric metabolic response of living systems to pathophysiological stimuli or genetic modification". The term takes it roots from the Greek words "meta" (change) and "nomos" (rules or laws) referring to chemometric models used to classify changes in metabolism. In contrast, the term metabolomics, although used widely is less well defined. Fiehn described it as the "comprehensive and quantitative analyses of all metabolites," which although more concise, does not appear to differ from the original definition of metabonomics. Some investigators have also used metabolomics to denote the measurement of metabolites in cells or cell systems. To confound and confuse the situation further, metabonomics and metabolomics have been described as subsets of each other. In this review, the term metabonomics is used, and is considered to represent a systems approach to the analysis of endogenous metabolites in biofluids or tissues using analytical methods and pattern recognition technology. From a practical perspective, metabonomics encompasses the application of NMR spectroscopy, HPLC, GC, and/or MS analyses coupled with pattern recognition tools and multivariate statistical methods to evaluate endogenous metabolites in biofluids and tissues. Regardless of terminology, the technology represents a potentially powerful method for determining the systemic response to toxicity or disease.

METABONOMIC PLATEFORMS

Just as transcriptomic and proteomic applications have used a variety of platforms and approaches, metabonomics also has utilized a variety of platforms, and the field continues to evolve. Historically, NMR spectroscopy has been the workhorse of the approach. Briefly, NMR spectroscopy is a characterization technique in which a sample is immersed in a strong, static magnetic field and exposed to an orthogonal low-amplitude, high frequency radio frequency. The most common application is ^1H (proton) NMR, and typically, chemical shifts, associated with various function groups are used to establish compound structure. For metabonomic applications, proton NMR spectroscopy is typically used, and it is a non-destructive and noninvasive method that offers the advantages of minimal sample preparation, as it requires only sample dilution, pH adjustment, and the addition of an internal standard. It is also broadly applicable to a variety of biofluids (including urine, plasma, saliva, etc.) and tissues. Sample throughput is high, with analysis time under 30 min. The analytical method is quantitative and provides detailed structural information. For analysis of biofluids, time course evaluations can be readily conducted, providing for assessment of baseline parameters and to follow the progression of toxic change from onset to resolution. Although thousands of metabolites are theoretically present, the most common metabolites identified by NMR analyses, especially in urine, are typically those associated with major endogenous metabolic pathways. In particular, major metabolites are those involved in the Kreb's cycle and include intermediates such as citrate, succinate, oxaloacetate, and α-ketoglutarate. Additional metabolites that are frequently detected include acetate, lactate, hippurate, glucose, creatine, creatinine, trimethylamine oxide, and taurine. The time-dependent changes in metabonomic provides an example of NMR spectra collected from urine of a rat prior to (control) and 72 hours following administration of the hepatotoxic agent, galactosamine.

The potential disadvantages of NMR spectroscopy include its recognition as a generally insensitive technique, often requiring at least 100 ng of mass for detection. The use of additional analytical methods, such as MS, can help to overcome this shortcoming. In all cases, the analytical tools are generally expensive, and for NMR, this includes both the instrumentation as well as the laboratory requirements to accommodate the instrument and its sensitive magnet (at least 600 MHz).

Recent research efforts have included the use of NMR coupled with MS, thereby enabling more complete identification of metabolites. The sensitivity of MS methods is a clear advantage over NMR and the ability to separate metabolites by HPLC or GC coupled with MS and/or NMR methods. The GC-based separation methods provide for analysis of volatile compounds or compounds made to be volatile by derivitization, whereas HPLC methods, although biased by solvent systems and columns, can accommodate a larger range of molecules. In both cases, the separation methods afford investigators the opportunity to increase resolution and separation of metabolites, and this enhancement in overall selectivity is particularly useful when novel biomarkers are sought.

Another useful and unique component of the NMR platform is the potential to analyze whole tissue by magic angle spinning (MAS). In this application, samples are spun rapidly at 54.7°, the so-called *magic angle*, relative to the applied magnetic field. In doing so, line-broadening effects that would normally obfuscate proton spectra of a solid sample are reduced. The MAS does not represent a rapid throughput procedure, but because there is no sample extraction or other manipulation prior to analysis, it represents an unbiased method in which changes in tissues can be studied, and as appropriate, compared to alterations observed in biofluids. In this manner, MAS is synergistic with and complimentary to analysis of biofluids by metabonomic applications. This method readily detects glucose and glycogen, choline and related metabolites and a variety of lipids, and fatty acids.

Metabonomic Data Analysis

As with any omics technology, the ability to generate large and complex data sets requires sophisticated methods to reduce and analyze data. In reality, the application of methods for data analysis is as important, if not more important, than the platform used to generate the data. Chemometrics is designated as the application of statistical methods to chemistry and with respect to metabonomics, includes approaches used to process NMR spectra and analyze peak alignments and normalize data.

Chemometrics is distinguished from bioinformatics, which involves the storage, retrieval, and analysis of biological information stored in computer databases. To date, chemometric methods for analysis of NMR data are more fully developed than for other separation techniques. This is largely because the NMR approaches have been used for many more years, enabling more comprehensive assessment of data analysis methods. Principal component analysis (PCA) is commonly used to identify those analytes that are most different from the control samples and provides for a visual characterization of the data set. Following data reduction, PCA is used to find linear combinations (eigenvectors) of the original resolved peaks most different from controls, and these vectors are used to create visually characterize data sets. The PCA Eigenvectors have several desirable properties, including: (a) the combinations are not correlated and (b) they can be rank-ordered (from most to least).

Chronic progressive nephropathy is an age-related phenomenon observed in rats, particularly males. It is characterized clinically by advancing proteinuria, and its histopathological features include degeneration of the renal tubular epithelium, glomerular lesions, interstitial inflammation, and fibrosis. The PCA plot provides a general illustration that urinary profiles obtained from male and female, young and old rats are metabolically different as they occupy very different three-dimensional space. Moreover, as shown in the plot, there is a young male rat that appears in the same space as the aging male rats, suggesting that this animal may have a renal defect.

As noted earlier, there is a common set of metabolites typically identified by NMR analyses, especially in urine, associated with major endogenous metabolic pathways. However, there is clear evidence that the pattern of changes noted, even with these commonly occurring metabolites, is altered in a toxicity- and tissue-specific manner, a feature that is extremely powerful with respect to the predictive utility of metabonomic data. As such, pattern recognition methods are as important as individual metabolite identification. For pattern recognition and predictive model development, additional multivariate statistical models are required. There are many examples of the application of pattern recognition techniques for characterizing and interpreting NMR spectral data, with most of these methods applied to the evaluation of toxicological responses or organ-specific toxicity. These data illustrate how metabonomic information and patterns of changes can be used to assess toxicity, and how it is essential to consider data sets from a multi-variate perspective rather than a univariate mindset. At the same time, there is the clear potential to identify unique and/or specific endogenous metabolites that are associated with a specific type of change, enabling the identification of biomarkers of toxic changes. Although this discussion represents a superficial overview of data analyses tools, it serves to emphasize that the successful application of metabonomic data to toxicology issues will always require the coordinated, multidisciplinary effort of toxicologists, analytical chemists, statisticians, chemometricians, and bioinformaticists.

Applying Metabonomics in Biological Sciences: Toxicological Research

Metabonomics has received considerable attention in the toxicological community, but based on published literature, metabonomic applications do not appear to be as widely used as transcriptomics (toxicogenomics). However, this is not a reflection on the utility of the approach, but more likely a consequence of the need to have a complex infrastructure, particularly with respect to data analysis and interpretation in order to carry out the technology. To date, a variety of work has been published which describes the metabonomic evaluation of urine of animals in response to toxicological insults, with some, albeit fewer investigators reporting analysis of plasma and tissues. In general, metabonomic analyses in toxicology have focused mainly on the identification of changes associated with liver or kidney toxicity. In this regard, changes detected in metabonomic patterns do not always directly correlate with histopathological changes and frequently precede those detected through clinical chemistry analyses. However, after extensive data analysis and application of pattern recognition tools, it is clear that metabonomic data can be used to accurately classify compounds as causing hepatic and/or kidney injury. More recently, investigations have also shown that metabonomic data can also be used to assess the development of vascular lesions and vasculitis in rats.

One potential issue with metabonomic analyses concerns its overall sensitivity to environmental and physiological changes. For example, age-dependent changes in renal function in rats, especially male rats, alters the typical urinary metabolite profile observed in untreated rats. In the example given, young and old rats were defined as 3 and 15 months of age. However, Robertson et al. showed that changes in renal function during the conduct of a typical subchronic toxicity study (13 weeks) could influence data interpretation. Similarly, variation in metabonomic patterns occurs during the normal estrus cycle, and any change in the general health status of the animals, most notably alterations in the resident flora within the gastrointestinal tract, can alter typical metabonomic profiles. On one hand this can be a disadvantage, but if carefully controlled, monitored and characterized, this sensitivity is easily dealt with. Conversely, as illustrated in the PCA plot shown in Figure 3, the sensitivity may be useful for identifying animals that are biochemically or physiologically outliers relative to a normal group distribution. With respect to preclinical studies, one interesting observation determined in metabonomic studies, is that vehicles used for compound administration are not biologically inert, and may influence the analysis of metabonomic data. In fact, some commonly used vehicles for compound administration are not compatible with metabonomics applications, most notably Labrofil and polyethylene glycol. Finally, because NMR is a non-discriminating tool, the profiles of compounds administered to animals to evaluate metabonomic changes can confound the interpretation of the NMR data. In this regard, the use of additional methods, including chromatography and MS detection can reduce or eliminate this potential interference.

Metabonomic evaluations have also been used to identify potential biomarkers of toxicity. One such example is the detection of phenylacetyl-glycine (PAG) as a potential useful biomarker for compound-induced phospholipidosis. As with any biomarker, careful validation is required to assess the overall utility of the biomarker (across species, sensitivity, and specificity) and efforts continue in this regard. However, a biomarker need not be a single metabolite. For example, the combination of changes in the urinary levels of four metabolites (trimethylamine-N-oxide, N,N-dimethyl-glycine, dimethylamine, and succinate) has been shown to accurately predict renal papillary necrosis. Prior to the application of metabonomics, the diagnosis of both phospholipidosis and renal papillary necrosis required histopathological evaluation. Accordingly, the ability to assess these toxicities in a non-invasive manner incorporating metabonomic analysis of urine represents an important scientific advancement.

A relevant and critical question regarding the utility of metabonomics concerns its overall comparison to other omic platforms, including transcriptomics and proteomics. This is an important consideration that has to date, not been fully evaluated. This is one of only a few examples of such a "*trans-platform*" comparison. The APAP is metabolized to a reactive intermediate that covalently modified macromolecules to cause severe centrilobular hepatic necrosis. The early events of necrotic cell death include mitochondrial defects, and the metabonomic data point to a shift in overall energy metabolism as a major change in the liver. In this particular example, the transcriptomic and proteomic results were only partial analyses, in that the investigators focused on changes in mitochondrial mRNAs and proteins. However, the results demonstrated an early change in specific genes and mitochondrial proteins that correlated with time-dependent changes in the metabonomic profiles. For example, down-regulation of the lipoprotein lipase gene, which catalyzes the hydrolysis of triglycerides, correlated with the increase in triglycerides in the liver. Similarly, the increase in mRNA for D-β-hydroxybutyrate dehydrogenase was reflected in the plasma metabonomic results in which D-β-hydroxybutyrate increased. These results suggest that the various platforms are likely to be complimentary to each other. Moreover, the results demonstrate how metabonomics provides the tools to evaluate the downstream or phenotypic effect of changes in gene and protein expression that may ultimately be more stable and, because plasma or urine samples are readily obtained, is likely to be more easily and more routinely evaluated.

As described herein, many metabonomic studies conducted to date have focused on assessing the patterns of change associated with toxicity and reporting the kinds metabolites that have been altered by chemical treatment or physiological alteration. These reports are extremely useful for establishing databases that can be used for predicting toxic liabilities. However, for all of its power, efforts to use metabonomics to identify mechanisms of toxicity are also important. For example, recent work from Mortishire-Smith et al. provided evidence of altered fatty acid metabolism as a mechanism of a novel drug-related hepatotoxicity and showed the potential for metabonomics to address mechanistically based hypotheses. This type of work, linking metabonomic results to better definition of mechanisms of toxicity will ultimately enhance this field by enabling more mechanistically founded predictive models to be evaluated and by providing the opportunity to translate findings in laboratory animals to the clinical situation.

APPLYING METABONOMICS TO BIOLOGICAL SCIENCES: CLINICAL APPLICATIONS

The NMR methods have been used in clinical medicine for many years, and metabonomic evaluation of human samples has been conducted for at least the past 10 years. Classical examples include the application of NMR to the evaluation of inborn errors of metabolism. More recent work has applied metabonomics to the evaluation of the clinical severity of coronary artery disease and to establish a relationship between serum metabolic profiles and hypertension. Because metabonomics is highly sensitive to environmental or dietary influences, concern has been raised that the natural variation in the human population would preclude the application of metabonomics to clinical problems. However, such concerns have been dealt with directly, and recently, Lenz et al. demonstrated that urine and plasma could be collected from human subjects and used successfully for metabonomic analyses. Furthermore, in addition to the disease states described above, metabonomics has been shown to a potentially useful tool for describing alterations associated with dietary and nutritional practices.

As the use of metabonomics advances, there are several challenges facing scientists using this tool that must be addressed in order to make it more mainstream and more relevant to predicting toxicity, and useful for hazard identification, human risk assessment and clinical medicine. First, advancing the use of metabonomics to identify mechanisms of toxicity is essential, and such efforts should help to increase the overall usefulness, validity, and relevance of toxicity prediction and biomarker development. Second, the use of metabonomic evaluations in the course of chronic toxicity rather than the heretofore emphasis on acute studies will help to establish its place in following the progression of toxicity or disease. Third, the application of metabonomics to biomarker identification from animal studies that can be translated to clinical use is an important challenge. To this end, rats have been the major animal model used in most metabonomic evaluations, but extension to other preclinical species, including non-human primates, is important. Ultimately, clinical evaluation of the technology is an important challenge and goal, and its use in clinical medicine is burgeoning. The technology will find even greater utility in clinical medicine when additional basic research has identified important biomarkers of toxicity or disease, or, as mechanistic information about toxicity or diseases is uncovered. Finally, although metabonomic data can be used independently to evaluate disease state or chemically induced insult, the integration of metabonomic data with other tools, particularly transcriptomics and proteomics, is necessary and critical and may also help to validate results obtained from these approaches.

21

FUTURE DIRECTIONS

We hope that the different chapters of this book will convey to anyone interested in pharmacogenomics some idea of the various themes and areas of specialized knowledge that will have to come together to convert expectations to reality. The expectations, which have been aroused by pharmacogenomics are substantial and involve the gradual development of personalized medicine or therapeutics, leaving behind the present statistically based medicine. There are variable estimates of the time, which these processes may require; perhaps it will take 15 to 20 years. Eventually, however, pharmacogenomics is hoped to be a major payoff for society from the scientific and technical revolution called *"genomics."* There is no doubt that some of the specialized techniques described in individual chapters are useful at the present time but may be outdated relatively fast as time goes on. This is always a danger for technical descriptions. In addition, the book covers many principles and problems, which will remain with us for a long time to come.

Pharmacogenetics and pharmacogenomics will have their impact on medicine, the biomedical sciences, and drug development in several ways. Variable responses to drugs and adverse events have always been observed. Modern genetic approaches have the promise of uncovering the genetic and molecular basis of such variability thereby identifying individuals who are non-responders to a drug or at risk for adverse drug reactions. Appropriate testing before a drug is used will often be possible and the potentially ineffective or offending drug can be avoided. For some drugs, pretesting may help in defining an appropriate dosage regimen that is effective and avoids toxicity. Drug development will be aided by finding effective medications whose design is based on disease-specific genomic and phenomic alterations. These scientific developments may lead to the elaboration of *"pharmacogenetic efficiency profiles"* for a given drug and more individualized therapy for the patient.

Clinical trials of new drugs will more frequently include only those individuals who on pharmacogenetic and pharmacogenomic grounds have a greater chance of favorably responding to the new drug. Adverse drug reactions are usually difficult to predict but better understanding of drug metabolism, drug response, and more data on genetic polymorphisms will provide occasional opportunities to screen out those at risk for currently unsuspected adverse events.

The best-understood pharmacogenetic examples relate to processes or reactions mediated by a single gene where a mutation grossly interferes with a crucial step in drug metabolism or drug response. However, while more such examples will be discovered, the more frequent role of genetics and genomics will involve multifactorial phenomena where multiple different genes affecting drug metabolism and drug action interact with the environment and with each other. The resultant bell-shaped curve (i.e., number of individuals plotted against a biologic endpoint such as drug half-life) is unlike the bimodal curve classically seen with monogenic drug reactions where "normals" and "abnormals" represent different populations. As knowledge augments, it will be increasingly possible to define the specific role of each of the various components of polygenic variation by genetic, molecular, and biochemical approaches with careful attention to fixed biologic characteristics (such as age and gender) as well as to various environmental factors.

Pharmacogenetics is not a new science. The role of genes in drug response had been known for about 50 years but recognition of a broader applicability of these concepts for drug therapy and drug discovery and development only occurred more recently, particularly as molecular techniques for in vitro studies became available and the need to administer a drug to healthy individuals and their family members no longer existed in pharmacogenetic studies. An additional reason for delay in the development of pharmacogenetics was the existence of only a few examples of pharmacogenetic variation that were not considered relevant for drug action in general. The demonstration that metabolism for many drugs as assessed by drug half-life differed among unrelated individuals but was very similar in identical twins as compared to non-identical twins pointed to an important role of genetic factors to explain variation of drug metabolism. Identical twins share all their genes while non-identical twins have only half of their genes in common.

Major emphasis in pharmacogenetics has remained on monogenic variation, which can be studied readily with a variety of modern techniques. In this regard, pharmacogenetics mirrors progress in medical genetics in general. While superb advances continue in unraveling the role of single- gene mutations in genetic diseases, success in isolating and elucidating the role of specific genes in the common multifactorial conditions has been much slower, even though considerable effort has been devoted to various approaches to find these genes. Chromosomal localizations of possibly involved genes have often been suggested. However, repeat studies have tended to be unsuccessful in confirming initial results. Few genes except those represented by the less common monogenic subtypes of a given common disease (such as the autosomal dominant breast and colon cancer genes) have been identified. Identification of the genes that contribute to "*polygenic pharmacogenetics*" may be simpler to achieve since the number of genes involved in drug disposal and drug response are likely to be fewer than in multifactorial diseases. The identification of genes in pharmacogenetics may therefore be less difficult.

A consortium of the pharmaceutical industry together with the Wellcome Trust and several academic institutions are now carrying out a search for common DNA variants known as single-nucleotide polymorphisms (SNPs) across the whole human genome in the hope that such DNA variants can be used as markers to signal the presence of very closely linked genes involved in pharmacogenetic processes. The likelihood of ultimate success in this endeavor is difficult to predict. If cSNPs and other DNA changes are detected and related to drug responses, one still has to (a) apply the classical techniques of cloning and identifying the entire gene, (b) express its protein products, and (c) study its function under physiological conditions. The population history, the evolutionary age, and possible selective factors of different SNPs as well as recombination rates between a SNP and the linked gene of interest will vary among populations. The total number of SNPs needed and the number of individuals requiring testing for identifying a relevant gene therefore will often vary between different genes and different populations. Use of genetically more homogeneous populations such as Icelanders in such studies may not necessarily be more helpful. However, data of successful narrowing the genetic region carrying the apo E4 allele (of interest in Alzheimer's disease) have been published by using the SNP approach. Linked sets of SNPs that are inherited together as a unique haplotype simplify the detection of linked genes affecting drug response. Efforts to construct the so-called hap-maps for different populations by this approach are under way, but the ultimate success of this methodology remains to be demonstrated.

Societal Problems

Fundamental research that led to potential practical applications of pharmacogenetics has usually been carried out in academic institutions. Together with a shift of more biomedical research to pharmaceutical and biotechnology companies, pharmacogenetic and pharmacogenomic approaches now occupy an important place in the research portfolio of such companies. With this shift and an interest of academic institutions to derive income from research discoveries, more patents are being applied for. Efforts have already been made to patent newly discovered human genes without any knowledge of their function. It appears now that the U.S. Patent Office is unlikely to issue such patents unless they describe a novel function or application that has utility such as the commercialization of a discovery. Since introduction of a new drug has become very expensive, granting of patents will make novel drugs more expensive still, increasing the cost of medical care, a major problem in much of the world.

The total impact of pharmacogenetics and pharmacogenomics on the pharmaceutical industry in the long run is hazardous to predict. However, even though some analysts on the business side of the pharmaceutical industry are concerned about reducing market size by targeting smaller segments of the population, most companies have placed large investments in genetic and genomic applications in the belief that these approaches will lead to ultimate success and profitability. The impact of pharmacogenetics and pharmacogenomics on the practice of medicine as compared with the development of new drugs should be considered separately. New drug development is of key interest to industry but of less importance to practicing physicians until a new drug becomes available for use. Genomic concepts and techniques together with the application of proteomics are likely to point out new targets for drug therapy based on better understanding of the biologic mechanism of disease. A more rational therapy is therefore likely to evolve. Effectiveness of a given drug in only some people is currently common. There may be environmental causes like food or smoking. In many cases, the reasons are pharmacogenetic differences between people, which may affect, e.g., the metabolism of a drug. Another reason may be the fact that a common disease to be treated is usually caused, or contributed to, by many genes; however, the set of genes contributing to an apparently identical disease often differs between subjects, thereby causing differences of therapeutic response. This is one factor calling for personalized medicine.

Pharmaceutical companies often want orphan drug status given to a new drug. Under current FDA rules, drugs for rare conditions affecting fewer than 200,000 people in the United States receive tax breaks on clinical trials and 7 years of marketing exclusivity. Drugs that currently have a larger market but that following pharmacogenetic testing would be predictably effective in $<200,000$ people might qualify under current rules. Will more drugs therefore be given orphan status? Developments in this area will be followed with much interest.

Ethical Problems

Not covered in this book are ethical issues, which may be harder to solve than some technical problems. Considering ethical issues, it is useful to start by contemplating the Hippocratic Code: the patient, after having agreed to be treated by a physician, trusts the physician to act in the patient's best interest; no other ethical problem arises. This is an entirely different situation from one in which a physician-scientist's interest is the promotion of knowledge. Protection of a patient's interest who participates in a research project has led to many statements and laws. A major start was the Nuremberg Code. In the United States, the Office of Protection from Research Risks (OPRR) has issued regulations known as the "Common Rule." Almost everywhere is institutional review boards, safeguarding the rights of the individuals. The point to be considered in the present context is that with the aim to create personalized medicine, most investigations will be designed to benefit the patient as well as to promote general knowledge. The logical consequence for the formulation of protective laws should be to combine the new rules with the spirit of the Hippocratic Code. It remains to be seen to which extent this will be possible.

If the medical choice of drug or drug dosage depends on a patient's genes, the prescriber has to know the genes of the patient, which may affect these choices; this requires a look into the patient's genetic privacy. However, it also requires the prescriber to know from a study of pharmacogenetics or pharmacogenomics which genotypes are compatible with which drug, necessitating a restructuring of medical education within the framework of the many other problems posed by developments in genetic and genomic medicine.

Many ethical and societal issues of pharmacogenetics and pharmacogenomics are not unique and raise issues similar to those brought up by the recent advances. While different human populations regardless of geographic origin of their ancestors share the vast majority of their genes, considerable genetic variation remains which renders everyone genetically unique. There is considerably more genetic variation within a given population (or "race") than among populations. Despite the universality of this finding in all studies, using non-coding DNA variants (such as microsatellites) and a novel statistical cluster technique, it has become possible to assign anonymous specimens from different populations to their correct geographic origin, such as Africa, East Asia, Europe, West Asia, etc. These designations correlate well with conventional racial classifications. The new method also allows assignment of the extent of admixture in hybrid populations. The frequencies of pharmacogenetic traits usually differ in populations from various parts of the world due to different selective factors but often for unknown reasons. Since such differences may cause adverse drug reactions or variable drug responses, knowledge of a patient's ethnic origin will often be useful to select appropriate pharmacogenetic tests for clinical trials or in medical practice. If a given allele (or set of alleles) that leads to different drug metabolism or variable drug response differs between ethnic groups, selection of the appropriate PCR reactions (or similar test) that is common in a given population can be made. However, it may often be difficult logistically to assign ethnic origin and ethnic mixture is increasingly common as well. All alleles of a given pharmacogenetic system rather than a population specific set may therefore need to be included in the test system. Utilization of biochemical tests such as measurement of enzyme activity may sometimes be more appropriate since it could detect low enzyme activity regardless of which one of multiple DNA alleles that reduce enzyme activity is involved. Molecular diagnosis, however, is currently simpler and more accurate, and can be more readily automated. The technical and population problems encountered will vary for different biochemical and molecular measurements of a given pharmacogenetic trait.

The DNA testing has raised public worries regarding privacy, and legislative initiatives have been proposed to restrict DNA testing in medical settings. Such trends often relate to failure of differentiating forensic DNA tests from DNA tests designed to diagnose various diseases or disease susceptibilities. Genetic testing in medicine raises problems of informed consent, privacy, confidentiality, stigmatization, and discrimination (health insurance and occupation), and requires appropriate guidelines and over-sight. Roses has pointed out, however, that pharmacogenetic testing which aims to detect genes and SNP profiles involved in drug metabolism and drug action is different by only searching for a "*pharmacogenetic efficiency*" or "*medicine response*" profile. He states that such a goal carries no special ethical or social problems and therefore should be considered differently than other kinds of genetic testing. Attempting to find the most appropriate drug for a patient is therefore considered similar to other diagnostic tests in medicine. However, an abnormal result is also relevant for drug therapy of relatives. As long as DNA specimens are only used for pharmacogenetic tests related to adverse events and effective drug responses, a good case can be made for treating such tests somewhat differently from more sensitive genetic tests with more serious implications.

Clinical trials on patients with a disease pose additional problems. Here, patients with variable disease mechanisms and often with a different natural history of their disease may require different treatments. Detailed descriptions of dietary habits, smoking, and other environmental exposures (depending on the condition under study) in addition to age, sex, and ethnic origin will be necessary in clinical trials to elucidate the interaction of environmental and genetic factors. Anonymity that strips a specimen of a name but retains demographic, genetic, and environmental information is one solution and allows additional investigation when new laboratory methodology and additional genetic and environmental markers for studies of the same disease become available. Retention of ethnic identity may be important for the reasons already mentioned. To prevent future abuses, it has been suggested to destroy DNA specimens after testing has been completed. Much valuable information in research studies would be lost under these circumstances, particularly if novel tests become available for the study of the same disease, thus causing problems in locating study subjects. Anonymity with retention of specimens therefore appears most appropriate but has the disadvantage that even a trial participant will not have access to his or her own specimen in the future.

Other problems arise. The intellectual property rights related to specimens from clinical trials are not always clear. Do the study participants whose SNPs lead to new drugs and more appropriate therapy own their DNA, or do all potential benefits go to the investigator or company who collect these specimens? Under what conditions could organizations that collect DNA for either clinical trials or other purposes sell this information to third parties?

INDEX